WITHDRAWN

Pediatric
Anaerobic
Performance

Emmanuel Van Praagh, PhD

Université Blaise-Pascal
Clermont-Ferrand, France

Editor

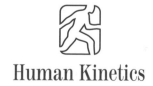

Human Kinetics

Library of Congress Cataloging-In-Publication Data

Pediatric anaerobic performance / Emmanuel Van Praagh, editor.
  p.   cm.
  Includes bibliographical references and index.
  ISBN 0-87322-981-9
  1. Exercise for children--Physiological aspects. 2. Motor ability
in children. 3. Children--Metabolism. 4. Sports for children-
-Physiological aspects. I. Praagh, E. van (Emmanuel van)
RJ133.P4   1998   97-38460
612' .044' 083--dc21   CIP

ISBN: 0-87322-981-9

Permission notices for material reprinted in this book from other sources can be found on pages xiii-xvi.

Developmental Editor: Andrew Smith; **Assistant Editor:** John Wentworth; **Editorial Assistant:** Laura Seversen; **Copyeditor:** Joyce Sexton; **Proofreader:** Pam Johnson; **Indexer:** Craig Brown; **Graphic Designer:** Stuart Cartwright; **Graphic Artist:** Joe Bellis; **Photo Editor:** Boyd LaFoon; **Cover Designer:** Jack Davis; **Illustrators:** Jennifer Delmotte and Joe Bellis; **Printer:** Braun Brumfield

Human Kinetics books are available at special discounts for bulk purchase. Special editions or book excerpts can also be created to specification. For details, contact the Special Sales Manager at Human Kinetics.

Printed in the United States of America

10 9 8 7 6 5 4 3 2 1

Human Kinetics
Web site: http://www.humankinetics.com/

United States: Human Kinetics, P.O. Box 5076, Champaign, IL 61825-5076
1-800-747-4457
e-mail: humank@hkusa.com

Canada: Human Kinetics, Box 24040, Windsor, ON N8Y 4Y9
1-800-465-7301 (in Canada only)
e-mail: humank@hkcanada.com

Europe: Human Kinetics, P.O. Box IW14, Leeds LS16 6TR, United Kingdom
(44) 1132 781708
e-mail: humank@hkeurope.com

Australia: Human Kinetics, 57A Price Avenue, Lower Mitcham, South Australia 5062
(088) 277 1555
e-mail: humank@hkaustralia.com

New Zealand: Human Kinetics, P.O. Box 105-231, Auckland 1
(09) 523 3462
e-mail: humank@hknewz.com

Contents

Preface

Readers interested in pediatric exercise physiology are always struck by the impressive accumulation of data relating to the cardiopulmonary system. Therefore, fitness testing has often become synonymous with the testing of aerobic fitness. However, anaerobic fitness has received much less research attention. This is a little surprising and quite illogical when one considers the activity patterns during the developmental years. These years are, as a matter of fact, characterized more by short-burst activities than by prolonged low-intensity exercises. Moreover, some recent research has shown that short-term intensive movements may optimize the anabolic effects of exercise in the growing child.

This type of short-term activity is observable not only when the child is playing during the kindergarten period, but also later on during participation in numerous games and sports activities. For example, among youth one may observe a huge increase in multiple-sprint sports such as tennis, squash, football, hockey, baseball, soccer, and the like. These activities all have a common denominator: they are based on short-term high-intensity skills. Most certainly our knowledge of the benefits and hazards of participation in sports by young people has increased markedly in recent years. However, since youth sports have been introduced at earlier and earlier ages, the same factors seen in adult sports—for example, precocious specialization, use of anabolic steroids, increased hours of training and year-round training—can be observed.

The purpose of this book is therefore to give the reader a state-of-the art appreciation of the development of anaerobic fitness and performance during growth and maturation. This goal is also to be examined as a fundamental aspect of the child's physical potential in sport. The approach of the book is necessarily multidisciplinary. *Pediatric Anaerobic Performance* is especially written for those involved in exercise and sport science, sports medicine, pediatrics, physical education, and coaching. The reader will undoubtedly be impressed by the overwhelming current information in this particularly interesting area.

Pediatric Anaerobic Performance is a compilation of up-to-date reviews written by prominent leaders in the field of developmental exercise physiology. It is the first time, to the editor's knowledge, that 28 leading researchers and practitioners have worked together in reviewing the principal developmental aspects of anaerobic performance. It must be emphasized that most of them belong to the European Group of Pediatric Work Physiology (EGPWP) and/or the North American Society of Pediatric Exercise Medicine (NASPEM). I am honored to have the chance to bring together this research and to move forward with the important work being done in this area.

Acknowledgments

Firstly, I am grateful to the participating authors for their contributions and the patience and understanding they have displayed throughout the editorial process. I am greatly indebted to my friends in the Department of Exercise Physiology, Drs. Jean Coudert, Mario Bedu, and Nicole Fellmann, who have supported me so much during about 15 years of studying children. Lastly, appreciation is extended to my developmental editor at Human Kinetics, Andy Smith, for his assistance and support in the editorial and production aspects of this volume.

Credits

Figures 1.1, 1.5, and 1.6: Simoneau, J.A., Lortie, G., Leblanc, C., et al. 1986. Anaerobic work capacity in adopted and biological siblings. In *Sport and human genetics,* ed. R.M. Malina and C. Bouchard, 165-171. Champaign, IL: Human Kinetics.

Figures 1.2, 1.4: Bouchard, C., Simoneau, J.-A., Lortie, G., et al. 1986. Genetic effects in human skeletal muscle fiber type distribution and enzyme activities. *Can. J. Physiol. Pharmacol.* 64: 1245-1251.

Figure 1.3: Simoneau, J.A., and Bouchard, C. 1995. Genetic determinism of fiber type proportion in human skeletal muscle. *FASEB J.* 9: 1091-1095.

Figure 1.5: Simoneau, J.-A., Lortie, G., Boulay, M.R., Marcotte, M., Thibault, M.-C., and Bouchard, C. 1986. Inheritance of human skeletal muscle and anaerobic capacity adaptation to high-intensity intermittent training. *Int. J. Sports Med.* 7: 167-171.

Figure 1.7: Simoneau, J.-A., Lortie, G., Boulay, M.R., and Bouchard, C. 1983. Tests of anaerobic alactacid and lactacid capacities: description and reliability. *Can. J. Sport Sci.* 8: 266-270. Simoneau, J.A., Lortie, G., Leblanc, C., et al. 1986. Anaerobic work capacity in adopted and biological siblings. In *Sport and human genetics,* ed. R.M. Malina and C. Bouchard, 165-171. Champaign, IL: Human Kinetics. Simoneau, J.-A., Lortie, G., Boulay, M.R., Marcotte, M., Thibault, M.-C., and Bouchard, C. 1986. Inheritance of human skeletal muscle and anaerobic capacity adaptation to high-intensity intermittent training. *Int. J. Sports Med.* 7: 167-171. Simoneau, J.A., Lortie, G., Boulay, M.R., Marcotte, M., Thibault, M.-C., and Bouchard, C. 1987. Effects of two high-intensity intermittent training programs interspaced by detraining on human skeletal muscle and performance. *Eur. J. Appl. Physiol.* 56: 516-521.

Figure 2.1: Timiras, R.S. 1972. *Developmental physiology and aging.* Macmillan: New York.

Figure 2.4: R.T. Harbourne, C. Guiliani and J. Mac Neela 1993, "A kinematic and electromyographic analysis of the development of sitting posture in infants," *Developmental Psychobiology,* 26:51-64.

Figure 2.5: G.J.P. Savelsbergh and J. van der Kamp, 1994, "The effect of body orientation to gravity on early infant reaching," *Journal of Experimental Child Psychology.* 58:510-528.

Figure 2.6: J.E. Clark, J. Whitall and S.J. Phillips, 1988, "Human interlimb coordination: The first 6 months of independent walking," *Developmental Psychobiology,* 21:445- 456.

Figure 2.7: K. Kamm, E. Thelen, and J.L. Jensen, 1990, "A dynamical systems approach to motor development," *Physical Therapy,* 70:763-775.

Figure 3.1: Bar-Or, O. 1983. *Pediatric sports medicine for the practitioner.* New York: Springer-Verlag. Docherty, D., and Gaul, C.A. 1991. Relationship of body size, physique and composition to physical performance in young boys and girls. *Int. J.*

Sports Med. 12: 525-532. Thorland, W.G., Johnson, G.O., Cisar, C.J., Housh, T.J., and Tharp, G.D. 1987. Strength and anaerobic responses of elite young female sprint and distance runners. *Med. Sci. Sports Exerc.* 19: 56-61. Delgado, A., Pérès, G., Allemandou, A., and Monod, H. 1993. Influence of cycle ergometer characteristics on the adolescents' anaerobic abilities testing. *Archiv. Int. Physiol. Biochim. Biophys.* 191: 145-148. Van Praagh, E., Fellmann, N., Bedu, M., Falgairette, G., and Coudert, J. 1990. Gender difference in the relationship of anaerobic power output to body composition in children. *Pediatr. Exerc. Sci.* 2: 336-348. Capranica, L., Cama, G., Fanton, A., Tessitore, A., and Figura, F. 1992. Force and power of preferred and non-preferred leg in young soccer players. *J. Sports Med. Phys. Fitness* 31: 358-363.

Figure 3.2: Falk, B., and Bar-Or, O. 1993. Longitudinal changes in peak aerobic and anaerobic mechanical power of circumpubertal boys. *Pediatr. Exerc. Sci.* 5: 318-331.

Figure 3.3: Malina, R.M., and Bouchard, C. 1991. *Growth, maturation, and physical activity.* Champaign, IL: Human Kinetics.

Figure 3.4: Saavedra, C., LaGasse, P., Bouchard, C., and Simoneau, J-A. 1991. Maximal anaerobic performance of the knee extensor muscles during growth. *Med. Sci. Sports Exerc.* 23: 1083-1089.

Figures 3.5 and 3.6: Maresh, M.M. 1970. Measurements from roentgenograms: heart size; long bone lengths; bone, muscle and fat widths; skeletal maturation. In *Human growth and development,* ed. R.W. McCammon, 155-200. Springfield, IL: Charles C Thomas.

Figure 3.7: Inbar, O., and Bar-Or, O. 1986. Anaerobic characteristics in male children and adolescents. *Med. Sci. Sports Exerc.* 18: 264-269. Docherty, D., and Gaul, C.A. 1991. Relationship of body size, physique and composition to physical performance in young boys and girls. *Int. J. Sports Med.* 12: 525-532. Naughton, G., Carlson, J., and Fairweather, I. 1992. Determining the variability of performance on Wingate anaerobic tests in children 6-12 years. *Int. J. Sports Med.* 13: 512-517. Falk, B., and Bar-Or, O. 1993. Longitudinal changes in peak aerobic and anaerobic mechanical power of circumpubertal boys. *Pediatr. Exerc. Sci.* 5: 318-331.

Figures 4.3 and 4.4: Fleishman, E.A. 1963. *The structure and measurement of physical fitness.* Englewood Cliffs, NJ: Prentice Hall.

Table 4.1: Veterans Administration Physicians Guide: Disability, Evaluation, Examination (1963); Moore (1978); and the American Academy of Orthopaedic Surgeons (1972).

Figure 5.2: Sargeant, A.J. 1989. Short-term muscle power in children and adolescents. In *Advances in pediatric sports sciences.* Vol. 3, *Biological issues,* ed. O. Bar-Or, chap. 2, 41-63. Champaign, IL: Human Kinetics.

Figure 5.5: Adapted with permission from Sargeant 1997 and Portland Press.

Figure 5.6: Sant'Ana Pereira, J.A.A., Sargeant, A.J., de Haan, A., Rademaker, A.C.H.J., and van Mechelen, W. 1996. Myosin heavy chain isoform expression and high energy phosphate content of human muscle fibres at rest and post-exercise. *J. Physiol.* 496(2): 1-6.

Figure 5.7: Zoladz, J.A., Rademaker, A., and Sargeant, A.J. 1995. Oxygen uptake does not increase linearly with power output at high intensities of exercise in humans. *J. Physiol.* 488(1): 211-218.

Figure 5.9: Beelen, A., and Sargeant, A.J. 1991. Effect of fatigue on maximal power output at different contraction velocities in humans. *J. Appl. Physiol.: Resp. Environ. Exerc. Physiol.* 71(6): 2332-2337.

Figure 5.10: Sargeant, A.J. 1987. Effect of muscle temperature on leg extension force and short-term power output in humans. *Eur. J. Appl. Physiol.* 56(6): 693-698.

Table 7.3: Armstrong, N., Welsman, J.R., and Kirby, B.J. 1997. Performance on the Wingate Anaerobic Test and maturation. *Pediatr. Exerc. Sci.* 9.

Figure 8.1: Van Praagh, E., Fellmann, N., Bedu, M., Falgairette, G., and Coudert, J. 1990. Gender difference in the relationship of anaerobic power output to body composition in children. *Pediatr. Exerc. Sci.* 2: 336-348.

Figure 8.2: Ferretti, G., Gussoni, M., di Prampero, P.E., and Cerretelli, P. 1987. Effects of exercise on maximal instantaneous muscular power of humans. *J. Appl. Physiol.* 62: 2288-2294.

Figure 8.3: Viitasalo, J.T., Rahkila, P., Österback, L., and Alén, M. 1992. Vertical jumping height and horizontal overhead throwing velocity in young male athletes. *J. Sports Sci.* 10: 401-413.

Figure 8.4: Moritani, T., Oddsson, L., Thorstensson, A., and Åstrand, P.O. 1989. Neural and biomechanical differences between men and young boys during a variety of motor tasks. *Acta Physiol. Scand.* 137: 147-155.

Figures 9.1, 9.2, 9.3, 9.4, 9.9, and 9.10: Blimkie 1989.

Figure 9.5: Faust, M.S. 1977. Somatic development of adolescent girls. Monograph. Society For Research In Child Development, 42(1): 1-90. Stolz, H.R., Stolz, L.M. 1951. Somatic development of adolescent boys. New York: Macmillan. Malina, R.M., Bouchard, C. 1991. Growth, maturation and physical activity. Champaign, IL: Human Kinetics.

Figures 9.6 and 9.12: Malina, R.M., Bouchard, C. 1991. Growth, maturation and physical activity. Champaign, IL: Human Kinetics.

Figures 9.7 and 9.8: Oertel, G. 1988. Morphometric analysis of normal skeletal muscles in infancy, childhood and adolescence. An autopsy study. *J. Neurol. Sci.* 88: 303-313.

Figure 9.11: T. Fukunaga and Y. Kawakami, personal communication.

Figure 9.13: Ramsay, J.A., Blimkie, C.J.R., Smith, K., Garner, S., MacDougall, J.D., Sale, D.G. 1990. Strength training effects in prepubescent boys. *Med. Sci. Sports Exerc.* 22: 605-614.

Figure 9.14: Pfeiffer, R.D., Francis, R.S. 1986. Effects of strength training on muscle development in prepubescent, pubescent, and postpubescent males. *Phys. Sportsmed.* 14: 134-143.

Figures 11.1, 11.2, and 11.3: Mero, A., Vuorimaa, T., and Häkkinen, K., eds. 1990. *Training in children and adolescents.* Jyväskylä, Finland: Gummerus Kirjapaino Oy.

Tables 11.1, 11.3, and 11.6: Mero, A., Vuorimaa, T., and Häkkinen, K., eds. 1990. *Training in children and adolescents.* Jyväskylä, Finland: Gummerus Kirjapaino Oy.

Tables 11.4 and 11.7: Semetka, M. 1982. Physical development and motor efficiency of 7 to 14 year old Slovak population. *Tréner* 26: 1.

Table 11.5: Mero, A., Lehtimäki, M., Mäkelä, J., Levola, M., Helander, E., Rajala, T., Aura, O., Peltola, E., Jouste, P., and Pullinen, T. 1992. Performance capacity of young speed and speed-strength athletes during two years of training. *Sprint Hurdle J.* 3-4: 20-33.

Figure 12.1: Ogden, J. 1987. Postnatal development and growth of the musculoskeletal system. In *The scientific basic of orthopaedics,* ed. J.A. Albright and R.A. Brand. Stamford, CT: Appleton & Lange Publishers.

Figures 13.1 and 13.2: Tirosh, E., Rosenbaum, P., and Bar-Or, O. 1990. A new muscle power test in neuromuscular disease: feasibility and reliability. *Am. J. Dis. Child.* 144: 1083-1087.

Figure 13.3: Bar-Or, O. 1993. Noncardiopulmonary pediatric exercise tests. In *Pediatric laboratory exercise testing: clinical guidelines,* ed. T.W. Rowland, 165-185. Champaign, IL: Human Kinetics.

Table 13.1: Tirosh, E., Rosenbaum, P., and Bar-Or, O. 1990. A new muscle power test in neuromuscular disease: feasibility and reliability. *Am. J. Dis. Child.* 144: 1083-1087.

Figure 14.6: Varray, A., Mercier, J., Ramonatxo, M., and Préfaut, C. 1989. L'exercice physique maximal chez l'enfant asthmatique: limitation aérobie et compensation anaérobie? *Sci. Sports* 4: 199-207.

Figure 15.1: de Jonge, R., Bedu, M., Fellmann, N., Blonc, S., Spielvogel, H., and Coudert, J. 1996. Effect of anthropometric characteristics and socio-economic status on physical performances of pre-pubertal children living in Bolivia at low altitude. *Eur. J. Appl. Physiol.* 74: 367-374.

Figure 15.3: Spurr, G.B., and Reina, J. 1995. Undernutrition, physical activity, and performance of children. In *New horizons in pediatric exercise science,* ed. C. Blimkie and O. Bar-Or. Champaign, IL: Human Kinetics.

Introduction

This volume is entirely devoted to anaerobic performance as it relates to the growth and maturation of children. It must be emphasized that most of what is known about human anaerobic function has come from research on adults. Classically, the adult model is simply adjusted for body dimensions and assumed to fit the child. This book reviews present knowledge concerning the various aspects of *Pediatric Anaerobic Performance*. Above all, it highlights new insights into genetics, development, and physiological and biomechanical aspects during short-term power activities. Therefore, for the reader's convenience this volume has been organized into four sections.

Part I, Biological Development and Anaerobic Performance, includes four chapters and deals with biological and biomechanical determinants of anaerobic fitness. In contrast to what we see in other areas of sport sciences, little has been written on the genetics of pediatric anaerobic performance. The first chapter, by Jean-Aimé Simoneau and Claude Bouchard, describes the genetic variation of anaerobic performance in adolescents. Chapter 2 by Jody Jensen and Krisanne Bothner gives new insight into infant motor development schedules from a biomechanical perspective. Developmental aspects of anaerobic performance related to age- and sex-associated variation are discussed in chapter 3 by James Martin and Robert Malina. A lack of flexibility during growth may not only influence the efficiency of short-term performance but also make the individual more susceptible to injury. This important and often neglected research purpose is addressed by David Brodie and Jon Royce in chapter 4.

Part II, entitled Assessment of Anaerobic Performance, contains four chapters. Here the reader is presented with the most recent information regarding current evaluation of anaerobic fitness, including a detailed description of measurement techniques and approaches. The first chapter in this section, by Anthony Sargeant, addresses fundamental considerations in the measurement of anaerobic muscle function in children. The accumulated oxygen deficit method as a measure of aerobic characteristics in children is discussed in chapter 6 by John Carlson and Geraldine Naughton. Chapter 7, by Joanne Welsman and Neil Armstrong, deals with blood lactate measurement and the interpretation of postexercise lactate. In the final chapter of this section, Emmanuel Van Praagh and Nanci França present current measurement techniques and the new technology available for evaluating short-term power capabilities during growth.

Part III, Anaerobic Trainability and Training, is composed of three chapters. Resistance training for children is still a controversial subject. In order to answer the question of whether resistance training can cause strength gains during childhood, Cameron Blimkie and Digby Sale in chapter 9 provide current information with respect to strength development and trainability during maturation. In children, it is possible to train and to assess maximal torque production through a complete range of motion while velocity of movement is maintained. Vasilios Baltzopoulos and Eleftherios Kellis in chapter 10 describe the variation of isokinetic strength observed during growth. It is often claimed that short-term activities are more suitable for the child than those of prolonged low intensity. Chapter 11, by Antti Mero, deals with the effects of power and speed training during growth and development.

Part IV, entitled Clinical and Environmental Limitations contains six chapters. This part of the book examines the anaerobic fitness limitations of chronically ill children with functional disabilities. Furthermore, the effects of some environmental constraints (malnutrition, high altitude) on anaerobic performance are reviewed. Educational, medical, and scientific professionals are often asked, Does resistance training harm children's skeletal systems? Chapter 12, by Lyle Micheli and Sig Berven, reviews the increasing occurrence of traumatic injuries and overuse syndromes in adolescents performing exercise that demands short and explosive bursts of maximal exertion. In chapter 13, Oded Bar-Or addresses research and clinical experience related to the anaerobic performance of young patients with neuromuscular disease; in chapter 14, François-Pierre Counil and Christian Préfaut present new insight regarding the participation of asthmatic children in anaerobic exercise and short-term sport events. In chapter 15, Nicole Fellmann and Jean Coudert address the relationship between malnutrition and anaerobic performance in children. Chapter 16, by Mario Bedu and Jean Coudert, deals with the effects of high altitude on anaerobic fitness in the growing child. Finally, chapter 17, by Emmanuel Van Praagh, discusses trends and future directions in pediatric anaerobic performance.

The volume consists of 17 topical chapters, each of which is a self-contained unit but all of which have a common theme: *Pediatric Anaerobic Performance*. At the end of each chapter, the contributors have also addressed the shortcomings of past research and suggested future research directions within their respective areas. The selection of the topics was one of the editor's responsibilities. Readers must judge for themselves the effectiveness of the choices.

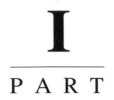

PART I

Biological Development and Anaerobic Performance

1

CHAPTER

The Effects of Genetic Variation on Anaerobic Performance

Jean-Aimé Simoneau
Claude Bouchard

This chapter focuses on the following objectives:

- The heritability of anaerobic performance
- The heritability of the major determinants of anaerobic performance
- Improvements in anaerobic performance due to training

There is no doubt that considerable human variation exists in the ability to perform maximally over a short period of time. Age, gender, body mass, and metabolic factors are recognized as determinants of maximal short-term performance. Elite athletes of a given age and sex group, such as sprinters or speed skaters, are able, on average, to accomplish more work during maximal exercise of short duration than age- and sex-matched athletes involved in endurance sport events or untrained persons (Serresse et al. 1989). Despite recent progress in understanding of the scientific basis of short-term high-intensity performance, it is not clear whether environmental or genetic factors contribute most to the differences observed in such performance phenotype. The present chapter will attempt to define the extent to which human variation in anaerobic performance can be attributed to genetic factors.

Heritability of Anaerobic Performance

Because of the complexity of the structural and functional determinants of human muscle performance under predominantly anaerobic conditions, it is essential to make a distinction between different types of anaerobic performance. Various tests are commonly used to quantify anaerobic performance levels. The present chapter will focus only on maximal short-term (about 10 s in duration) and long-term (about 90 s in duration) anaerobic performance and will review the evidence for a role of inheritance in such performances.

Maximal Short-Term Anaerobic Performance

Values previously reported concerning the total genetic effect in maximal short-term performance are widely divergent, ranging from almost zero to almost 100% of the variance (Komi, Klissouras, and Karvinen 1973; Komi and Karlsson 1979; Simoneau et al., "Anaerobic Work Capacity," 1986). This variability in the heritability estimates can be accounted for by various factors, but primarily by the small sample size of most studies. Only two types of cross-sectional studies have been reported so far—those based on comparison of the phenotype in sibships of brothers and sisters by adoption or descent or in the classical twin study design.

In one of our studies (Simoneau et al., "Anaerobic Work Capacity," 1986), a total of 328 individuals belonging to adopted sibships (n = 19), regular biological sibships of brothers and sisters (n = 55), dizygotic (DZ) twin sibships (n = 31), and monozygotic (MZ) sibships (n = 49) were tested for maximal working capacity during 10 s of cycling exercise. The intraclass correlations for these types of sibships are summarized in figure 1.1. Adopted children living together did not exhibit similarity in performance, since the intraclass coefficient between these sibships was close to zero. For biological sibships, significant resemblances were found for maximal short-term performance. The intraclass coefficient in pairs of brothers and sisters living together reached 0.46. In a study of sibling similarities in running (35 yd dash) among 114 black and 101 white sibling pairs aged 6-12 years, Malina and Mueller (1981) noted no differences in sibling correlations by race, but greater sibling similarities among brothers than among sisters. These results suggest that sharing about one-half of the genome and living together translate into an enhanced resemblance over that found in cohabitating sibs who have no genes in common by immediate descent. Intraclass correlations among biological sibs and DZ twins (r = 0.58) are also quite similar, suggesting that increased environmental similarity (as is the case when DZ twins and regular brothers and sisters are contrasted) does not translate into increased phenotypic resemblance for maximal short-term performance (Simoneau et al., "Anerobic Work Capacity, 1986).

Using the classical twin study design, Komi, Klissouras, and Karvinen (1973) found an intrapair variance in DZ twins that was about five times higher than in MZ twins for a measurement of maximal anaerobic power (Margaria test). Intraclass

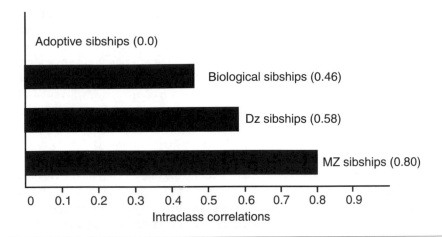

Figure 1.1 Intraclass coefficients for maximal 10 s cycle ergometer performance test determined in adoptive, biological, dizygotic twin, and monozygotic twin sibships. Data are expressed in Joules per kilogram of body mass.

Data from Simoneau et al. 1986.

coefficients computed from the data in their original paper for maximal short-term power, expressed per kilogram of body mass, reached 0.69 and 0.80 for DZ and MZ twin sibships, respectively. These latter results are fairly similar to those obtained for maximal short-term performance in our own study (Simoneau et al., "Anaerobic Work Capacity," 1986; figure 1.1), since the intraclass coefficients reached 0.58 and 0.80 for the DZ and MZ sibships, respectively. Heritability estimates of a variety of running, jumping, and throwing tasks have been reported in several studies with use of the twin experimental model (Kovar 1975; Sklad 1972; Weiss 1979; Wolanski, Tomonari, and Siniarska 1980). Heritability coefficients for dashes of different distances (20-60 m) ranged between 0.45 and 0.91. Wolanski, Tomonari, and Siniarska (1980) suggested that heritability was highest for the shorter dashes (10 m) and decreased with the longer dashes (60 m). Sklad (1972) published a report concerning the similarity of movements during 60 m runs in DZ and MZ twins. The movement structures, the tempo of the runs, the time components, and the length and number of steps recorded on film revealed that the kinetic structure of a run was more similar in MZ twins than in DZ twins. These results suggest that speed and tempo of movements, which are potential determinants of maximal short-term performance, are strongly genetically influenced.

　　Resemblance in maximal short-term performance among members of a sibship increases with the proportion of the genes shared by descent. We therefore conclude that such performances are characterized by a significant genetic component. It can be estimated that the total genetic effect in maximal short-term performance is about 50% of the age-, gender-, and body mass-adjusted phenotype variance.

Two other approaches in the study of the contribution of the genes to variation in a phenotype are to test for associations between the phenotype and polymorphism at specific genetic markers, or to screen regions of the genome in which genes affecting that phenotype may reside, by using sib-pair linkage analysis. Association analyses are performed to establish whether there is a correlation between a particular phenotype and genotypes at a specific locus, whereas a sib-pair linkage analysis is a method to screen for genetic linkage between a quantitative trait and polymorphic genetic markers. We have used these approaches for the maximal 10 s ergocycle performance test phenotype with several polymorphic loci related to blood groups and red blood cell enzymes in a total of 250 subjects, including 55 pairs of brothers and sisters and 31 pairs of DZ (unpublished results). No evidence for either association or linkage was found between the polymorphism in ABO, Rh, MN, SS, Kell, and Duffy erythrocyte antigenic systems, or in phosphoglucomutase-1, acid phosphatase, adenosine deaminase, adenylate kinase, and esterase D red blood cell enzymes, and maximal 10 s cycle ergometer performance test. Notwithstanding these negative findings, it is clear that further investigations are needed, since a very small fraction of the human genome has been screened until now.

Maximal Long-Term Anaerobic Performance

There is a dearth of data regarding the genetics of anaerobic performance of longer duration. Klissouras (1973) has reported on the performance time for a 1000 m run in twins. The MZ intraclass correlation reached .98 with a low 5% mean intrapair difference. In the DZ twin pairs, the figures were .69 and 30%, respectively. These results would support the notion that genes contribute to the long-term anaerobic running performance variance. One additional study undertaken by Klissouras (1971) is interesting in relation to long-term anaerobic working capacities. Maximal blood lactate values were characterized by high twin intraclass correlations (MZ = 0.93; DZ = 0.76). It cannot be concluded that high levels of circulating lactate are an indicator of success in maximal long-term anaerobic performance, but the ability to resist acidosis could increase performance. To our knowledge, these are the only published studies that have covered this topic. These estimates could suggest that maximal long-term performance is also influenced by genetic factors, but more research is clearly warranted.

Heritability of the Major Determinants of Anaerobic Performance

Multiple factors contribute to maximal anaerobic performance. A favorable combination of several determinants (e.g., large muscle mass, high muscle fiber recruit-

ment, high proportion of fast-twitch muscle fibers, large muscle fibers, high glycolytic metabolic profile, etc.) would be expected to correlate with the exceptional
ability of some individuals to reach high levels of anaerobic performance.

Muscle Mass

Skeletal muscle atrophy following immobilization or hypertrophy as a result of
exercise training are examples of interindividual variation in muscle mass that can
be attributed to environmental influences. Muscle mass is an important component
of body composition and physique at all ages and represents one of the important
determinants of muscle force and power. Skeletal muscle mass is commonly ap-
proximated by measurements of fat-free mass obtained with a variety of procedures
or is estimated from imaging techniques applied to specific sites or regions of the
body. Few genetic studies have been performed on muscle mass phenotypes or on
surrogate measurements. Radiographic measurements of calf muscle diameter in
young siblings (Hewitt 1957), as well as parent-child correlations for estimated
muscle diameters of the arm and calf (arm and calf circumferences corrected for the
thickness of the triceps and medial calf skinfolds, respectively; Bouchard 1991),
suggest that muscle size is influenced by genetic characteristics.

Fat-Free Mass

The purpose of one of our previous studies was to determine the heritability of fat-
free mass (Bouchard et al., "Inheritance," 1988). Underwater weighing estimates of
body density were determined in a cohort of 1698 members of 409 families in order
to derive total body fat-free mass. This cohort of subjects included the following
pairs of family members for whom fat-free mass estimates were available: spouses
(maximum number of pairs = 166), foster parent-adopted child (252), siblings by
adoption (104), first-degree cousins (37), uncle/aunt-nephew/niece (29), parent-
natural child (531), full sibs (152), DZ twins (58), and MZ twins (76). The degree
of resemblance in fat-free mass within these pairs of family members revealed that
the genetic inheritance accounted for about 30% of the age- and gender-adjusted
phenotype variance (see figure 1.2). More recently, no major gene effect could be
identified by segregation analysis using the data of the same cohort of subjects (Rice
et al. 1993); but, in contrast, about 60% of the variance in fat-free mass was accounted for by a non-Mendelian major effect. This latter finding was recently confirmed in a sample of Mexican American subjects (Comuzzie et al. 1994). It may be
inferred, on the basis of these results, that undetermined genetic characteristics
contribute to individuality in estimated muscle mass.

Estimated Muscle Mass

In sets of midparent-natural child and foster midparent-adopted child (Bouchard
1991), the upper-arm circumference corrected for the triceps skinfold, and the calf

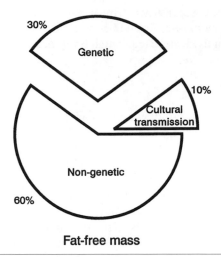

Fat-free mass

Figure 1.2 Major affectors of human variation in fat-free mass as assessed with the BETA path analysis technique.

Data from Bouchard et al. 1986.

circumference corrected for the contribution of the medial calf skinfold (Brozek 1961), were used as estimates of muscle mass on the limbs. The correlations for both estimated muscle diameters were not significantly different from zero in the relatives by adoption, but they reached 0.3 in the biological relatives. These results are compatible with the previous observation that the genotype contributes significantly to variations in densitometrically estimated fat-free mass.

Skeletal Muscle Characteristics

As already mentioned, successful anaerobic performance is dependent on many factors, and investigation of characteristics such as muscle fiber type proportion, muscle fiber size, and glycolytic and aerobic-oxidative capacities of skeletal muscle has been the concern of exercise physiologists interested in the function and capacity of muscle during anaerobic conditions. The literature demonstrating the extent to which these characteristics are genetically determined is, however, rather scarce.

Muscle Fiber Type Proportion

In humans, as well as in most mammals, skeletal muscle is composed in varying proportions of two major categories of fibers exhibiting specific contractile properties. These skeletal muscle fiber categories have been commonly named slow-twitch (ST) and fast-twitch (FT) fibers because of the time they require to reach peak isometric tension in response to a single twitch. In humans, ST and FT muscle fibers have an approximate mean time to peak tension of 90 and 45 ms, respectively (Gollnick 1982; Saltin and Gollnick 1983). Several studies reveal that human skeletal muscle can exhibit substantial variation in its fiber type proportion (Saltin and Gollnick 1983; Simoneau and Bouchard 1989). On the basis of a large sample (more than 400), we have shown that the vastus lateralis muscle of about 25% of North American Caucasian men and women has either less than 35% or more than 65% of type I fibers (Simoneau and Bouchard 1989), thus demonstrating that the number of individuals in the population with a low or a high proportion of muscle type I fibers is not negligible. Not only is it possible to find that vastus lateralis muscle of sedentary women exhibits, on average, slightly more type I fiber and less type IIB fiber proportions than that of sedentary men (Simoneau et al. 1985), but we have also reported that the vastus lateralis muscle of sedentary Black African subjects from western and central African countries has slightly more type II fibers than in sedentary White subjects (Ama et al. 1986).

An important question is, to what extent is skeletal muscle fiber type proportion under the control of genetic factors? The data available are few, and the results are widely divergent. In 1977, Komi et al. reported heritability coefficients of 0.995 in male subjects and of 0.928 in female subjects for the distribution of muscle fiber types on the basis of data derived from a small sample of DZ and MZ twins. Such high heritability coefficients suggest that the fiber type proportion phenotype is almost exclusively genotype dependent and is not affected by any error variance or by nongenetic factors, which is, of course, hard to accept. For instance, determination of the skeletal muscle fiber type proportion in human subjects is influenced by tissue-sampling and technical errors. Repeated measurements within the vastus lateralis muscle revealed that sampling and technical error combined (standard deviation for repeated measurements) represented about 15% of the mean value of each fiber type category (Simoneau and Bouchard 1995).

Two studies of interest have appeared on this topic during the past 10 years. Nimmo, Wilson, and Snow (1985), using inbred strains of mice, showed that genetic factors accounted for about 75% of the variation in fiber type I proportion of the soleus muscle with 95% confidence intervals ranging from 55% to 89%. Our own study based on a sample of brothers (n = 32 pairs), DZ twins (n = 26 pairs), and MZ twins (n = 35 pairs) indicated that the heritability of muscle fiber type proportion was much lower than previous estimates (Bouchard et al. 1986). Intraclass correlations for the percentage of type I fibers were significant and reached 0.33 in brothers, 0.52 in DZ twins, and 0.55 in MZ twins. Broad heritability estimates can be obtained from twice the biological sib correlation (66%), from twice the difference between MZ and DZ correlations (6%), or directly from the MZ twin sibship correlation (55%) (Falconer 1960). Although brothers and DZ twins share about one-half of their genome by descent, comparison of their correlations suggests that increased environmental similarity (i.e., DZ twins experience more similar environmental circumstances than regular brothers) appears to translate into increased phenotypic resemblance for the proportion of skeletal muscle type I fibers (i.e., the intraclass coefficients of 0.52 vs. 0.33). We have summarized the data in a recent paper

Pediatric Anaerobic Performance

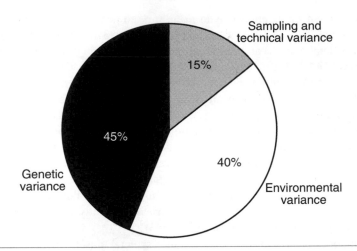

Figure 1.3 Estimates of the sampling and technical, environmental, and genetic variance in the proportion of type I fibers of human skeletal muscle.

Data from Simoneau and Bouchard 1995.

(Simoneau and Bouchard 1995) as follows. A fraction (about 15%) of the total variance in the proportion of type I muscle fibers in humans is explained by the error component related to muscle sampling and technical variance; about 40% of the phenotype variance is influenced by environmental factors; and the remaining part of the variance (about 45%) is associated with inherited factors (see figure 1.3). If these estimates are approximately correct, a difference of about 30% in type I fibers among individuals could be potentially explained exclusively by differences in the local environment and level of muscular contractile activity. However, unidentified genetic factors would have to be invoked to account for the observation that the skeletal muscle of about 25% of the North American Caucasian population has either less than 35% or more than 65% of type I fibers.

Muscle Fiber Areas

Similar to the situation with fiber type proportion, substantial variation exists in the size of skeletal muscle fibers. An almost fourfold difference is seen between the lowest and highest values found in samples taken from the vastus lateralis muscle of sedentary subjects (Simoneau and Bouchard 1989). This variation is noticeable within each category of fibers and is even more striking when muscle fiber areas of men are compared to those of women. Type II fibers are generally smaller by about 25% in sedentary women compared to sedentary men (Simoneau et al. 1985). To our knowledge, the only study that has reported heritability estimates for skeletal muscle fiber area in humans is from our laboratory (Bouchard et al. 1986). No correlation pattern coherent with a genetic effect for any of the muscle fiber type areas was found. The MZ intraclass coefficients were quite erratic, ranging from –0.09 to 0.30. None of the within-pair or among-pair estimates of genetic variance reached significance or were even close to significance. In general, these results are in agreement with the observations that muscle fiber size is altered by exercise training (Simoneau 1995) or more evidently by disuse (Roy, Baldwin, and Edgerton 1991).

Muscle Enzyme Activities

The importance of interindividual variability in the enzyme activity profile of human skeletal muscle confirms that one may find high and low activity levels of enzyme markers regulating the catabolism of different substrates in skeletal muscle of healthy sedentary and moderately active individuals (Simoneau and Bouchard 1989). For instance, women exhibit, on average, lower skeletal muscle glycolytic capacities than men (Simoneau et al. 1985), whereas sedentary Black African subjects from western and central African countries have higher skeletal muscle glycolytic capacities than sedentary Caucasian subjects (Ama et al. 1986). Numerous factors are undoubtedly involved in accounting for the large interindividual variations observed. Little has been reported about the heritability of different metabolic enzyme markers of human skeletal muscle. Howald (1976) showed that muscle hexokinase (HK) and succinate dehydrogenase activities were identical in DZ as well as MZ twins, while muscle glyceraldehyde-3-phosphate dehydrogenase (GAPDH) and 3-hydroxyacyl-CoA dehydrogenase (HADH) activities were significantly more variable within DZ than within MZ twin pairs. Even though this could be indicative of a genotype influence, there were significant mean differences within both sets of twins for GAPDH and HADH enzymes, and a there was a significant difference in variance for GAPDH between twin types. On the other hand, in the study reported by Komi et al. (1977), there was no evidence of significant genetic variation in activities of muscle ATPases, creatine kinase (CK), myokinase, phosphorylase, and lactate dehydrogenase (LDH) from DZ and MZ twin comparisons.

These studies were extended further by us when maximal enzyme activity of CK, HK, phosphofructokinase (PFK), LDH, malate dehydrogenase (MDH), HADH, and oxoglutarate dehydrogenase (OGDH) was determined in brother, DZ twin, and MZ twin sibships (Bouchard et al. 1986). Resemblances in muscle enzyme activities were systematically significant in MZ twins but less consistently so in DZ twins and brothers. When comparisons were made between DZ twins and brothers, large discrepancies in intraclass coefficients were observed for HK, LDH, MDH, and HADH. More extensive analyses of the twin data revealed that a significant genetic variance could be detected for PFK, LDH, MDH, OGDH, HADH, and the PFK/OGDH ratio. Heritability reached about 60% and more for LDH, MDH, and HADH enzyme activity. The genetic effect was low for CK (about 16%) and moderate for PFK, OGDH, and the PFK/OGDH ratio (ranging from 25% to 50%). Because both PFK and OGDH are key enzymes of their respective metabolic pathways (Newsholme 1980), these data suggest that genetic factors are involved in the variation of regulatory enzymes of the glycolytic and citric acid cycle capacities as well as in the variation of the glycolytic to aerobic-oxidative enzyme ratio. The intraclass correlation patterns for the glycolytic (PFK) to aerobic-oxidative (OGDH) enzyme capacities observed in brothers and in DZ and MZ twin sibships suggest that about 50% of the phenotype variance is influenced by genetic factors whereas about 35% is associated with environmental factors (see figure 1.4).

One possible explanation as to how genetic factors contribute to the variation in enzyme activity levels of skeletal muscle could be the presence of mutations affecting the amino acid sequence of proteins that could impact favorably or not on the efficiency of a metabolic pathway. To investigate the hypothesis that protein polymorphism could be involved in the genetic effect identified for muscle enzyme activities, samples were obtained from the vastus lateralis muscle of a cohort of about 300 men and women and analyzed for the presence of charge variation as revealed by isoelectrofocusing analyses (Bouchard et al., "Charge Variants," 1988; Marcotte et al. 1987; Bouchard et al. 1989). No charge variant was found in the muscle extract of these individuals for any of the 11 enzymes of glycolysis (Bouchard et al., "Charge Variants," 1988) or 9 enzymes of the tricarboxylic acid cycle (Marcotte et al. 1987), while 6 individuals exhibited a CK muscle enzyme variant and 21 individuals were heterozygotes for an inherited form of the adenylate kinase muscle enzyme (Bouchard et al. 1989). However, human variation in the maximal 10 s cycle ergometer performance test could not be accounted for by the genetic polymorphism of the two kinase enzymes (Bouchard et al. 1989). It is clear that this

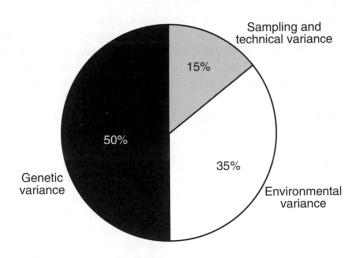

Figure 1.4 Estimates of the sampling and technical, environmental, and genetic variance in the ratio of glycolytic to aerobic-oxidative enzyme capacity of human skeletal muscle.

Data from Bouchard et al. 1986.

work is still in its infancy. More research on amino acid sequence variation of key regulatory enzymes and its potential association with variation in performance is needed.

Improvements in Anaerobic Performance Due to Training

Untrained subjects or even athletes can progressively improve their anaerobic performance in response to several weeks of specific training. Previous studies from our laboratory revealed, however, that these training-induced improvements in anaerobic performance are not similar for every individual even when the training regimen is clamped for all subjects. Accordingly, there are considerable individual differences in the response to exercise training; some people exhibit a high-responder pattern while others are almost nonresponders. Human variation in trainability is considerable for both maximal short-term and long-term anaerobic performance phenotypes. This was shown when we submitted 19 sedentary subjects to 15 weeks of high-intensity intermittent exercise training (Simoneau et al. 1987). Maximal short-term and long-term performance phenotypes improved significantly with training (about 30%), but with a range of about 40% between the lowest and highest performance gains.

The major causes of human variation in the response to training are the current phenotype level, that is, the pretraining status of the trait considered, and a genetically determined capacity to adapt to exercise training that is probably unique for each biological characteristic or family of phenotypes (Bouchard et al. 1992). The latter represents the so-called role of heredity in trainability or, more rigorously, the genotype-training interaction. The role of the genotype in determining the response of predominantly anaerobic performance phenotypes to training has been studied with 14 pairs of MZ twins subjected to a 15-week high-intensity intermittent training program (Simoneau et al., "Inheritance," 1986). Results have shown that the training response of short-term anaerobic performance capacity was little affected by the genotype of the individuals when the scores were expressed in absolute terms or per kilogram of body mass. However, when the results were expressed in Joules per milliliter of thigh volume, the training response was higher and was characterized by a high resemblance among MZ twins (see figure 1.5). The intraclass correlation for the response pattern reached 0.57, which suggests that genetic factors were contributing to individual differences in the capacity to improve maximal short-term performance.

These observations reveal that the range of training changes in the 10 s performance test was about 0.4 J/ml of thigh volume and that the maximal difference in the 10 s performance test between subjects in either the untrained or the trained state reached about 1.5 J/ml. On the other hand, about 60% of the variation in response to training appears to be genetically determined based on the intraclass correlation reported

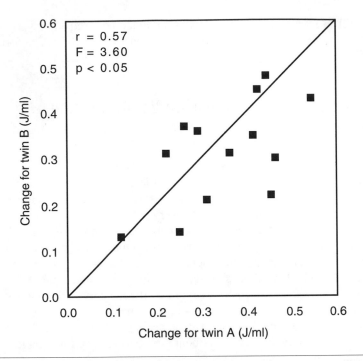

Figure 1.5 Changes in 10 s cycle ergometer performance test, expressed in Joules per milliliter of thigh volume, in monozygotic twins following 15 weeks of high-intensity intermittent exercise training. The intraclass coefficient reflecting the intrapair resemblance for the changes in performance reached 0.57.

Data from Simoneau et al. 1986.

above. However, this value not only includes the genotype-training interaction effects; it is also likely affected by inherited differences in initial performance level.

Similarly, the response of long-term anaerobic performance phenotype is highly comparable among members of MZ pairs. Thus, trainability of the 90 s work output test per kilogram of body mass was characterized by an intraclass coefficient explaining about 70% of the training response variance. When the results were expressed per milliliter of thigh volume, the intraclass coefficient for the training response was even higher, reaching 0.79, as shown in figure 1.6. These data clearly indicate that there are high and low responders to training and that this trainability characteristic is found in close association with the genotype of the individual.

Directions for Future Research

The conclusions proposed in this chapter also constitute a set of hypotheses amenable to testing. Major advances are continuously made in the development of

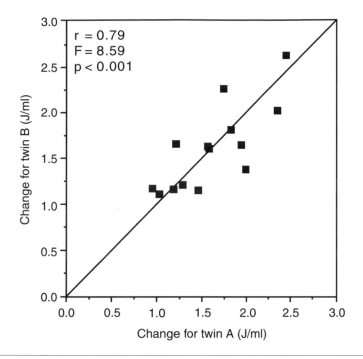

Figure 1.6 Changes in 90 s cycle ergometer performance test, expressed in Joules per milliliter of thigh volume, in monozygotic twins following 15 weeks of high-intensity intermittent exercise training. The intraclass coefficient reflecting the intrapair resemblance for changes in performance reached 0.79.

Data from Simoneau et al. 1986.

molecular biology tools and experimental design that can be used in the genetic dissection of complex human multifactorial traits such as the performance phenotypes. Anaerobic performance involves several determinants that are likely influenced primarily by polygenic systems. Because of the complexity of the phenotype, identification of the genes becomes an enormously difficult task. The challenges include those of generating an appropriate phenotype database and of obtaining a dense set of polymorphic markers typed on a large number of phenotyped individuals. This would allow researchers to begin the task of detecting the contribution of polymorphic markers linked to the variation in anaerobic performance. Another avenue of research is that of defining the genes responsible for the high or low response pattern to training. This task is, however, even more complex, since it requires exposing a large number of biologically diverse individuals to a standardized training program. This approach is the one used in the Heritage project, a family study of health-related variables and their response to endurance training (Bouchard et al. 1995). It is quite clear that such research is beyond the capability of a single laboratory. It requires a concerted effort on the part of several well-developed units.

Although it is utopian at the moment to consider using genetic markers to identify young people who are well endowed for anaerobic performance, this situation may change in the coming decades. When one considers the enormous financial stakes surrounding high-performance events, such as those of the World Championships or the Olympic Games, it would not be surprising if the necessary human and material resources to undertake the genetic dissection of anaerobic performance phenotypes became available in the near future.

Summary

Considerable variation exists in the ability to perform maximally over a short period of time, and this heterogeneity can to a large extent be attributed to genetic factors. As summarized in figure 1.7, we propose that (a) genetic factors account for approximately 50% of the total variance in maximal anaerobic performance phenotype (Simoneau et al., "Anaerobic Work Capacity," 1986), (b) exercise training and other alterable causes represent about 30% of the variance (Simoneau et al. 1987), and (c) a fraction—about 5%—of the variance can be attributed to technical and other sources of error related to the measurement of performance phenotype (Simoneau et al. 1983). From the preceding, one may conclude that the

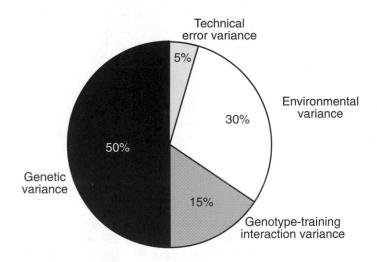

Figure 1.7 An estimate of the contribution of technical error, training, genetic, and genotype-training interaction variance components to the total phenotypic variation in human maximal anaerobic performance phenotypes.

Data from Simoneau et al. 1983; Simoneau et al. 1986; Simoneau et al. 1986; and Simoneau et al. 1987.

genotype-training interaction effects (which are significant, as shown previously) account for the remaining fraction (about 15%) of the total variance in maximal short-term anaerobic performance. Important determinants of anaerobic performance such as fiber type proportion and glycolytic enzyme capacity of skeletal muscle are also influenced by genetic factors, and variation in these and other relevant characteristics can be partly responsible for high and low anaerobic performance phenotypes and training potential.

References

Ama, P.F.M., Simoneau, J.A., Boulay, M.R., et al. 1986. Skeletal muscle characteristics in sedentary Black and Caucasian males. *J. Appl. Physiol.* 61: 1758-1761.

Bouchard, C. 1991. Genetic aspects of anthropometric dimensions relevant to assessment of nutritional status. In *Anthropometric assessment of nutritional status,* ed. J. Himes, 213-231. New York: Liss.

Bouchard, C., Chagnon, M., Thibault, M.-C., et al. 1988. Absence of charge variants in human skeletal muscle enzymes of the glycolytic pathways. *Hum. Gen.* 78: 100.

Bouchard, C., Chagnon, M., Thibault, M.-C., Boulay, M.R., Marcotte, M., Côté, C., and Simoneau, J.-A. 1989. Muscle genetic variant and relationship with performance and trainability. *Med. Sci. Sports Exerc.* 21: 71-77.

Bouchard, C., Dionne, F.T., Simoneau, J.-A., and Boulay, M.R. 1992. Genetics of aerobic and anaerobic performances. In *Exerc. Sport Sci. Rev.* 20, ed. J.O. Holloszy, 27-58. Baltimore: Williams & Wilkins.

Bouchard, C., Leon, A.S., Rao, D.C., Skinner, J.S., Wilmore, J.H., and Gagnon, J. 1995. The Heritage Family Study. Aims, design, and measurement protocol. *Med. Sci. Sports Exerc.* 27: 721-729.

Bouchard, C., Pérusse, L., Leblanc, C., et al. 1988. Inheritance of the amount and distribution of human body fat. *Int. J. Obes.* 12: 205-215.

Bouchard, C., Simoneau, J.-A., Lortie, G., et al. 1986. Genetic effects in human skeletal muscle fiber type distribution and enzyme activities. *Can. J. Physiol. Pharmacol.* 64: 1245-1251.

Brozek, J. 1961. Body measurements including skinfold thickness, as indicators of body composition. In *Techniques for measuring body composition,* ed. J. Brozek and A. Henschel. Washington, DC: National Research Council.

Comuzzie, A.G., Blangero, J., Mahaney, M.C., Mitchell, B.D., Stern M.P., and MacCluer, J.W. 1994. Genetic and environmental correlations among skinfold measurements. *Int. J. Obes.* 18: 413-418.

Falconer, D.S. 1960. *Introduction to quantitative genetics.* New York: Ronald Press.

Gollnick, P.D. 1982. Relationship of strength and endurance with skeletal muscle structure and metabolic potential. *Int. J. Sport Med.* 3: 26-32.

Hewitt, D. 1957. Sib resemblance in bone, muscle and fat measurements of the human calf. *Ann. Hum. Genetics* 22: 213-221.

Howald, H. 1976. Ultrastructure and biochemical functions of skeletal muscle in twins. *Ann. Hum. Biol.* 3: 455-462.

Klissouras, V. 1971. Heritability of adaptive variation. *J. Appl. Physiol.* 31: 338-344.

Klissouras, V. 1973. Prediction of potential performance with special reference to heredity. *J. Sports Med. Phys. Fitness* 13: 100-107.

Komi, P.V., and Karlsson, J. 1979. Physical performance, skeletal muscle enzyme activities and fiber types in monozygous and dizygous twins of both sexes. *Acta Physiol. Scand. Suppl.* 462: 1-28.

Komi, P.V., Klissouras, V., and Karvinen, E. 1973. Genetic variation in neuromuscular performance. *Int. Zeitschrift für Angewandte Physiol.* 31: 289-330.

Komi, P.V., Viitasalo, H.T., Havu, M., et al. 1977. Skeletal muscle fibres and muscle enzyme activities in monozygous and dizygous twins of both sexes. *Acta Physiol. Scand.* 100: 385-392.

Kovar, R. 1975. Motor performance in twins. *Acta Genet. Med. Gemellolol.* 24: 174.

Malina, R.M., and Mueller, W.H. 1981. Genetic and environmental influences on the strength and motor performance of Philadelphia school children. *Hum. Biol.* 53: 163-179.

Marcotte, M., Chagnon, M., Côté, C., et al. 1987. Lack of genetic polymorphism in human skeletal muscle enzymes of the tricarboxylic acid cycle. *Hum. Gen.* 77: 200.

Newsholme, E.A. 1980. Use of enzyme activity measurement in studies of the biochemistry of exercise. *Int. J. Sports Med.* 1: 100-102.

Nimmo, M.A., Wilson, R.H., and Snow, D.H. 1985. The inheritance of skeletal muscle fibre composition in mice. *Comp. Biol. Physiol.* 81A: 109-115.

Rice, T., Borecki, I.B., Bouchard, C., and Rao, D.C. 1993. Segregation analysis of fat mass and other body composition measures derived from underwater weighing. *Am. J. Hum. Genetics* 52: 967-973.

Roy, R.R., Baldwin, K.M., and Edgerton, V.R. 1991. The plasticity of skeletal muscle: effects of neuromuscular activity. *Exerc. Sports Sci. Rev.* 19: 269-312.

Saltin, B., and Gollnick, P.D. 1983. Significance for metabolism and performance. In *Handbook of physiology.* Sec. 10, *Skeletal muscle,* ed. L.D. Peachey, R.H. Adrian, and S.R. Geiger, 555-631. Bethesda, MD: American Physiological Society.

Serresse, O., Ama, P.F.M., Simoneau, J.A., et al. 1989. Anaerobic performances of sedentary and trained subjects. *Can. J. Sport Sci.* 14: I46-52.

Simoneau, J.A. 1995. Adaptation of human skeletal muscle to exercise-training. *Int. J. Obes.* 19: S9-S13.

Simoneau, J.A., and Bouchard, C. 1989. Human variation in skeletal muscle fiber-type proportion and enzyme activities. *Am. J. Physiol.* 257: E567-E572.

Simoneau, J.A., and Bouchard, C. 1995. Genetic determinism of fiber type proportion in human skeletal muscle. *FASEB J.* 9: 1091-1095.

Simoneau, J.-A., Lortie, G., Boulay, M.R., and Bouchard, C. 1983. Tests of anaerobic alactacid and lactacid capacities: description and reliability. *Can. J. Sport Sci.* 8: 266-270.

Simoneau, J.-A., Lortie, G., Boulay, M.R., Marcotte, M., Thibault, M.-C., and Bouchard, C. 1986. Inheritance of human skeletal muscle and anaerobic capacity adaptation to high-intensity intermittent training. *Int. J. Sports Med.* 7: 167-171.

Simoneau, J.A., Lortie, G., Boulay, M.R., Marcotte, M., Thibault, M.-C., and Bouchard, C. 1987. Effects of two high-intensity intermittent training programs interspaced by detraining on human skeletal muscle and performance. *Eur. J. Appl. Physiol.* 56: 516-521.

Simoneau, J.-A., Lortie, G., Boulay, M.R., Thibault, M.-C., Thériault, G., and Bouchard, C. 1985. Skeletal muscle histochemical and biochemical characteristics in sedentary male and female subjects. *Can. J. Physiol. Pharmacol.* 63: 30-35.

Simoneau, J.A., Lortie, G., Leblanc, C., et al. 1986. Anaerobic work capacity in adopted and biological siblings. In *Sport and human genetics,* ed. R.M. Malina and C. Bouchard, 165-171. Champaign, IL: Human Kinetics.

Sklad, M. 1972. Similarity of movements in twins. *Wychowanie Fizyczne i Sport* 16: 119-141.

Weiss, V. 1979. Die Heritabilitäten sportlicher Tests, berechnet aus den Leistungen zehnjähriger Zwillingspaare. *Leistungssport.* 9: 58-61.

Wolanski, N., Tomonari, K., and Siniarska, A. 1980. Genetics and the motor development of man. *Hum. Ecol. Race Hyg.* 46: 169-191.

2

CHAPTER

Infant Motor Development: The Biomechanics of Change

Jody L. Jensen
Krisanne E. Bothner

This chapter focuses on the following objectives:

- To document changes in mass, mass distribution, and the forces associated with these changing mass characteristics in the first year of life
- To demonstrate the impact of changing inertial characteristics and gravitational context on the performance of fundamental motor skills
- To document how relief from biomechanical demands leads to precocious movement behavior
- To show the integration of muscular and non-muscular forces in the expanding motor repertoire
- To demonstrate the importance of kinetic analyses in revealing developmental change

It is during the first two years of life that infants begin to express, and master, the fundamental motor skills of sitting, reaching, standing, walking, and running. Traditional developmental theories have posited neuromaturational, cognitive, and interactive explanations for the order of appearance and the time scale for the emergence of these motor skills. Depending on the perspective, the physical properties of the neuromotor system have been either ignored, or acknowledged only in a cursory way. The literature is replete with descriptions of growth changes throughout early childhood and adolescence (e.g., Malina and Bouchard 1991; Tanner and Whitehouse 1982). Only recently, however, have attempts been made to quantify the impact of such growth changes on the force requirements for the production of functional movement in the context of a gravity-defined environment and the changing inertial characteristics of the musculoskeletal system.

Consider the tasks assessed by developmental schedules. Such schedules are typically organized around reflexive behaviors, balance skills, non-locomotor and locomotor skills, and tasks involving object reception and projection (e.g., Bayley Scales of Infant Development, 2nd Ed., 1993, Psychological Corp; Frankenburg, Dodds, Archer, Shapiro, and Bresnick 1992). Rather than classify the developmental skills by function performed, we could create a new classification system based on the mechanics mastered. In such a scheme, tasks would be characterized by increasing demands on a) the ability to stabilize a larger proportion of total body mass, b) the ability to oppose and, when appropriate, exploit the forces of gravity, and c) the ability to exploit the passive/reactive forces associated with multi-segmented motion.

In this chapter we will revisit the "developmental schedule" from the perspective of biomechanics. There will be four parts to our discussion. First, we will discuss physical growth changes in mass, resultant changes in mass distribution, and the forces associated with these changing mass characteristics. In the second section we will discuss the impact of changing inertial characteristics of the moving system and the gravitational context on the performance of fundamental skills. The third section addresses how relief from biomechanical demands leads to precocious movement behavior. In the fourth section we explore how expansion of the infant motor repertoire is, in part, a function of the infant's changing ability to combine muscular and non-muscular (inertial and gravitational) forces. In the final section on future directions for research, we discuss kinetic analyses as important tools in exploring developmental change. Sitting, reaching, kicking, and locomotor tasks acquired in the first year of life will be our windows on the infant's mastery of the physical properties of the motor system in a context defined by gravity.

Changes in Mass, Mass Distribution, and the Forces Associated With Moving Masses

The first year of life is characterized by dramatic change in body size and shape. Consider these elements of development: (a) birth weight typically doubles before 6 months of age; (b) by the end of the first year, body weight is nearly three times the birth weight; (c) body length increases by approximately 30% in the first 6 months; and (d) a 50% increase in body length is reached by the end of the first year (Payne and Isaacs 1995). The importance of the changing mass and length characteristics of the developing infant lies in the concomitant changes in factors that define the inertial characteristics of the moving body and limbs. In addition to the mass of the system, the other important characteristics are the location of the segment (or limb) center of gravity and the moment of inertia.

Changes in Mass

Growth means an increase in size and mass, but the pattern of growth is not uniform across all body segments. At birth, the mass is concentrated in the head and trunk segments. At this age, the head makes up a full quarter of total body length, and the extremities are disproportionately short relative to the trunk (Timiras, 1972). After birth, head growth slows while growth of the trunk continues at a moderate rate, with the fastest rate of growth occurring in the extremities. Figure 2.1 shows data on lower extremity segmental changes in mass between 2 weeks and 11 months of age. These data are based on body mass, segment length, and segment circumference measures made on a total of 33 infants. Individual segment inertial parameters (segment mass, location of segment center of gravity, and moment of inertia) were calculated using the regression equations of Schneider and Zernicke (1992) (1). Greater gains are made in the more proximal segments. In this sample, the respective average gains in the thigh, leg, and foot segments were 0.48, 0.26, and 0.08 kg per month during the first year (see also Sun and Jensen 1994). Thus it is not only mass, but also the proportions that change over the course of infancy and early childhood.

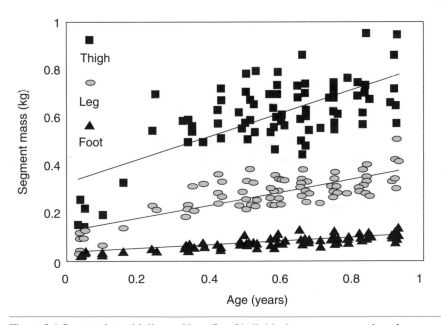

Figure 2.1 Scatter plot, with lines of best fit, of individual segment masses based on anthropometric measurements from infants between 2 weeks and 11 months of age. Figure includes repeated measures on 26 of 33 infants.

Data from Timiras 1972.

Location of the Center of Gravity (2)

The center-of-gravity (COG) is a single point in the rigid body that we use to represent the balanced distribution of body's mass. One of the assumptions we make in the determination of mechanical demands is that the limb is a rigid body, like a stiff rod of uniform density. This assumption allows us to fix the point of application of the gravitational force at the COG. Thus, the weight of the segment (mass · gravity) acts at the center of gravity. The position of the COG for limb segments is generally expressed as a percentage of the segment length from the proximal end (e.g., Schneider and Zernicke 1992; Sun and Jensen 1994).

As a consequence of growth in length, the segment COG will move away from the joint, or rotational axis. The perpendicular distance between the axis of rotation and the vertical line of action of gravity as it passes through the limb COG is referred to as the moment arm. Thus, growth in segment length increases the moment arm for the weight of the limb. The consequence of increasing the moment arm is in its effect on the resultant torque, or the turning effect of a force. Torque is the product of the force and the moment arm. Thus increasing the gravitational moment arm increases the effect of gravity on creating rotation at a joint. This increase in the gravitational torque has a profound effect on the mechanics of movement. The task becomes one of gaining a mechanical advantage over this longer, heavier limb, subject to the limitations of available muscle strength and short moment arms for the muscle force line of action (see Jensen, Sun, Treitz, and Parker 1997).

Moment of Inertia

Inertia (I) is a function of mass and its distribution and refers to an object's resistance to a change in rotational motion ($I = mr^2$ for a long rigid body; where m = mass and r = distance between the COG and the axis of rotation). The greater the mass, the more difficult it is to set the mass in motion, or to stop it once it is moving. Distributing the mass away from an axis of rotation also increases the system's resistance to change in rotational motion. Thus as the infant grows, the gains in mass and segment length make the initiation and cessation of motion more effortful.

A two-dimensional representation of combined changes in mass and length is presented in figure 2.2. The two leg models reflect the anthropometric characteristics of the lower extremity at 2 weeks of age (shaded model) and 3 months of age (unshaded model). The change in inertial characteristics produced by this growth in length and mass is clear. Based on measurements on representative infants, the moment of inertia for the thigh segment of a 2-week-old infant (depicted in figure 2.2) is $4.91 \cdot 10^{-4}$ kg-m^2. At 3 months of age, the thigh moment of inertia increases to $10.39 \cdot 10^{-4}$ kg-m^2. This is a 210% increase. By 6 months of age, the magnitude of change in the thigh is on the order of 350% of the inertia value at 2 weeks. The implication is, of course, that increasing the resistance to motion requires a corresponding increase in forces applied to the system to produce motion.

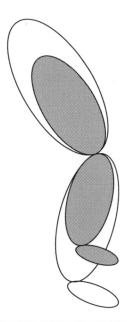

Figure 2.2 Representation of infant leg mass based on measurements taken at 2 weeks (shaded) and 3 months of age (unshaded). The area of each ellipse is scaled to the infant's calculated mass for that segment. The length of each ellipse is scaled to the infant's measured limb length.

The dramatic changes in body mass, total body length, and proportionality that occur in the first year of life mean significant changes in the dynamic characteristics of the moving system. The consequences of these inertial changes can be seen in changes in muscle torque required to lift the limb or move a body defined by larger mass and increased moments of inertia. As an example of the consequences of segment mass and length changes on the infant's ability to move the leg, consider the torque at the hip if the child performs a leg lift. Figure 2.3 shows a typical lower extremity configuration for a 2-week-old and a 3-month-old kicking in a supine posture. The filled circle marks the COG for the system of thigh, shank, and foot. D1 and d2 identify the gravitational moment arms for each system. Using the inertial characteristics of two representative infants we can determine the changes in the gravitational moment created by the changes in the inertial characteristics. For the 2-week-old infant, the moment created by gravity is 0.31 Nm; for the 3-month-old the value is 0.85 Nm, a 280% increase in required torque. The leg lift position shown in figure 2.3 is not an uncommon leg position for young infants. To maintain this posture requires a flexor muscle torque that matches the torque due to gravity. The calculation of the gravitational torque experienced by each infant in this static posture directly reveals the influence of growth in mass and length on the force requirements for performance of the task.

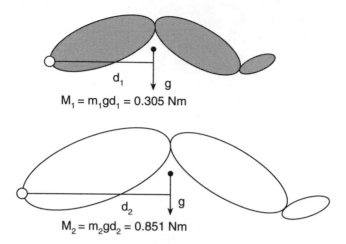

$$M_1 = m_1gd_1 = 0.305 \text{ Nm}$$

$$M_2 = m_2gd_2 = 0.851 \text{ Nm}$$

Figure 2.3 Graphic illustration of the effect of segment length increases between 2 weeks (shaded) and 3 months of age (unshaded) on the moment arm of the leg system. Filled circle represents approximate position of the total limb's center of gravity. These static hip joint moments, calculated from the anthropometrics for two representative infants, and based on a defined posture and orientation to gravity, show the effect of increases in length and mass on required muscle torque.

The Shaping of Motor Skills

Movement is constructed in a world defined by gravity. Certainly one of the constraints on the appearance of new motor skills is the infant's ability to generate sufficient force to oppose this damping gravitational force field.

The Ubiquity of Gravity

In the previous section we quantified the effect of growth in a gravity environment. Here we present developmental evidence for the shaping of motor outcomes by the external force environment.

Sitting

The course to independent sitting begins with the ability to lift the head and hold it erect on the trunk, while a care giver holds the infant about the trunk and provides the upright orientation. To remove the external support would result in an immediate forward fall of the head and trunk. As increasing control (sufficient strength for stabilization) of the head, neck, and trunk develops, the infant adopts a "prop-sit" strategy. Here the arms are used as a brace to constrain the forward lean of the trunk (4-5 months of age). The consequence, of course, is that the arms are involved in the postural task, not exploratory and manipulative tasks. Such use of the arms comes only after the development of appropriate postural muscle activation for pelvic and trunk control (5-6 months of age).

The alignment of the head and trunk above the support surface is directly related to the muscle activation patterns used by infants to maintain stability. Evidence for this claim comes from the identification of two predominant muscle activation combinations in response to a natural perturbation created by releasing the infant from supported sitting in a vertical posture (Harbourne, Guiliani, and Mac Neela 1993). One activation pattern was a combination of the lumbar paraspinals and quadriceps. The lumbar paraspinals and hamstrings constituted the second pattern. With an initial anterior tilt to the pelvis and lower trunk at the time of release (see figure 2.4, left), the most effective compensation for the resultant forward motion of the trunk and head is activation of the musculature on the posterior aspect of the body, the lumbar paraspinals and hamstrings. A posture with an initial posterior tilt to the pelvis and lower trunk, but anterior tilt in the upper trunk (see figure 2.4, right) leads to activation of the lumbar paraspinals and the quadriceps to facilitate upper trunk extension and stabilization, and flexion of the pelvis on the thigh. The recruitment of the quadriceps in this case serves to pull the trunk forward, in fact contributing to the overall destabilization of the infant's upper body over the support

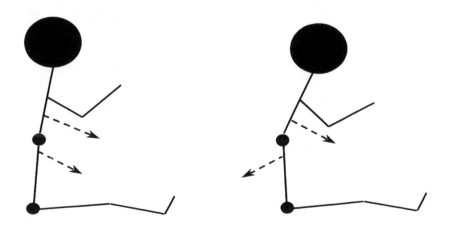

Figure 2.4 Simplified model of a sitting child. Two possible orientations of the pelvis and trunk determine the muscle activation pattern observed. Arrows indicate the direction of initial segmental collapse when postural support is removed from the infant. Left: Initial posture is one of anterior tilt of the pelvic and trunk segments. Right: Pelvic segment shows an initial posterior tilt, trunk segment is in a position of anterior tilt.

Data from R.T. Harbourne, C. Guiliani, and J. Mac Neela 1993.

surface. When this combination of muscles is activated together, the resultant forward movement of the trunk is larger in amplitude and has higher velocity than other responses. The biomechanics of the sitting posture, specifically the initial orientation with respect to gravity, thus plays a significant role in shaping the kinematics as well as the electromyographic patterns observed in response to this postural disturbance (3).

Reaching

Research on the development of reaching skills also demonstrates the infant's sensitivity to working in an environment of forces. For example, opposing forces due to gravity may be maximized or minimized, depending on one's posture. Initiation of the reach in any posture requires that muscular forces must be developed to overcome the opposition presented by gravity. An analysis of stylized versions of the supine and vertical postures reveals the posture-dependent force requirements induced by gravity (see figure 2.5).

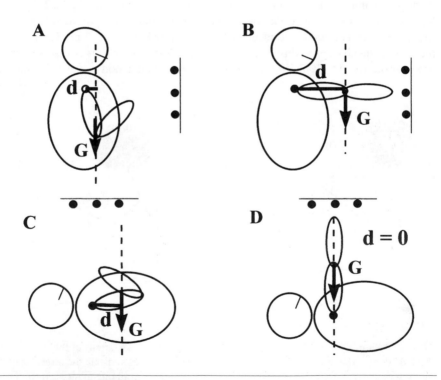

Figure 2.5 Representation of gravitational moment arms in vertical (a, b) and supine (c, d) reaching postures. *d* represents the gravitational moment arm; G represents the line of action for gravity. The gravitational torque is the product of *d* and G.

Data from G.J.P. Savelsbergh and J. van der Kamp 1994.

As previously described, the magnitude of the gravitational opposition to movement is the product of the gravitational moment arm (d), and the acceleration due to gravity. Since the acceleration is a constant (-9.81 m/s^2), the factor of interest, and the factor that may be manipulated, is d. In figure 2.5 a-d, we can see that, for initiation, d is smallest in the vertical posture when compared to supine (compare figures 2.5a and b). As the reaching movement progresses, d changes and the gravitational torque increases. Thus, the vertical posture facilitates initiation of the reach, but the gravitational torque increases as the hand closes on the target (figure 2.5b). In contrast, d decreases during the course of a reach performed in the supine position (compare 2.5c and 2.5d).

If gravity plays a functional role in the construction and expression of infant movement, then one would argue that the initiation of reaching is facilitated when d is small, and this condition is met most often in the vertical posture. Following the logic, one would further argue that while the initiation of reaching is facilitated by the vertical posture, the effect of gravity makes reaching for high targets more problematic. Thus an infant reaching for targets of different heights while seated in a vertical position is more likely to reach for lower targets than for higher targets. These hypotheses were proposed by Savelsbergh and van der Kamp (1994).

In a series of experiments, Savelsbergh and van der Kamp (1994) explored the effect of orientation to gravity on reaching behavior of infants between 12 and 27 weeks of age. As depicted in figure 2.5, the infants were enticed to reach for objects while seated in vertical, reclined (30° from the vertical: not shown), and supine positions. The results followed the predictions. Younger infants (12-19 weeks of age) were particularly sensitive to posture and initiated more reaches in the vertical position than in either the reclined or supine postures. (Posture had no effect on reach initiation for the older infants, 20-27 weeks of age. This result may point to the role of increasing strength — a particularly troublesome measure to gain from infants.) More reaches were initiated when the arms were close to the body (when d was small), than when the arms were held in an extended posture away from the body. When placed in the reclined and vertical postures, infants (regardless of age) were less likely to contact balls in the top row of the display. These results are consistent with our understanding of the effort required to produce the movement based on the mechanical demands.

Kicking

A similar sensitivity to gravitational constraints was observed in the kicking behaviors of 3-month-old infants (Jensen, Ulrich, Thelen, Schneider, and Zernicke 1994). A comparison of kinematic and kinetic characteristics of kicks performed in supine, reclined and vertical postures revealed a distinct postural effect. Hip joint flexion decreased successively from supine to reclined, and reclined to vertical postures. Just as Savelsbergh and van der Kamp (1994) found in movements of the upper extremity, these infants did not lift the mass of the lower extremity as high (relative to the body) in those postures in which gravity provided the greatest opposition.

Lifting the leg against gravity appeared to be more effortful in the vertical posture. This "effort" was apparent in the increased synchrony of hip and knee joint angle changes (Jensen et al. 1994). In the supine posture, gravitational resistance to the *initiation* of motion was high, but the resistance decreased during the course of motion as the gravitational moment arm decreased. This reduction of the external constraints was associated with greater independence in hip and knee joint actions.

Artificial Manipulations of Inertial Characteristics

Artificial manipulations of inertial characteristics have been achieved by adding mass to or subtracting it from the body or moving limbs. These manipulations explicitly demonstrate the sensitivity of the neuromotor system to inertial constraints, both in their effects on the perturbed limb and on interlimb coordination.

Kicking

The sensitivity of the infant neuromotor system to the mechanical and gravitational demands of the task has been studied explicitly by manipulating the mass of the limb and observing the motor response. In a now classic study, Thelen, Fisher, and Ridley-Johnson (1984) offered the hypothesis of a reduced strength-to-weight ratio as an explanation for the disappearance of the infant stepping reflex. Previously hypothesized to be the result of cortical maturation, Thelen and colleagues argued for a physical, rather than neural, explanation. As infants gain weight, predominantly adipose versus muscle tissue, the legs may simply become too heavy to lift. If this is the case, then "making" the legs lighter should facilitate the performance of the stepping reflex. The test of this hypothesis was to manipulate the weight of the legs of young infants. Submerging an object, or limb, in water, functionally lightens the object as the downward pull of gravity is partially offset by an upward buoyant force. If the weight of the limb is the constraint on stepping, then reduction in limb weight should result in the "reappearance" of the stepping behavior. Thelen, Fisher, and Ridley-Johnson (1984) found that upon submersion in water, these 4-week-old infants, with a decreased tendency to step on dry land, increased both the number of steps performed and the amplitude of the movement (i.e., higher leg lift). Theoretically, Savelsbergh and van der Kamp (1994) would find infants reaching to the top row of the object display if they, too, were submerged in chest deep water.

It is intuitively obvious that strapping an additional mass on to an arm or leg changes the inertial characteristics of the limb. What is not obvious is the effect of this perturbation on the movement outcome. Mechanically, the task demands have increased. The intriguing question is how will the neuromotor system deal with this constraint? The application of external weights to the limbs of infants has been used as an experimental intervention to study the strength of interlimb coordination. Thelen, Skala, and Kelso (1987) weighted one leg of 6-week-old infants and recorded their kicking behaviors. As might be expected, the weighted leg kicked less frequently. However, the overall kick rate was maintained at the unweighted level by an increase in the kicks performed by the non-weighted leg. Thelen and colleagues argued that this result demonstrated a dynamic bilateral coupling between the limbs. (See also Corbetta and Thelen, 1994, for an example of the dynamic coupling between unilaterally weighted arms.)

Locomotion

The addition of an external mass has also been shown to reduce performance variability. When first learning to walk, infants have a gait pattern all their own. While it is true that infant gait and the mature adult gait share such features as an alternating pattern and 50/50 phasing (one limb starts the gait cycle half way through the other limb's cycle), high variability characterizes both interlimb and intralimb spatial and temporal patterns of the new walker. By adding mass to the system, some of this variability can be reduced.

Clark and Phillips (1993) weighted one leg of new walkers with an ankle weight equivalent to 5% of the infant's body weight. The newest walkers (capable of three independent steps) would not take a step with one limb weighted. For the toddler with four weeks of walking experience, the added weight was not disruptive. The inertial forces of the weight led to better swing limb dynamics, the result of which was measured by the appearance of a more mature pattern in the timing of reversals in thigh and leg segment motion. In fact the weight allowed the 4-week walker to express an intralimb timing pattern typical of the mature walker.

Precocious Movement Behavior

Adding a mass to the limb or body is one way of assessing the susceptibility of the neuromotor system to mechanical demands of the task. An alternative paradigm is to provide varying degrees of external support. Numerous examples exist in which the provision of postural support relieves a significant mechanical burden and allows for the appearance of otherwise hidden movement patterns — hidden behind the overwhelming mechanical demands of controlling the body's mass, its orientation, and acceleration. In each case, what is being provided is a) a release of constraints applied to the body by its own configuration and/or inertial characteristics, or b) the application of constraints to control unwanted accelerations of the body or its segments.

Sitting

As the infant makes the transition from pushing up on the hands from a prone position to independent sitting, the tasks may be viewed as tasks of lifting and balancing large, multi-articulated masses. Once the balance task of head and trunk control has been mastered, the arms are no longer required as props, and reaching and manipulation skills emerge. For example, Rochat and Goubet (1995) studied the relationship between sitting independence and manipulative skill in three groups of infants: nonsitters (unable to sit independently for 30 s), near-sitters (able to sit independently for 30 s but with the hands used as props or with the trunk folded forward over the legs), and sitters (able to sit independently for 30 s with hands above the ground). The infants were presented with a 15-ball display with balls arranged in central and peripheral regions, high and low. The results revealed that sitting control was positively correlated with increasing access to wider reaching zones.

Mastery of head and trunk postural control means more than just the ability to balance the masses in a static posture. Mastery means that movement between the segments is effectively controlled, with movements in concert — not in opposition. For example, to reach an object just at the edge, or just out, of arm's reach, a forward lean of the trunk provides the mechanism of displacement to successfully contact the object. Independent sitters typically demonstrate a coordinated pattern of trunk and arm movement with extension of the arm towards the toy and a definitive forward lean of the trunk during the final seconds of acquisition (Rochat and Goubet 1995). Unlike the sitters, the non-sitters showed no such coordinated pattern. If there was forward lean of the trunk it typically occurred at the start of the trial, just after the infant had been positioned in a trunk-vertical posture and released. The timing of this trunk motion suggested that the infant fell forward, after which the arm extended towards the toy. If sufficient external trunk support is provided to a non-sitter, however, the coordination differences between the sitter and non-sitter can be eliminated. This was the follow-up study done by Rochat and Goubet after observing the differences in the trunk-arm coordination pattern of sitters, near-sitters, and non-sitters. To provide the postural support, Rochat and Goubet (1995) placed an inflatable bladder around the hips and lower trunk of the infant. When provided with a high degree of postural support, the frequency of coordinated reaches by non-sitters was similar to that of independent sitters.

Locomotion

Mature gait is characterized by right and left steps of equal distance (distance phasing) and right and left steps of equal duration and with 50/50 phasing. From the onset of independent locomotion, mean temporal and distance phasing measures are 50/50 (see Clark, Whitall, and Phillips 1988; and figure 2.6a). The same cannot be said for temporal and distance phasing variability. The less experienced in independent locomotion, the more variable the locomotor pattern. But hold the hands of a new walker and this variability will be significantly reduced. Compare temporal phasing variability of the "new supported" walker (capable of three independent steps, but lightly supported at the hands) and infants with 2 weeks, 1 month, 3

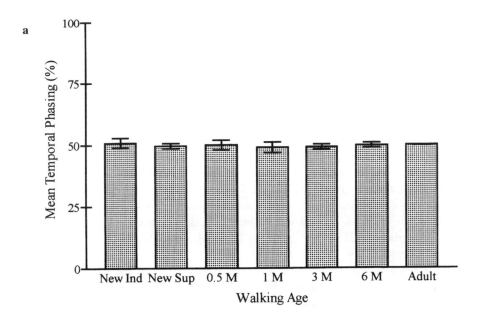

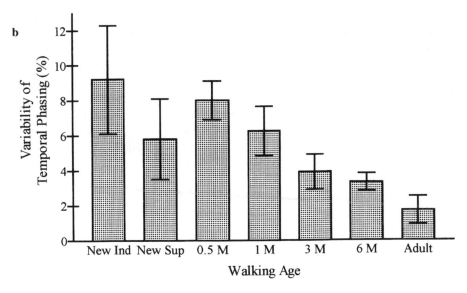

Figure 2.6 (a): Mean temporal phasing for children with different walking experience, and the adult comparison. (b): Variability in temporal phasing between subjects with different walking experience, with the adult comparison.

Data from J.E.Clark, J. Whitall, and S.J. Phillips 1988.

months and more walking experience (see figure 2.6b). When given postural support, new walkers performed with reduced variability similar to that of a walker with 3 months of experience.

Exploiting Nonmuscular and Gravitational Forces

Developmental schedules for motor skills reflect the increasing ability of the infant to oppose and counterbalance the force of gravity. Independent sitting and independent stance, as static postures, are built upon the infant's ability to create a finely tuned balance between muscular forces and the pull of gravity. Movement, however, introduces another set of forces to be controlled — motion-dependent forces, or the forces associated with the mechanical interaction of linked segments (e.g., Hollerbach and Flash 1982; Hoy and Zernicke 1986; Schneider and Zernicke 1990). Consider, for example, the difference in the control of a kick of small amplitude and low velocity compared to a more vigorous kick of larger amplitude. Figure 2.7 shows the muscular (MUS), gravitational (GRA), and motion-dependent torques (MDT) associated with each type of kick. Control at the hip for the slower kick (see figure 2.7a) is predominantly a balancing act between a flexor muscle torque and the tendency towards hip extension created by gravity. MDT is comparatively small, oscillating about zero. Notice that MUS is a flexor torque during the entire course of the kick. Muscle is the motive force for the flexion phase, and eccentrically controls the gravity-driven extension. The vigorous kick (see figure 2.7b) is characterized by greater acceleration of the segments and, consequently, larger motion-dependent torques. In this case, MDT provides the flexor torque during the terminal flexion phase (0.2 - 0.3 s). Muscle, in concert with gravity, initiates and drives hip extension (0.3 s) by creating an extensor torque to counterbalance the large flexor MDT influence. With motions involving large MDTs, the need for muscular force may be reduced as the non-muscular torques provide the drive behind parts of the action.

Using muscular forces to complement and counterbalance gravity and motion-dependent forces is a hallmark of motor skill. This complementary use of forces, however, is also a skill that infants must acquire. Just because infant movements create motion-dependent forces, does not mean that these forces are being functionally and adaptively exploited in the achievement of the task. A comparison of early infant and adult locomotion provides an example of how behavioral similarities are constructed from quite different kinetic patterns.

Long before infants are capable of independent locomotion, they are capable of performing alternating stepping on a motorized treadmill when provided with postural support (Thelen 1986; Thelen and Ulrich 1991; see also Forssberg 1985). This is another example of a functional behavior that may be expressed early in development under the proper support conditions.

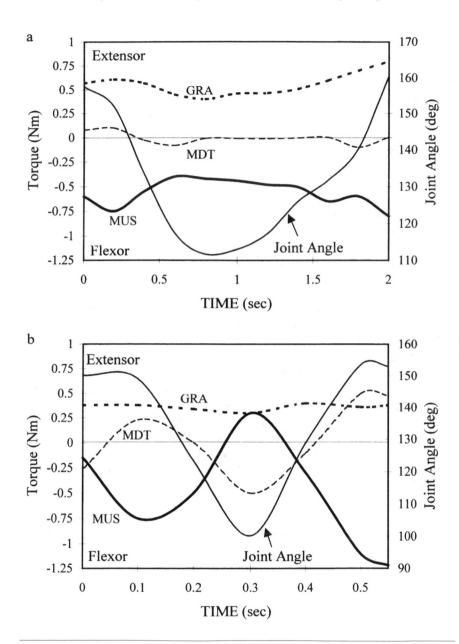

Figure 2.7 Hip joint torques for representative slow (a) and fast (b) kicks performed by a 3-month-old infant. The NET torque (not shown) has been partitioned to show the separate contributions of motion-dependent (MDT), gravitational (GRA), and muscular (MUS) torques to the control of these kicks at the hip. See text for discussion.

Data from K.Kamm, E. Thelen, and J.L. Jensen 1990.

The infant stepping is clearly an immature form of the adult pattern. Infants demonstrate greater variability in lower extremity joint range of motion, step cycle times, and swing/stance ratios. Despite the kinematic differences between adult and infant treadmill stepping, we still recognize the lower extremity movement pattern of these infants as the same macroscopic behavior that ultimately serves us in the performance of independent locomotion. While alternating stepping is recognized as a distinguishing characteristic of independent locomotion, infants and adults do not perform this movement in the same way. It is in the kinetic description of the two steps that interesting differences, and a developmental story, may be found.

For the adult, swing is initiated with a flexor muscle torque at the hip. Midway through the swing, however, the MDTs begin to generate a large flexor torque. In fact, continued flexion of the thigh at the hip is driven by MDT. In the later half of the swing, an extensor muscle torque opposes the motion and acts with gravity to slow the forward rotation of the thigh in preparation for the next heel strike. This is a classic example of exploitation of swing limb dynamics. While muscle initiates the action, its subsequent role is to complement the work done by gravity and other non-muscular forces.

Little exploitation of non-muscular forces is seen in the infant. Like the adult step, swing initiation is driven by muscle. Motion-dependent torques may contribute to hip joint flexion, but they are typically of insufficient magnitude to carry the motion. The muscle torque is remains flexor throughout much of the swing. Gravity is the dominant contributor to hip joint reversal. Ulrich and colleagues reported that hip reversal at the end of swing in 85% of all analyzed trials by 7-month-old treadmill steppers was driven by gravity. In 60% of the trials, the muscle torque was flexor throughout the swing (Ulrich et al. 1994).

Directions for Future Research

The emphasis of past research has been on qualitative aspects of motor behavior in infancy and early childhood. Motor milestones have been described in terms of what they look like and when they occur, and yet we are left with the most interesting of all questions: *Why do these behaviors emerge when they do?* The answer to this question requires assessment at multiple levels of analysis.

Developmental schedules originated from behavioral observations, providing a time line for the appearance of new behaviors. More exacting descriptions of movement topography are the result of kinematic analyses, the quantification of movement amplitudes, velocities and accelerations. Electromyographic studies add another level to the analysis, providing a window on central nervous system strategies for the control of movement. The information provided by these analyses is copious and allows for elaborate description of movement and developmental change. What they do not provide is an understanding of cause. At the level of biomechanics, questions of causation must be answered by kinetic analyses.

Underlying the maintenance of posture or the initiation and cessation of move-ment is an intricate balance of muscular and non-muscular forces. To understand how the nervous system controls movement requires an understanding of this ki-netic strategy. Electromyography typically has been used as our window on central nervous system control of movement, but as Winter (1995) argues "the moments-of-force [joint torques]... are net effects of all agonist and antagonist muscles ... and in spite of their mechanical units (N-m) they must be considered to be neurological signals" (p. 112).

Limited work on joint torque analyses of infant motor performance has appeared in the literature to date, but this preliminary work has been quite informative (e.g., Jensen et al. 1994; Schneider et al. 1990; Thelen et al. 1993). One important outcome of this research is an appreciation of how the infant constructs the motor performance out of muscular, inertial, and gravitational force components, and how this construction differs from the mature pattern. Determination of these individual components informs us about developmental changes in the structure of the perfor-mance. It is at this level of analysis that compelling observations may be made regarding the infant's changing capabilities in force generation and control of the complex interplay of movement dynamics. The subtle (and not so subtle) qualitative differences in task performance that do not make it into the Bayley Scales of Infant Development (e.g., sits alone momentarily *with less head instability,* or sits down gently *rather than sits down with a drop*) are likely to be the result of improvement in muscular force management skills. For example, Roncesvalles (1997) has revealed the increasingly task-appropriate modulation of muscle torques about the ankle, knee, and hip that underlies the improvement in standing balance control in infants and young children. Thus torque analyses provide a level of understanding previously unexplored in the study of infant motor development.

Kinetic analyses need not be restricted to torques variables. Mechanical energy and power analyses are specifically suited to the assessment of energy efficiency, interlimb coupling, and the rate at which work can be done. Previous discussion of torque analyses introduced the consideration of motion-dependent torques — those torques resulting from the mechanical interaction of linked segments. We can take advantage of the MDTs, thus relieving the muscle from having to do work on the system. If the MDTs can sustain hip joint flexion during the swing cycle of locomo-tion, why activate the hip joint flexors? Here, the passive forces contribute to an increase in the energy of a limb or limb segment. Alternatively, it may be necessary to constrain MDTs if they would otherwise cause inappropriate motion. In this case, limb segment energy is reduced, or absorbed, as muscle torques are generated to counterbalance MDT.

The absorption of energy is not necessarily a negative outcome. When the muscle torque opposes the direction of motion (e.g., a hip extensor muscle torque during hip joint flexion), energy is absorbed. The associated physiological event is an eccen-tric, or lengthening, contraction. This is a metabolically effective way of reducing the momentum of the limb. It is also a mechanism that can serve as a conduit of energy from one segment to another, or as an energy storage device for later use (potential energy). Determining whether, and/or when, infants use energy conservation and energy transfer, will reveal greater detail about the development of control processes.

Power analyses may also be used to inform us about interlimb coupling. Jensen et al. (1995) documented a developmental course of increasing stiffness modulation in the hip and knee joints during kicks performed by infants between 2 weeks and 7 months of age. Comparison of power generation at the hip and knee revealed a hip dominance of the order of 20:1 for 2-week-old infants. Kicks for these young infants were under proximal control with little independent motion allowed at the knee. Seven-month-olds demonstrated a more adult-like pattern (4-to-1 ratio). These power changes showed a developing independence in hip and knee joint actions, and an ability to transfer energy between proximal and distal segments. Use of these mechanisms for energy transfer is critical to the development of task-appropriate and functionally adaptive patterns of movement.

Summary

The biomechanics of the neuromotor system, the interaction of biological and mechanical constraints, plays an important role in shaping an infant's motor performance. The inertial properties of the limbs — mass, COG location, and moments of inertia — are significant contributors to the movement topography and thus become logical parameters for experimental manipulation. We manipulate the mechanics of the task to elicit or suppress the expression of selected motor behaviors. These manipulations may lead to a) a shortening of the gravitational moment arm, thus reducing muscular effort, b) a redistribution of the limb or whole body center of mass, exploiting a decrease or increase in the system's inertia, or c) a reduction in the effective mass; that is, a reduction in the mass that must be stabilized or maintained by the mover. What we gain from this kind of manipulation is an understanding of developing movement control and the changing interaction between the biological and mechanical constraints that affect the performer and ultimately define the performance. The expression of new behaviors in the infant's motor repertoire must be viewed not just as a sequence of skills waiting solely on maturation of the nervous system. Expansion of the motor repertoire reflects, as well, the infant's increasing ability to functionally employ and exploit muscular and non-muscular forces.

Kinetic analysis, as an addition to the tools of kinematic and electromyographic analysis, is critical to the exploration and explanation of the construction of developmental sequences. *Why do these behaviors emerge in this sequence, at this time?* Our greatest advances in understanding infant motor skill development will come from kinetic analyses that reveal and quantify 1) muscular and non-muscular force contributions to movement, and 2) the infant's changing capacity to exploit the dynamics of gravity and interlimb coupling.

Acknowledgments

K.E. Bothner was supported by a fellowship awarded through the National Institutes of Health Systems Physiology Training Program, GM07257

Notes

1. Dynamic analyses require data regarding the mass of segments, locations of the segment centers of mass, and the moments of inertia. Most reported values for anthropometric parameters are based on cadaver studies of adult males. There are obvious limitations to such studies and the inappropriateness of adult models for infants is clear. Here we used the regression model for infant anthropometric inertial characteristics developed by Schneider and Zernicke (1992). Inertial parameters for infants and children also may be derived from the regression equations developed by Sun and Jensen (1994).

2. When considering the location of the center of mass in only one dimension, which is defined by the direction of gravity, the center of mass may be referred to as the center of gravity.

3. See also Hirschfeld and Forssberg (1994). Hirschfeld and Forssberg approached the development of independent sitting as an issue of the maturation of central pattern generators for postural control. While the sensitivity of the infant system to mechanical manipulations (postural orientation) was not explicitly tested, they observed dominant postural configurations (see figure 2.4) similar to those observed by Harbourne, et al. (1993). Unlike Harbourne and colleagues, however, Hirschfeld and Forssberg reported that no consistent pattern of muscle activation could be identified in those conditions in which forward sway of the sitting infant was induced. Insufficient information is present in the Hirschfeld and Forssberg article to determine if the variability in the muscle activation patterns was a function of initial body configuration though the authors acknowledge the potential role of mechanical constraints. A recent study by Hirschfeld (1997) has confirmed, however, adaptation of the neuromotor response dependent upon postural orientation.

References

Clark, J.E., and S.J. Phillips. 1993. A longitudinal study of intralimb coordination in the first year of independent walking: A dynamical systems analysis. *Child Development* 64, no. 4: 1143-1157.
Clark, J.E., J. Whitall, and S.J. Phillips. 1988. Human interlimb coordination: The first 6 months of independent walking. *Developmental Psychobiology* 21: 445-456.

Pediatric Anaerobic Performance

Corbetta, D., and E. Thelen. 1994. Interlimb coordination in the development of reaching. *In Motor development: Aspects of normal and delayed development, ed.* J.H.A. van Rossum and J.L. Laszlo, 11-24. Amsterdam: VU University Press.

Forssberg, H. 1985. Ontogeny of human locomotor control. I. Infant stepping, supported locomotion and transition to independent locomotion. *Experimental Brain Research* 57: 480-493.

Frankenburg, W. K., J. B. Dodds, P. Archer, H. Shapiro, and B. Bresnick. 1992. The Denver II: A major revision and re-standardization of the Denver developmental screening test. *Pediatrics* 89: 91-97.

Harbourne, R.T., C. Guiliani, and J. Mac Neela. 1993. A kinematic and electromyographic analysis of the development of sitting posture in infants. *Developmental Psychobiology* 26: 51-64.

Hirschfeld, H. June, 1997. Influence of postural orientation on postural responses to surface translations during sitting in diplegic cerebral palsy. Paper presented at the 13th International Symposium: Multisensory Control of Posture & Gait. Paris, France.

Hirschfeld, H., and H. Forrsberg. 1994. Epigenetic development of postural responses for sitting during infancy. *Experimental Brain Research* 97: 528-540

Hollerbach, J.M., and T. Flash. 1982. Dynamic interactions between limb segments during planar arm movement. *Biological Cybernetics* 44: 67-77.

Hoy, M.G., and R.F. Zernicke. 1986. The role of intersegmental dynamics during rapid limb oscillations. *Journal of Biomechanics* 19: 867-877.

Jensen, J.L., B.D. Ulrich, E. Thelen, K. Schneider, and R.F. Zernicke. 1994. Adaptive dynamics of the leg movement patterns of human infants: I. The effects of posture on spontaneous kicking. *Journal of Motor Behavior* 26: 303-312.

————. 1995. Adaptive dynamics of the leg movement patterns of human infants: III. Age-related differences in limb control. *Journal of Motor Behavior* 27: 366-374.

Jensen, R.K., H. Sun, T. Treitz, and H.E. Parker. 1997. Gravity constraints in infant motor development. *Journal of Motor Behavior* 29: 64-71.

Kamm, K., E. Thelen, and J.L. Jensen. 1990. A dynamical systems approach to motor development. *Physical Therapy* 70:763-775.

Malina, R.M., and C. Bouchard. 1991. *Growth, maturation, and physical activity.* Champaign, IL: Human Kinetics.

Payne, V.G., and L.D. Isaacs. 1995. *Human motor development.* 3rd ed. Mountain View, CA: Mayfield.

Rochat, P. 1992. Self-sitting and reaching in 5- to 8-month-old infants: The impact of posture and its development on early eye-hand coordination. *Journal of Motor Behavior* 24: 210-220.

Rochat, P., and N. Goubet. 1995. Development of sitting and reaching in 5- to 6-month-old infants. *Infant Behavior and Development* 18: 53-68.

Roncesvalles, M.N.C. 1997. "The development of kinetic strategies for balance control in infants and young children." University of Oregon.

Savelsbergh, G.P., and J. van der Kamp. 1994. The effect of body orientation to gravity on early infant reaching. *Journal of Experimental Child Psychology* 58: 510-528.

Schneider, K., and R.F. Zernicke. 1990. A FORTRAN package for the planar analysis of limb intersegmental dynamics from spatial coordinate-time data. *Advances in Engineering Software* 12: 123-128.

———. 1992. Mass, center of mass, and moment of inertia estimates for infant limb segments. *Journal of Biomechanics* 25: 144-148.

Schneider, K., R.F. Zernicke, B.D. Ulrich, J.L. Jensen, and E. Thelen. 1990. Understanding movement control in infants through the analysis of limb intersegmental dynamics. *Journal of Motor Behavior* 22: 493-520.

Sun, H., and R. Jensen. 1994. Body segment growth during infancy. *Journal of Biomechanics* 27, no. 3: 265-275.

Tanner, J.B., and R.H. Whitehouse. 1982. *Atlas of children's growth: Normal variation and growth disorders.* New York: Academic Press.

Thelen, E. 1986. Treadmill-elicited stepping in seven-month-old infants. *Child Development* 57: 1498-1506.

Thelen, E., D. Corbetta, K. Kamm, J.P. Spencer, K. Schneider, and R.F. Zernicke. 1993. The transition to reaching: Mapping intention and intrinsic dynamics. *Child Development* 64: 1058-1098.

Thelen, E., D.M. Fisher, and R. Ridley-Johnson. 1984. The relationship between physical growth and a newborn reflex. *Infant Behavior and Development* 7: 479-493.

Thelen, E., K.D. Skala, and J.A.S. Kelso. 1987. The dynamic nature of early coordination: Evidence from bilateral leg movements in young infants. *Developmental Psychology* 23: 179-186.

Thelen, E., and B.D. Ulrich. 1991. Hidden skills: A dynamic systems analysis of treadmill stepping during the first year. *Monographs of the Society for Research in Child Development* 56(1) (Whole Serial No. 223).

Timiras, P. S. 1972. *Developmental physiology and aging.* New York: Macmillan.

Ulrich, B.D., J.L. Jensen, E. Thelen, K. Schneider, and R.F. Zernicke. 1994. Adaptive dynamics of the leg movement patterns of human infants: II. Treadmill stepping in infants and adults. *Journal of Motor Behavior* 26: 313-324.

Winter, D. A. 1995. Kinetics: Our window into the goals and strategies of the central nervous system. *Behavior and Brain Research* 67: 111-120.

Developmental Variations in Anaerobic Performance Associated With Age and Sex

James C. Martin
Robert M. Malina

This chapter focuses on the following objectives:

- Defining the key terms necessary to understand developmental variations in anaerobic performance
- Discussing testing procedures for children and adolescents
- Assessing peak anaerobic power results in young people
- Comparing anaerobic performance in children and adults
- Discussing the determinants of anaerobic performance

The majority of activities of children and youth ordinarily involve bursts of energy expenditure that are primarily dependent upon anaerobic energy production mechanisms. The development of anaerobic power during growth and maturation is thus an important consideration. Changes in anaerobic power with age during childhood and adolescence may provide insights into the development of underlying metabolic mechanisms. This chapter provides an overview of age- and sex-associated variation in anaerobic performance during childhood and adolescence.

Defining Key Terminology

Three terms are often used interchangeably in discussions of short-term maximal power output: peak anaerobic power, mean anaerobic power, and anaerobic capacity. Each has a quite different meaning, however (Green 1994).

Peak anaerobic power is defined as the highest value measured over a short period, usually 1 to 5 s. Methods used to measure peak power include cycle ergometry, running, jumping, and repetitive muscle flexions and extensions (Bouchard et al. 1990). Mean anaerobic power is often assessed using the 30 s Wingate Anaerobic Test on a cycle ergometer (Bar-Or, Dotan, and Inbar 1977), but is also measured using the other tasks just mentioned. The subject performs maximally throughout the duration of the test, and a pacing strategy is not permitted. With this protocol, power is highest for the first few seconds and then declines for the remainder of the test. Mean power is calculated as the total work done divided by the total time. The majority of studies of children and youth report peak anaerobic power and mean anaerobic power. Several groups of investigators have attempted to quantify anaerobic capacity as the total amount of work performed independent of aerobic metabolism. The two most notable methods are the maximum accumulated oxygen deficit (Medbo et al. 1988) and critical power (Moritani et al. 1981). Both methods predict the potential for anaerobic work and employ steady state bouts at workloads that are 10% to 50% above the subject's maximum aerobic work rate. The methods have not been extensively applied to children and adolescents.

In all three measures of anaerobic performance, values of peak power, mean power, and capacity are ordinarily expressed per unit body mass. Several studies have expressed results per unit estimated fat-free mass or per unit estimated thigh cross-sectional area (muscle plus bone).

Testing Children and Youth

Specifics of anaerobic testing of children and youth are discussed in more detail in Part II in this volume. It is a task substantially different from the measurement of power in adults. The majority of data for children and youth are derived from cycle ergometry. The Wingate Anaerobic Test (Bar-Or, Dotan, and Inbar 1977; Bar-Or 1987) requires a standard mechanically braked cycle ergometer. During friction load tests, flywheel resistance is provided by a friction belt and is assumed to remain constant, and peak power is evaluated at a maximum pedaling rate reached by the subject for a short period. The Wingate test recommends the use of a single body mass-dependent load (75 g/kg). This single load may or may not elicit a subject's peak power because it may identify a submaximal point on the power-velocity relationship, and power varies parabolically with velocity or pedaling rate (Dotan and Bar-Or 1983; Nadeau, Cuerrier, and Brassard 1983; Vandewalle et al. 1985). A modified method, a force-velocity protocol, uses repeated bouts at different loads (Vandewalle et al. 1985). This method accounts for the interaction of power and velocity and determines the optimal load for each individual.

The isokinetic method, in which velocity is held constant and the force exerted on the pedals is measured (Sargeant, Hoinville, and Young 1981), has been used less extensively with children and adolescents. The method accounts for the interaction of power and velocity and allows identification of peak power by taking repeated measures at several velocities.

There are other considerations specific to the measurement of peak power in children besides the interaction between power and velocity. The general layout of a cycle ergometer is designed to fit an adult. Although ergometers are adjustable, they may not properly accommodate smaller children. The crank on most cycle ergometers is 170 mm in length. It is appropriate for the leg length of adults but may be longer than optimal for shorter children (Inbar et al. 1983). These cranks are not adjustable, and changing the length involves substantial mechanical overhaul of the ergometer.

The inertia of the ergometer flywheel may induce errors in measurement of peak power up to 50% (Lakomy 1986). The error may be even larger in children because the inertial load component represents a larger portion of total power for children than for adults.

Studies of peak power in children and youth should be compared within a given method. Presently available data on anaerobic power are limited largely to boys. Other tests that incorporate data for boys and girls from late childhood through adolescence include a 10 s all-out ride on a cycle ergometer (Bouchard et al. 1990) and repetitive maximal knee flexions and extensions for 10, 30, and 90 s, that is, short-, intermediate- and long-term "anaerobic" performance (Saavedra et al. 1991).

Peak Anaerobic Power of Children and Youth

Peak power per unit body mass based on the Wingate protocol (Bar-Or, Dotan, and Inbar 1977), the force-velocity protocol of Vandewalle et al. (1985), and the isokinetic method of Sargeant, Hoinville, and Young (1981) is summarized in figure 3.1. The data are derived largely from studies of boys. Peak power per unit mass generally increases with age from middle childhood into adolescence, but results of some studies are variable.

The Wingate Protocol

Although absolute peak power increases with age, differences between age groups in peak power per unit body mass are greatly reduced. In the study of Inbar and Bar-Or (1986), the estimated peak power per unit mass increased from about 6.8 W · kg^{-1} in boys < 10 years of age to about 8.0 W · kg^{-1} in boys 10.0-11.9 years of age. The latter value is not substantially different from that for 18.0-24.9-year-old young adults, which was 8.7 W · kg^{-1}. It should be noted, however, that these values were estimated from a graph. Naughton, Carlson, and Fairweather (1992) noted that peak power per unit body mass did not differ among boys 6, 8, and 10 years of age (respectively, 6.2 ± 0.4 W · kg^{-1}, 7.0 ± 0.3 W · kg^{-1}, and 7.1 W · kg^{-1}), but was greater among 12-year-

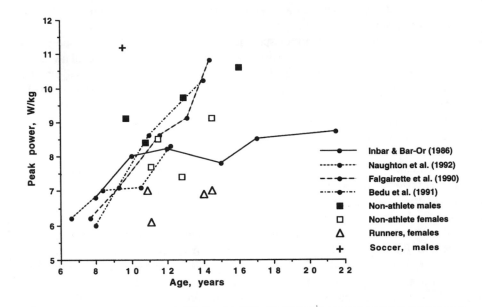

Figure 3.1 Peak power per unit body mass during childhood and adolescence in males and females. Data are based on the Wingate, force-velocity, and isokinetic protocols. Studies with several adjacent age groups include only boys, and sources are indicated.

Data from Bar-Or 1983; Docherty and Gaul 1991; Thorland et al. 1987; Delgado et al. 1993; Van Praagh et al. 1990; Capranica et al. 1992.

old boys (8.3 ± 0.5 W · kg^{-1}). The age trends suggest that peak power increases during middle childhood (6-10 years) largely as a function of increased body size; the onset of puberty perhaps contributes to the increase in 12-year-old boys.

Among boys grouped as prepubertal, midpubertal, and late pubertal, peak anaerobic power increased, on average, with pubertal status (see figure 3.2), which may suggest qualitative changes in muscle tissue associated with pubertal development. There was, however, no clear trend for age-associated gains in peak power with age within each pubertal group in this short-term longitudinal study (Falk and Bar-Or 1993). It should be noted that the prepubertal boys apparently experienced a significant learning effect from the first to the second test session.

Absolute peak power and mean power (W) with the Wingate protocol increased with stage of pubertal development in boys and girls (Williams et al. 1994). Unfortunately, the results were not considered relative to body mass, and it is well known that stature and weight increase with stage of pubertal development. Youth in different pubertal groups also differ in chronological age (see figure 3.2), so that age per se may be a factor influencing peak anaerobic power independent of pubertal status, perhaps reflecting neural maturation of recruitment (neuromuscular activation) and motor coordination. Thus, chronological age should be statistically con-

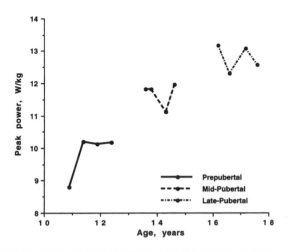

Figure 3.2 Peak power per unit mass in three longitudinal samples of boys grouped on the basis of pubertal status.

Data from Falk and Bar-Or 1993.

trolled in comparisons of subjects in different pubertal status groups. A more appropriate evaluation of the influence of puberty on anaerobic performances may be obtained by comparing children of different pubertal status but of the same chronological age.

Comparison of 11-year-old boys and girls indicates no sex difference in absolute peak power, 313 ± 61 W for boys and 315 ± 66 W for girls. However, expressing peak power per unit mass indicates greater anaerobic power in boys, 8.4 ± 1 W$\cdot$kg^{-1}, than in girls, 7.7 ± 1 W $\cdot$ kg^{-1} (Docherty and Gaul 1991).

Data for female sprint (<400 m) and middle distance (<3200 m) runners in an Olympic Development Camp indicate small differences in peak power per unit body mass between younger (9.6-11.7 years) and older (11.7-17.7 years) runners in each event; similar trends are apparent for mean anaerobic power (Thorland et al. 1987). However, when expressed per unit estimated fat-free mass, the older sprinters appear to have greater peak power than the other three groups (Thorland et al. 1987). Given the age range of the older sample and the potentially confounding effects of selection for sprinting and training, it is difficult to interpret the influence of age per se. Nevertheless, the peak power of reasonably elite young runners is not different from that of nonathletic girls.

The Force-Velocity Method of Vandewalle et al. (1985)

Several studies have used the force-velocity method, which has the potential to elicit higher peak power by identifying the optimal load, in children and youth. Among boys 6-15 years of age, peak power increased, on average, gradually with age (Falgairette et al. 1991). Salivary testosterone also increases with age from 6 to 15 years, leading the authors to suggest that the increase in peak anaerobic power with age is associated with gonadal (sexual) maturation in boys. Among boys 7-15 years of age, peak power did not vary with altitude of residence in boys of French ancestry in France and Bolivia, but increased with age in the combined sample: 6.0 ± 0.2 W · kg⁻¹ at 7-8 years, 8.6 ± 0.3 W· kg⁻¹ at 11-12 years, and 10.2 ± 0.3 W · kg⁻¹ at 14-15 years (Bedu et al. 1991).

The effect of ergometer characteristics on peak anaerobic power in 23 adolescent males 14-17 years of age was considered by Delgado et al. (1993). Two flywheels with masses of 18.0 kg and 6.3 kg were used. Flywheel mass did not significantly affect peak power (10.6 ± 0.5 W· kg⁻¹ for the 6.3 kg flywheel and 10.2 ± 0.4 W · kg⁻¹ for the 18.0 kg flywheel). While these results appear to minimize the importance that might be placed on energy transfered to the flywheel, such an interpretation needs further study. The important measure for evaluating the rotational dynamics of an ergometer flywheel is moment of inertia and not mass. Moment of inertia is defined by the distribution of mass about the axis of rotation, and it is possible for a 6.3 kg flywheel to have a moment of inertia that is the same as, or even greater than, that of a flywheel of 18.0 kg. Therefore, the data do not completely address the issue of the influence of flywheel inertia on peak power.

Peak anaerobic power per unit mass was found to be greater in 12-year-old boys than girls, 9.7 ± 0.6 W · kg⁻¹ vs. 7.4 ± 0.3 W · kg⁻¹; however, when expressed per unit estimated fat-free mass, the sex difference was reduced, 11.5 ± 0.6 W · kg⁻¹ in boys and 10.0 ± 0.4 W ·kg⁻¹ in girls (Van Praagh et al. 1990).

In a comparison of prepubertal male swimmers and boys classified as active or nonactive, peak anaerobic power (force-velocity protocol) did not significantly differ among the three groups: 8.1 ± 1.4 W · kg⁻¹, 8.4 ± 1.4 W · kg⁻¹, and 8.1 ± 1.4 W · kg⁻¹, respectively (Falgairette et al. 1993). Corresponding values with the Wingate protocol were 5.8 ± 1.0 W ·kg⁻¹, 6.3 ± 1.7 W · kg⁻¹, and 5.0 ± 1.1 W · kg⁻¹ in the swimmers, active boys, and nonactive boys, respectively (Falgairette et al. 1993). Thus, systematic training and habitual physical activity are apparently not significant factors affecting peak anaerobic power in prepubertal boys, which is consistent with the data for elite young female runners described earlier.

The Isokinetic Method

A comparison of 9-year-old male soccer players and a control sample indicates greater peak anaerobic power in the former, 11.3 W· kg⁻¹ versus 8.7 W ·kg⁻¹ (Capranica et al. 1992). It is perhaps worth noting that the mean peak powers of the two samples (mean age 9.6 years) estimated with the isokinetic protocol of Sargeant, Hoinville, and Young (1981) were higher than those for other samples of 9- and 10-year-old boys based upon friction-braked ergometers (6.8 to 8.0 W · kg⁻¹). The higher peak power may be due to methodological factors, because isokinetic testing is not confounded by acceleration of the ergometer flywheel. The higher peak power in the young soccer players as compared to the control subjects is in contrast to that for male swimmers and active boys (Falgairette et al. 1993) and for female runners (Thorland et al. 1987), who have peak powers that are not different from those for nonactive boys and girls, respectively.

Maximum Accumulated Oxygen Deficit Protocol

One study of boys and girls with a mean age of 10.6 and 10.7 years, respectively, shows a sex difference in the anaerobic capacity (Carlson and Naughton 1993). In absolute (liters) and relative (ml · kg^{-1}) terms, the accumulated oxygen deficit decreased with an increase in the intensity of supramaximal exercise from 110% to 130% to 150% in girls: 1.7, 1.6, and 1.3 L, respectively, and 40.4 ± 2.4, 37.8 ± 2.2, and 31.8 ± 2.3 ml · kg^{-1}, respectively. Boys, on the other hand, showed minimal changes with increase in intensity of exercise: 1.3 L for each intensity and 35.3 ± 4.3, 37.1 ± 3.7, and 36.8 ± 3.2 ml · kg^{-1}, respectively, for 110%, 130%, and 150% (Carlson and Naughton 1993). The standard error for absolute accumulated oxygen deficit was 0.1 in both sexes and at each exercise intensity. The biological maturity status of the subjects was not indicated. Assuming that the children were drawn from the general population, the girls were maturationally advanced compared to the boys, and this may underlie in part the observed sex difference.

Total Work Output in 10 Seconds

The Quebec 10 s all-out (maximal) ride on a cycle ergometer provides a measure of total work output. Absolute and relative total work output in 10 s increases with age from 10 to 19 years in boys and girls (see figure 3.3a and b). Absolute total work output (Joules) increases to 14 years in girls and then remains rather constant, while it increases linearly with age in boys. Thus, the sex difference in absolute work output is negligible to about 14 years of age, and then is clearly apparent. The qualitative appearance of the growth curve for total work output in 10 s is similar to that for body mass, fat-free mass, and muscle mass (Malina and Bouchard 1991). The growth curve for relative work output (J · kg^{-1}) is similar to that for absolute output, but the sex difference is already apparent at 10 years of age and is especially marked in later adolescence.

Repetitive Maximal Knee Flexion and Extension

Total work output in 10 and 30 s bouts of repetitive maximal knee flexion and extension in males and females 9 through 19 years of age is shown in figure 3.4a-c. Total work output (Joules) is expressed per unit body mass (figure 3.4a), per unit fat-free mass (figure 3.4b), and per unit estimated thigh cross-sectional muscle area (figure 3.4c). Total work output (Joules) increases with age, more so for total work output per unit mass in 30 s than in 10 s. Sex differences are more apparent in

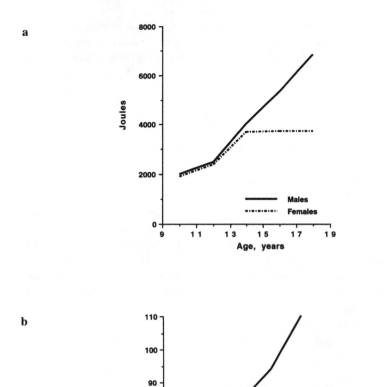

Figure 3.3 Absolute (a) and relative (b) total work output on a 10 s all-out cycle ergometer test in a cross-sectional sample of French Canadian youth.

Unpublished data of C. Bouchard and J-A. Simoneau. Data from Malina and Bouchard 1991.

the 30 s task and are somewhat greater in later adolescence. The patterns of age- and
sex-associated variation in total work output per unit body mass and per unit thigh
cross-sectional area are similar, but the sex difference is reduced, especially in later
adolescence, when total work output is expressed per unit fat-free mass.

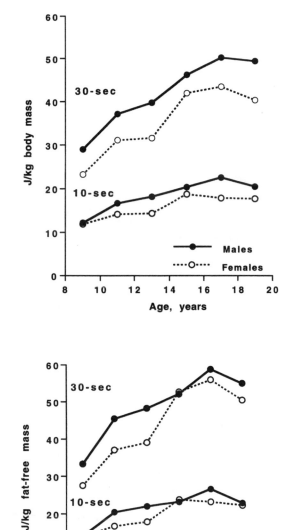

Figure 3.4 Total work output per unit body mass (a), per unit fat-free mass, (b) and per unit mid-thigh muscle cross-sectional area (c) on 10 and 30 s bouts on a repetitive knee flexion and extension test in a cross-sectional sample of French Canadian youth.

Data from Saavedra et al. 1991.

(continued)

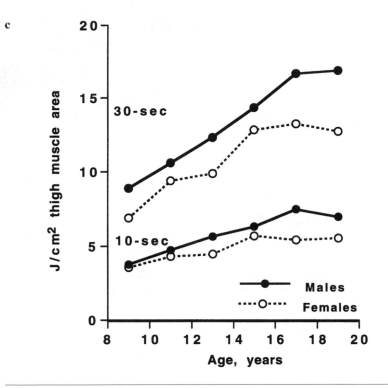

Figure 3.4 (continued)

Overview of Age and Sex Differences

Peak anaerobic power per unit body mass in boys shows, in general, an increase with age from childhood into adolescence. However, results of some individual studies yield mixed results. Corresponding data for girls are quite limited. Total work output per unit mass in a 10 s maximal cycle ergometer task and in a 10 s repetitive maximal knee flexion-extension task increases with age from 9-10 years to 19 years in boys and from 9-10 years to 14-15 years in girls. Sex differences are evident in late childhood and early adolescence, and are magnified later in adolescence. The several measures of anaerobic performance considered previously thus show somewhat different patterns of age- and sex-associated variation, emphasizing the specificity of results to the test protocol used.

Child-Adult Comparisons

Mean peak power per unit body mass, based upon the Wingate, force-velocity, and isokinetic protocols, for children and youth range from 6.0 W · kg^{-1} to 10.8

W · kg⁻¹ (figure 3.1). Although there is some overlap, the values for children and adolescents are lower than those of adults, $10.5\ W \cdot kg^{-1}$ to $14.7\ W \cdot kg^{-1}$ (Dotan and Bar-Or 1983; Nadeau, Cuerrier, and Brassard 1983; Vandewalle et al. 1987; Sargeant, Hoinville, and Young 1981; Sargeant 1987). The maximum accumulated oxygen deficits observed in 10-year-old girls, 32 to 40 ml · kg⁻¹, and boys, 35 to 37 ml · kg⁻¹ (Carlson and Naughton 1993), are considerably less than comparable values reported for adults, 52 ml · kg⁻¹ to 90 ml· kg⁻¹ (Medbo et al. 1988; Scott et al. 1991). These differences in anaerobic work capacity are larger than those observed in short-term anaerobic performances, and cannot be accounted for by differences in muscle size. Rather, they probably lie in the specific components of anaerobic metabolism and anaerobic glycolysis (Medbo et al. 1988). The $ADP+CP \rightarrow ATP+C$ cycle may be limited by stored creatine phosphate (CP). Creatine phosphate was lower in children than in adults in one study (Inbar and Bar-Or 1986), while values reported for children were similar to those for adults in another study (Hirvonen et al. 1994). However, the main determinant of anaerobic capacity is believed to be phosphofructokinase (PFK), which catalyzes anaerobic glycolysis. Phosphofructokinase in 11-year-old boys, 8 µmol · g⁻¹ · min⁻¹ (Eriksson, Karlsson, and Saltin 1971), is considerably less than that in 16-year-old males, 29 µmol · g⁻¹· min⁻¹ (Fournier et al. 1982), and in adult males, 25 µmol· g⁻¹ · min⁻¹ (Saltin and Gollnick 1983). Further, PFK is highly adaptive to training.

Evidence from total work output on the 10 s maximal cycle ergometry task (figure 3.3) and on the 10 and 30 s knee flexion-extension task (figure 3.4) indicates lower levels of short-term anaerobic power in boys and girls than in young adults. Similar to child-adult differences obtained with the maximum accumulated oxygen deficit method, child-adult differences in total work output per unit mass between 10-year-old children and 19-year-old young adults are larger than those observed with the Wingate and force-velocity protocols.

Determinants of Anaerobic Performance

The factors that limit human muscular performance under predominantly anaerobic conditions are still under debate. There is a dearth of data on the metabolic aspects of skeletal muscle in children and adolescents. Consequently, questions relating to developmental aspects of anaerobic performance remain largely unanswered. Peak anaerobic power, mean anaerobic power, anaerobic capacity, and total work output in 10 s are related to body size, and especially to estimated fat-free mass or thigh muscle cross-sectional area. Age- and sex-associated variation in anaerobic performance during childhood and youth are apparently related more to variation in muscle mass than to other factors.

Determinants of anaerobic performance include muscle quantity (length and cross-sectional area), muscle quality (fiber type, substrate availability), muscle architecture (alignment of muscle fibers), musculoskeletal architecture (joint geometry), neuromuscular activation (recruitment and coordination), muscular endurance (glycolytic enzymes, CP stores), and fatigue resistance (buffering capacity). Three of these determinants are to be considered in the context of growth and maturation.

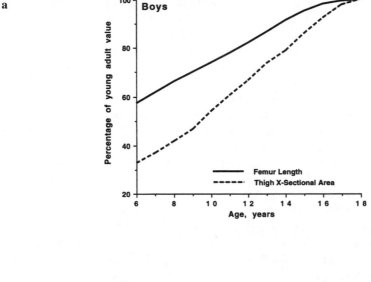

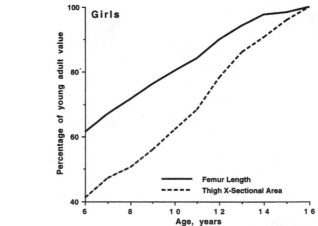

Figure 3.5 Femur length (a proxy for muscle length) and estimated mid-thigh cross-sectional area in boys (a) and girls (b). Values are expressed as a percentage of young adult dimensions, 18 years in boys and 16 years in girls.

The data are calculated from radiographic dimensions in the mixed-longitudinal series of children from the Child Research Council (Denver) growth study: Maresh 1970.

Muscle Quantity

Power is the product of force and velocity; hence, it is reasonable to expect the force and velocity characteristics of skeletal muscle tissue to be determinants of peak power. Force generated by a muscle is related to the cross-sectional area of the active muscle, while velocity of muscle contraction is related to muscle fiber length. Each sarcomere in a muscle fiber contracts to about one-half of its resting length. A longer fiber, composed of more sarcomeres in a series, will thus have a higher contraction velocity than a shorter muscle fiber. Based on these considerations, it is reasonable to assume that muscle power scales to the product of cross-sectional area and muscle length.

Since most studies of anaerobic performance in children and youth involve the thigh muscle mass, changes in femur length (a proxy for muscle length) and estimated midthigh cross-sectional area are shown in figure 3.5a and b. Values are expressed as a percentage of young adult dimensions, at 18 years in boys and 16 years in girls. Femur length and thus estimated muscle length is associated with overall skeletal growth in length and is closer to adult values at all ages than estimated muscle cross-sectional area. This is consistent with growth of the muscle mass and strength in general. Growth in muscle widths of the arm and static muscular strength of the shoulder, for example, reach maximum velocities, on average, about 6 months after peak height velocity during adolescence (Beunen and Malina 1988).

Since power is the product of force and velocity, the product of estimated muscle area and length may serve to estimate thigh muscle mass and in turn provide insight into anaerobic power during growth. The ratio of the product of estimated midthigh muscle area and femur (estimated muscle) length per unit body mass (L/kg) for boys and girls is shown in figure 3.6. The ratio increases linearly with age in both sexes. Girls appear to have greater thigh muscle mass per unit body mass in childhood, but in early adolescence and subsequently, males have greater estimated thigh muscle mass per unity body mass. Expressing this ratio as a percentage of the ratio in young adulthood may provide some insight into growth in peak power. This is shown in figure 3.7, which is based on estimated thigh muscle mass, peak anaerobic power, and mean anaerobic power per unit body mass in boys from 6 to 16 years. Values are expressed as a percentage of young adult values (18 years). Ten-year-old boys, for example, have attained about 80% of the thigh muscle mass per unit body mass in young adulthood; hence, the ratio of peak power to body mass of 10-year-old boys might be expected to approximate 80% of the young adult value. This is suggested by the composite data. Peak power and mean power track reasonably well with estimated thigh muscle mass in boys, suggesting that the development of muscle mass accounts for a major portion of the variation in age-related changes in these indicators of anaerobic performance. Corresponding data for girls across the age continuum are not available.

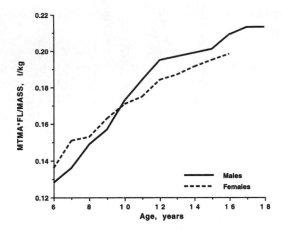

Figure 3.6 The ratio of the product of estimated mid-thigh muscle area (MTMA) and femur (estimated muscle) length (FL) per unit body mass (L/kg) in boys and girls during childhood and adolescence.

The data are calculated from radiographic dimensions in the mixed-longitudinal series of children from the Child Research Council (Denver) growth study: Maresh 1970.

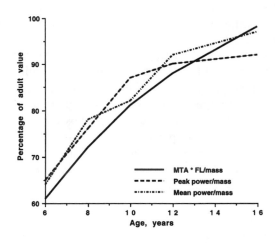

Figure 3.7 Estimated thigh muscle mass, peak anaerobic power, and mean anaerobic power per unit body mass in boys from 6 to 16 years. Values are expressed as a percentage of young adult values (18 years).

The estimates for muscle mass are based on Denver children, while the estimates for peak power and mean power are based on mean values with the Wingate test from Inbar and Bar-Or 1986; Docherty and Gaul 1991; Naughton, Carlson, and Fairweather 1992; Falk and Bar-Or 1993.

Neuromuscular Activation and Motor Coordination

Skeletal muscles do not contract spontaneously; they are recruited by impulses from the brain to efferent motor neurons. The timing of muscular recruitment must also be coordinated among the specific muscles and joints involved in the movement. Therefore, both neural drive and skill development are determinants of anaerobic power.

Speed of impulse transmission (motor nerve conduction velocity) improves rapidly during infancy and early childhood, approaching adult levels between 3 and 8 years of age with small gains subsequently (Gamstorp 1963). There is, of course, variation among nerves.

Mature movement patterns of basic motor skills (run, kick, throw, hop, skip, etc.) are generally in place by 6 to 8 years of age, although some patterns attain mature status a bit later (Seefeldt and Haubenstricker 1982). Jumping patterns attain mature status, on average, somewhat later. Longitudinal observations indicate that 60% of children reach the mature pattern for the standing long jump at about 9-10 years of age (Seefeldt and Haubenstricker 1982), which means that a significant percentage of children have not yet mastered this basic movement. Corresponding data for the vertical jump, which is occasionally used as an indicator of peak power (Sargent 1921; Davies 1971; Ferretti et al. 1994), indicate that only about 40% of fourth- and seventh-grade children (approximately 9-13 years) perform the vertical jump with a mature pattern (Reuschlein and Haubenstricker 1985, see Notes). However, performances (distance or height) in both jumping tasks improve linearly with age during childhood in boys and girls; boys perform, on average, slightly better than girls. During adolescence, jumping performances of girls reach a plateau, while those for boys show evidence of an adolescent spurt (Malina and Bouchard 1991). The standing long jump and vertical jump show maximum growth velocity, respectively, during the interval of peak height velocity and after peak height velocity in boys (Beunen and Malina 1988). The apparent differences in the timing of the growth spurts in the two jumping tasks may be related to analytical strategies. The estimate for the former is based on annual velocities, while that for the latter is based on semiannual velocities. If the vertical jump is accepted as an estimation of anaerobic power, changes in neuromuscular coordination per se and the timing of the growth spurt may influence power independent of muscular potential.

Musculoskeletal Architecture

Muscles do not exert force or power directly; rather, they create torque about skeletal joints. The torque generated by a muscle is dependent on both the force produced by the muscle and that produced by the lever arm about the joint. The lever arm is defined by the perpendicular distance from the line of action of the muscle force to the center of rotation of the joint. This distance is affected by the location of the attachment point of the tendon and by the angle of the joint. Muscle force and velocity must be delivered to a joint and then transmitted as torque and angular velocity to the outside environment. If a muscle has a relatively longer lever arm about a joint, it will tend to produce more torque but less velocity about that joint. Conversely, a shorter lever arm will tend to produce lower torque but higher velocity. Therefore, all of the muscles that span a given joint will combine to form patterns of power production that are influenced by characteristics of the muscles and the musculoskeletal architecture.

Bone growth in length occurs at the epiphyses, and in the major long bones with epiphyses at each end the growth rates are not the same. Each major long bone undergoes a growth spurt during adolescence. The spurts occur earlier in girls than in boys, and earlier in the long bones of the lower extremity than in those of the upper extremity (Roche 1974). Tendon attachment points are located on the shafts of long bones; hence, tendon origin/insertion points undergo remodeling during growth of a bone in length. This remodeling in turn influences the lever arm of a muscle at each joint. Although these processes are not well defined in growing children, they may have a significant influence on the torque-angular velocity relationship independent of the muscle force-velocity relationship.

Directions for Future Research

There is a need for further refinement of methods to accurately measure peak power, especially in the context of developing and refining procedures to meet the characteristics of children and youth. This should permit more accurate assessment of the effects of growth and maturation on the development of anaerobic power and capacity.

Compared to information on the anaerobic power of boys, the information available for girls is rather limited. There is a need to refine the data on age- and maturity-associated variation in the anaerobic performances of girls.

Information on maturity-associated variation in anaerobic performances is extremely limited. Two studies indicate maturity-associated variation in boys (Falgairette et al. 1991; Falk and Bar-Or 1993). The data are cross-sectional, and numbers of subjects are limited. Given the importance of body mass and muscle mass in anaerobic performance, maturity effects are probably mediated through the influence of maturity status on body size and muscle mass. A question that needs study is the specific influence of variation in the timing and tempo of pubertal maturation on the development of anaerobic performances independent of chronological age, body size, and muscle mass.

There is a need for longitudinal study of anaerobic performances that span childhood and adolescence to estimate the tempo (progress) of development as well as the timing and tempo of the adolescent spurt in anaerobic performances. Muscle mass, static strength, submaximal power output, and maximal aerobic power show adolescent spurts in both sexes, while functional (flexed arm hang) and dynamic (standing long jump, vertical jump) strength show well-defined adolescent spurts in boys; corresponding data for girls are lacking (Beunen and Malina 1988; Malina 1997).

Information on the determinants of performance under anaerobic conditions is derived largely from adults and athletes. Data for growing and maturing children and youth are limited. Although it may be reasonable to assume that the determinants of anaerobic performances are somewhat similar in children, adolescents, and adults, there is a need for information on the morphological, biomechanical, physiological, and biochemical (metabolic) determinants of anaerobic performances during childhood and adolescence. The role of heredity and training are additional concerns.

Summary

Peak anaerobic power per unit body mass increases with age from childhood into adolescence in boys, but some studies yield mixed results. Corresponding data for girls are limited. Total work output per unit mass in a 10 s maximal cycle ergometer task and in a 10 s repetitive maximal knee flexion-extension task increases with age from late childhood to 14-15 years in girls and 19 years in boys. Sex differences are evident in late childhood and early adolescence and are magnified later in adolescence. Variability in results among several studies emphasizes the specificity of results to the test protocol used.

Although there is some overlap, mean peak power per unit body mass, based upon the Wingate, force-velocity, and isokinetic protocols, in children and adolescents is lower than that of adults. Total work output on 10 s maximal cycle ergometry and on 10 s and 30 s knee flexion-extension tasks indicates lower levels of short-term anaerobic power in boys and girls than in young adults. Child-adult differences in total work output per unit mass between 10-year-old children and 19-year-old young adults are larger than those observed with the Wingate and force-velocity protocols.

Notes

The mature pattern of the vertical jump is described as follows:

1. A preparatory movement: Arms with elbows at or near full extension po sitioned behind the trunk just prior to the time that the knees are reaching maximum flexion ($90 \pm 10°$).
2. An upward swing of both arms (to at least shoulder height) coordinated with full extension of legs and reaching arm at take-off.
3. Continuous swing of one arm with the hand touching the wall at the apex of the jump. Simultaneously, the opposite arm is swinging downward.

4. Balanced landing incorporating both hip and knee flexion.
5. Little or no horizontal displacement at landing (at least one foot landing within a 2 ft circle drawn around the take-off spot).

From Reuschlein and Haubenstricker (1985, 33), with permission.

References

Bar-Or, O. 1983. *Pediatric sports medicine for the practitioner.* New York: Springer-Verlag.

Bar-Or, O. 1987. The Wingate Anaerobic Test: an update on methodology, reliability and validity. *Sports Med.* 4: 381-394.

Bar-Or, O., Dotan, R., and Inbar, O. 1977. A 30 s all out ergometry test: its reliability and validity for anaerobic capacity. *Israel J. Med. Sci.* 13: 326-327.

Bedu, M., Fellmann, N., Spielvogel, H., Falgairette, G., Van Praagh, E., and Coudert, J. 1991. Force-velocity and 30-s Wingate tests in boys at high and low altitudes. *J. Appl. Physiol.* 70: 1031-1037.

Beunen, G., and Malina, R.M. 1988. Growth and physical performance relative to the timing of the adolescent spurt. *Exerc. Sport Sci. Rev.* 16: 503-540.

Bouchard, C., Taylor, A.W., Simoneau, J-A., and Dulac, S. 1990. Testing anaerobic power and capacity. In *Physiological testing of the high-performance athlete,* ed. J.D. MacDougall, H.A. Wenger, and H.J. Green (2nd ed.), 175-221. Champaign, IL: Human Kinetics.

Capranica, L., Cama, G., Fanton, A., Tessitore, A., and Figura, F. 1992. Force and power of preferred and non-preferred leg in young soccer players. *J. Sports Med. Phys. Fitness* 31: 358-363.

Carlson, J.S., and Naughton, G.A. 1993. An examination of the anaerobic capacity of children using maximal accumulated oxygen deficit. *Pediatr. Exerc. Sci.* 5: 60-71.

Davies, C.T.M. 1971. Human power output in exercise of short duration in relation to body size and composition. *Ergonomics* 14: 245-256.

Delgado, A., Pérès, G., Allemandou, A., and Monod, H. 1993. Influence of cycle ergometer characteristics on the adolescents' anaerobic abilities testing. *Archiv. Int. Physiol. Biochim. Biophys.* 191: 145-148.

Docherty, D., and Gaul, C.A. 1991. Relationship of body size, physique and composition to physical performance in young boys and girls. *Int. J. Sports Med.* 12: 525-532.

Dotan, R., and Bar-Or, O. 1983. Load optimization for the Wingate Anaerobic Test. *Eur. J. Appl. Physiol.* 51: 409-417.

Eriksson, B.O., Karlsson, J., and Saltin, B. 1971. Muscle metabolites during exercise in pubertal boys. *Acta Paediatr. Scand.*(suppl.)217: 154-157.

Falgairette, G., Bedu, M., Fellmann, N., Van Praagh, E., and Coudert, J. 1991. Bioenergetic profile in 144 boys aged from 6 to 15 years with special reference to sexual maturation. *Eur. J. Appl. Physiol.* 62: 151-156.

Falgairette, G., Duche, P., Bedu, M., Fellmann, N., and Coudert, J. 1993. Bioenergetic characteristics in prepubertal swimmers: comparison with active and nonactive boys. *Int. J. Sports Med.* 14: 444-448.

Falk, B., and Bar-Or, O. 1993. Longitudinal changes in peak aerobic and anaerobic mechanical power of circumpubertal boys. *Pediatr. Exerc. Sci.* 5: 318-331.

Ferretti, G., Narici, M.V., Binzoni, T., Gariod, L., Le Bas, J.F., Reutenauer, H., and Cerretelli, P. 1994. Determinants of peak muscle power: effects of age and physical conditioning. *Eur. J. Appl. Physiol.* 68: 111-115.

Fournier, M., Ricci, J., Taylor, A.W., Ferguson, R.J., Montpetit, R.R., and Chairman, B.R. 1982. Skeletal muscle adaptation in adolescent boys: sprint and endurance training and detraining. *Med. Sci. Sports Exerc.* 14: 453-456.

Gamstorp, I. 1963. Normal conduction velocity of ulnar, median and peroneal nerves in infancy, childhood and adolescence. *Acta Paediatr. Scand.*(suppl.)146: 68-76.

Green, S. 1994. A definition and systems view of anaerobic capacity. *Eur. J. Appl. Physiol.* 69: 168-173.

Hirvonen, J., Nummela, A., Rusko, H., Rehunen, S., and Harkonen, M. 1994. Fatigue and changes in ATP, creatine phosphate, and lactate during the 400 m sprint. *Can. J. Sport Sci.* 17: 141-144.

Inbar, O., and Bar-Or, O. 1986. Anaerobic characteristics in male children and adolescents. *Med. Sci. Sports Exerc.* 18: 264-269.

Inbar, O., Dotan, R., Trousil, T., and Dvir, Z. 1983. The effect of bicycle crank length variation upon power performance. *Ergonomics* 26: 1139-1146.

Lakomy, H.K.A. 1986. Measurement of work and power using friction load cycle ergometers. *Ergonomics* 29: 509-517.

Malina, R.M. 1997. Prospective and retrospective longitudinal studies of the growth, maturation, and fitness of Polish youth active in sport. *Int. J. Sports Med.* 18(suppl. 3): S1-S7.

Malina, R.M., and Bouchard, C. 1991. *Growth, maturation, and physical activity.* Champaign, IL: Human Kinetics.

Maresh, M.M. 1970. Measurements from roentgenograms: heart size; long bone lengths; bone, muscle and fat widths; skeletal maturation. In *Human growth and development,* ed. R.W. McCammon, 155-200. Springfield, IL: Charles C Thomas.

Medbo, J.I., Mohm, A.C., Tabata, I., Bahr, R., Vaage, O., and Serjersted, O.M. 1988. Anaerobic capacity determined by maximal accumulated O_2 deficit. *J. Appl. Physiol.* 64: 50-60.

Moritani, T., Nagata, A., DeVries, H.A., and Muro, M. 1981. Critical power as a measure of physical work capacity and anaerobic threshold. *Ergonomics* 24: 339-350.

Nadeau, M., Cuerrier, J.P., and Brassard, A. 1983. The bicycle ergometer for muscle power testing. *Can. J. Appl. Sport Sci.* 8: 41-46.

Naughton, G., Carlson, J., and Fairweather, I. 1992. Determining the variability of performance on Wingate anaerobic tests in children 6-12 years. *Int. J. Sports Med.* 13: 512-517.

Reuschlein, S., and Haubenstricker, J., eds. 1985. *1984-1985 Physical education interpretive report: Michigan Educational Assessment Program.* Lansing, MI: Michigan Department of Education.

Roche, A.F. 1974. Differential timing of maximum length increments among bones within individuals. *Hum. Biol.* 46: 145-157.

Saavedra, C., LaGasse, P., Bouchard, C., and Simoneau, J-A. 1991. Maximal anaerobic performance of the knee extensor muscles during growth. *Med. Sci. Sports Exerc.* 23: 1083-1089.

Saltin, B., and Gollnick, P.D. 1983. Skeletal muscle adaptability: significance for metabolism and performance. In *Handbook of physiology.* Sec. 10, *Skeletal muscle,* ed. L.D. Peachey, 555-631. Washington, DC: American Physiological Society.

Sargeant, A.J. 1987. Effect of muscle temperature on leg extension force and short-term power output in humans. *Eur. J. Appl. Physiol.* 56: 693-698.

Sargeant, A.J., Hoinville, E., and Young, A. 1981. Maximal leg force and power output during short term dynamic exercises. *J. Appl. Physiol.* 51: 1175-1182.

Sargent, D.A. 1921. The physical test of a man. *Am. Phys. Ed. Rev.* 26: 188-194.

Scott, C.B., Roby, F.B., Lohman, T.G., and Bunt, J.C. 1991. The maximally accumulated oxygen deficit as an indicator of anaerobic capacity. *Med. Sci. Sports Exerc.* 23: 618-624.

Seefeldt, V., and Haubenstricker, J. 1982. Patterns, phases, or stages: an analytical model for the study of developmental movement. In *The development of movement control and coordination,* ed. J.A.S. Kelso and J.E. Clark. New York: Wiley.

Thorland, W.G., Johnson, G.O., Cisar, C.J., Housh, T.J., and Tharp, G.D. 1987. Strength and anaerobic responses of elite young female sprint and distance runners. *Med. Sci. Sports Exerc.* 19: 56-61.

Vandewalle, H., Pérès, G., Heller, J., and Monod, H. 1985. All out anaerobic capacity tests on cycle ergometers: a comparative study of men and women. *Eur. J. Appl. Physiol.* 54: 222-229.

Vandewalle, H., Pérès, G., Heller, J., Panel, J., and Monod, H. 1987. Force-velocity relationship and maximal power on a cycle ergometer: correlation with the height of a vertical jump. *Eur. J. Appl. Physiol.* 56: 650-656.

Van Praagh, E., Fellmann, N., Bedu, M., Falgairette, G., and Coudert, J. 1990. Gender difference in the relationship of anaerobic power output to body composition in children. *Pediatr. Exerc. Sci.* 2: 336-348.

Williams, C.A., Armstrong, N., Welsman, J., and Kirby, B. 1994. Anaerobic performance of boys and girls related to sexual maturation. *J. Sports Sci.* 12: 155-156 (abstract).

4

CHAPTER

Developing Flexibility During Childhood and Adolescence

David A. Brodie
Jon Royce

This chapter focuses on the following objectives:

- Importance of flexibility
- The options for measuring flexibility
- The range of available devices and procedures
- Research in pediatric flexibility

Anaerobic performance ultimately depends on the efficiency of the human musculature, which represents some 40% of the mass of the body. Muscular efficiency is optimal when the appropriate range of motion is available. This illustrates the direct relevance of flexibility to anaerobic performance.

Flexibility has generally been identified as one of the components of physical fitness. In introducing a review of literature on the subject, Humphrey (1981) states that leaders in physical education and human performance include flexibility among the essential components of physical fitness and performance.

Irrespective of whether athletes, laymen, or children are the subject of our attention, physiologists, physiotherapists, and coaches generally agree that "the importance of flexibility and its contribution to individuals is no longer disputed" (Cornelius and Hinson 1989, 75). Schultz (1979) decries the lack of education and the insufficient emphasis on this important aspect of physical fitness and identifies flexibility as "the overlooked sibling of strength, endurance and speed."

Research within the field of joint range of motion has covered many areas of concern, but experimentation has been fairly spasmodic. The polio epidemic at the start of the century and the need to rehabilitate soldiers from their injuries during the two World Wars brought flexibility into the forefront of research. Despite periods of great activity in this field, many questions remain partially or wholly unanswered. Indeed, a good deal of confusion still abounds concerning the nomenclature alone. Experimenters have often used flexibility, range of motion, mobility, suppleness, and joint laxity interchangeably. Quite understandably, this has led to some confusion within physical education, and as a result professionals are "convinced that trainers and physical educators are confused and unsure how to improve flexibility." Some range of motion exercises are described as "sometimes amusing, often horrifying" (Carter 1978).

Over recent years, flexibility has deservedly received more attention. Before publication of a research paper entitled "The Report That Shocked the President" in *Sports Illustrated* in the 1950s, Weber and Kraus (1949) reported that large numbers of American children could not undertake simple strength and flexibility tasks. One of the first large-scale tests for schools, the American Alliance for Health, Physical Education and Recreation Youth Fitness Test of 1958, incorporated tests of strength, endurance, speed, power, agility, and cardiorespiratory endurance. In spite of the interest in flexibility developed by Weber and Kraus, no flexibility test was included in the 1958 draft. In 1980 the test was revised as the American Alliance for Health, Physical Education, Recreation and Dance Health Related Fitness Test. This included a test of flexibility in the form of the popular sit and reach test.

Some authorities would argue that too great an emphasis is now being placed on flexibility. One outspoken critic, particularly of the static method of stretching, believes that many recreational athletes have been swept up in what he calls "a cult of flexibility" (Shyne and Dominguez 1982, 138).

The Importance of Flexibility

In recent years many publications have established the importance of flexibility, yet the benefits are still a contentious issue, with a review of literature revealing contradictory evidence with regard to the effect of flexibility on performance. Beaulieu (1981) claimed that flexible athletes are usually the better performers. His claims may have been overstated, since Beaulieu drew only on evidence from Cureton (1933) based on swimmers in the 1932 Olympic Games, two limited theses using simple gymnasium tests, and a recent paper on girls' grade school running patterns. Clark (1975) provided evidence of improved performance with increased flexibility during laboratory experiments in children 6-13 years of age. Improvements were found in standing broad jump, softball distance throw, and an obstacle race. It has been stated that "flexibility influences performance by increasing the distance over which force can be applied resulting in greater impulse, or by allowing the best possible body position to perform an effective motor pattern" (Hoshizaki and Bell 1984, 97). Thus, all other factors being equal, a javelin thrower who pulls the implement through a greater range of motion will throw a greater distance.

Humphrey (1981) suggested that in gymnastics, dance, ice skating, and diving, a full range of motion was necessary for peak aesthetic performance, although it should be noted that, as Corbin and Noble (1980) state, "Additional flexibility may not enhance performance providing that the necessary body positions can be comfortably achieved" (57). This last consideration may explain why it is difficult to predict performance from flexibility tests. Marshall et al. (1980) found a significant negative correlation between joint looseness and performance in sprints and various gymnastic tests. More experimentation is necessary to reveal the relationship between range of motion and performance. Basic flexibility requirements in many activities have yet to be identified—information that would be invaluable to coaches. Corbin and Noble (1980) quite correctly warn that claims of increased performance "may be generalised beyond the facts" (57).

It has been widely claimed that the flexible individual is less susceptible to injury, but evidence is indirect and few longitudinal studies have been undertaken. The problem of a suitable experimental design, and the time such a study would take to complete, make this particular question an extremely difficult one to address. The role of preventative stretching is also very important. Wiktorsson-Moller et al. (1983) estimate that the cost of sports injuries to Swedish society in 1970 was 25 million crowns. If it were possible to reduce injuries by stretching, the potential savings would be considerable. Many authorities, among them Hartley-O'Brien (1980), Beaulieu (1981), Humphrey (1981), and Surburg (1981), have claimed that soft tissue injuries are reduced by stretching and by possessing adequate amounts of flexibility, although it is important not to extrapolate beyond the groups studied. Flexibility is also of considerable importance in contact sports, where joints are often forced to the extreme. Sufficient flexibility is necessary to avoid injury, yet Nicholas (1970) took the view that too much flexibility may make a joint unstable. These contradictory findings may in part be due to the confusion in the nomenclature indicated earlier. An athlete with a large range of motion does not necessarily have a loose joint suggesting instability. Clear, concise terminology would undoubtedly help in allowing conclusions to be drawn from these experiments.

Corbin and Noble (1980) state that clinical and theoretical evidence has also been found establishing a link between back problems, poor posture, and a lack of flexibility. Dysmenorrhea may also be prevented, or partly relieved, by adequate flexibility in the pelvic area (Mathews and Fox 1976, 153). Once injury has occurred, an adequate amount of flexibility must be maintained or established for rehabilitation from injury. Without such flexibility, injury often recurs on the recommencement of athletic performance.

Warm-Up

Many sport participants use flexibility exercises as part of a warm-up routine to prevent injury. Inclusion of such exercises within the warm-up has been challenged by few authorities. Shyne and Dominguez (1982) suggests that joggers should start their runs slowly and finish with a gentle "warm down." They believe in a gentle 15 min warm-up before explosive activities such as sprinting, but is particularly critical of the present emphasis on static stretching; they believe participants set themselves up for an injury by "overstretching muscle and ligaments around the joint" (Shyne and Dominguez 1982, 138). This view has been hard to substantiate, there being little evidence to support it, although Nicholas' (1970) data may do so. Nicholas classified American football players as either "tight" or "loose" depending on their ability to perform three out of five mobility tests. Of the loose group, 72% suffered major ligamentous disruption.

While the vast majority of authorities firmly believe that flexibility exercises should be included within a warm-up routine, their place within the total structure has been a question of some debate. Beaulieu (1981) and Sapega et al. (1982) believe that flexibility exercises should be placed relatively late in the warm-up for several reasons. "1) Stretching muscles that have not been warmed can result in injuries. 2) Warming the muscle increases extensibility, which results in immediate gains in flexibility. 3) Stretching after a warm-up allows the athlete to make greater gains in flexibility" (Beaulieu 1981, 61). The inclusion of warm-up exercises before flexibility testing is important, with Clark (1975) noting that even one pretest trial results in an improved score. Stretching has also been used in a warm-up as a panacea for nervous excitement. A nervous state has also been found to restrict range of motion, making an adequate range even more important.

Stretching Methods

Researchers do not know for certain which type of stretching is best to use to develop flexibility. Static stretching has largely taken the place of ballistic stretching because bobbing and bouncing stretching movements can injure tissue.

Relatively recently, proprioceptive neuromuscular facilitation techniques (PNF) have been used following exploratory research on the rehabilitation of patients who have paralysis. Preliminary research suggests that PNF may be the most efficient technique for improving flexibility. The results of PNF research studies must be viewed with caution, as few of them have used the same procedures and consequently results vary considerably. Although some authorities consider PNF the most efficient technique, under certain circumstances it can be unsuitable. Physiotherapists learn to develop the correct touch and sense for the desired stretching force. Unless specialist training has been undertaken it is probably wisest to continue with static methods. The PNF techniques can also take time to implement, especially if a large number of movement patterns are used.

Limitations of Flexibility

Johns and Wright (1962), using cat wrists, provided data on the relative contribution of the joint capsule, muscle, tendons, and skin; the authors argued that the cat wrist is similar in structure to the human metacarpophalangeal joint. Johns and Wright's data are taken from the midrange of motion and are concerned as much with joint stiffness as with range of motion. Other authors such as Hutton and Nelson (1986) have concentrated their research on the neuromuscular constraints of range of motion. Sapega et al. (1982), in a biophysical analysis of range of motion, examined the role of the connective tissue found in tendons, ligaments, joint capsules, aponeuroses, and fasciae. Sapega et al. (1982) have highlighted the effect of temperature on the state of connective tissue.

It has been found that individuals vary considerably in their flexibility. Marshall et al. (1980) investigated the possibility that "it may be possible to validly array individuals on a looseness scale". Extensive research has tended to lead to the conclusion that flexibility is joint specific (Mathews and Fox 1976; De Vries 1986; Garfield in Burke, Hagbarth, and Lofstedt 1978). Individuals may be tight in one joint and loose in another. The trait pattern, if indeed one exists, may be further masked by participation in a particular sport.

To date, sport scientists and coaches have failed to identify the levels of flexibility required in a given sport. One of the more common beliefs has been that heavily muscled athletes are likely to be "muscle bound" (Cureton 1941) and therefore likely to have poor flexibility. Holland (1949), Rasch and Burke (1978), and Weber and Kraus (1949) are in agreement with Ekstrand that "habitual postures and chronic heavy labour through restricted ranges of motion have been reported to lead to adaptive shortening of muscles and connective tissue" (Ekstrand et al. 1982, 171).

Provided that exercises are carried out through a full range of motion, even heavy weight training need not cause restricted range of motion. Indeed, such athletes have been found to be superior in many articulations (Leighton 1957). It is generally accepted that the idea that weight training causes a "muscle-bound" condition is a myth.

The effect of certain anthropometric parameters on range of motion has been investigated. Cureton (1941) spoke of the necessity of "eliminating the needless fat around the joints and in the muscles" (382). Once again this seems to have little scientific justification. Laubach and McConville (1966) found that body fat yielded significant negative correlations with the flexibility measures. Whether the correlations were causative remains uncertain, especially as the best relationship (between subscapular skinfold and knee flexion extension) explained only 26% of the variance. Laubach and McConville (1966), in a study designed to compare two flexibility measures with 30 different anthropometric measurements, concluded that correlations were generally low and statistically nonsignificant. In the same study the authors correlated two flexibility measurements with somatotype; once again little relationship could be identified.

Measurement of Single-Joint Range of Motion

A review of the literature reveals two basic types of measurement. On the one hand there are single-joint measures and on the other, composite joint measures. The former may require some further explanation and might be better termed "movements visible at a single joint." For example, regarding the movement of the shoulder, the Cybex II manual (1982) notes, "The three primary joints of the shoulder girdle (the sternoclavicular, acromioclavicular and glenohumeral) move together each making a critical contribution to any specific movement" (31).

It has been common to term movement visible at the shoulder as a single-joint measure, and the specific combinations of joint movements within the body have been ignored in classifying the movement. Measurements visible at a single joint can be assessed in three ways: by goniometers, by visual means, and by mathematical calculation. Goniometers involve the measurement of joint range of motion in degrees and can be of two types, universal or joint specific.

Universal Goniometers

This group includes such instruments as the universal goniometer, Leighton flexometer, and Cybex dynamometer. The origin of the goniometer is unknown, but its value has been discussed in English and American literature since the turn of the century. The two World Wars brought about periods of intensive and extensive use, with much work being pioneered by the French in their rehabilitation programs. Moore (1949) divides universal goniometers into two basics models, double-armed instruments and instruments in which one arm is movable and two are stationary. Instruments with two stationary arms on the base of a goniometer enable one "to measure joints on the right and left side of the body with equal ease." They also provide "a long line for sighting in placing the device, this can be of great assistance in measuring joints characterised by long anatomical levers" (Moore 1949, 196). The simple double-armed goniometer has been a more popular instrument. Cave and Roberts (1936), who developed the neutral zero method chosen by the Committee of the American Academy of Orthopaedic Surgeons to form the basis for a new guide to measuring joint range of motion, used such a device. The modified neutral zero method was revised and approved in principle by the Executive Committee of the Academy in 1961. In 1962 publication was approved, and in 1964 it was unanimously accepted by representation of the Orthopaedic Association of all English-speaking countries.

The final draft was used in 1965 and was entitled *Joint Motion Method of Measuring and Recording* (American Academy of Orthopaedic Surgeons 1965). The guidelines in this manual have been used in many studies, including the works of Brodie et al. (1982) and Bell and Hoshizaki (1981).

Schlaaf (quoted in Russe and Gerhardt 1971) proposed a different approach to the problem of standardization by advocating universal measurements, the standard application of measuring devices, and a universal recording and standardization of terminology. All joint movements were described in three basic planes: sagittal, frontal, and transverse. Gerhardt recognized the value of this work and combined both methods to form the SFTR method (S = sagittal, F = frontal, T = transverse, R = rotational). The method was first published in 1963. Russe introduced the method to Europe, where it has received wide acceptance. Its authors claim that "it provides in the shortest possible way full information of joint measurements. It is simple and easily understandable. It is easily comprehensive by all without confusion as to discipline, language and terminology. It is a method read by everyone in the same way so that accurate comparisons may be made. By virtue of its clear, precise, concise and short recording the SFTR method is the most suitable for computer use" (Russe and Gerhardt 1971, 6). The reliability of a double-armed goniometer varies according to the body joint being examined. Bird et al. (1979), using a universal goniometer and the method of the American Academy of Orthopaedic Surgeons, calculated an overall reliability of 0.91. This, however, excluded movements where there was little difference between subjects, measurements that varied by less than 10° between subjects, measurements made by eye, and movements reflecting body and muscular contour rather than ligamentous joint laxity. Boone et al. (1978), from a study of four physical therapists measuring six different ranges of motion weekly for a period of 4 weeks, concluded that the same tester should measure flexibility when evaluating the effect of treatment or in a longitudinal study. The authors also found that one measurement per session was as accurate as an average over a number of trials. They advised that if different testers measured the same motion, changes in range of motion should exceed 5° in the upper and 6° in the lower extremity. A 4-week training period was suggested as necessary to reduce learning effects and intertester variation. A recent text edited by Eston and Reilly (1996) devotes almost the whole of the chapter on flexibility to the double-armed goniometer. For details of use of this instrument in a practical context, this reference is strongly recommended.

Leighton Flexometer

The Leighton flexometer measures the flexibility of the shoulder, wrist, hip, knee, and ankle. It uses a 360° dial and a weighted pointer in a case. The dial and pointer operate freely and independently; the movement of each is controlled by gravity. The instrument will record movement while in any position that is 20° or more from the horizontal. The zero mark on the dial and the top of the pointer move freely to a position of rest and coincide when the instrument is placed in any position from the horizontal. Independent working devices are provided for the pointer and the dial that stop all movement of either at any given position. While in use the flexometer is strapped to the segment being tested. When the dial is locked at one extreme position (e.g., a full extension of the elbow), the direct reading of the pointer on the dial is the arc through which the movement has taken place.

In addition to the flexometer, a projecting wall corner, a long bench or table, and a low-backed armchair are also required. Detailed procedures for all main joint complexes are available from other texts (e.g., Leighton 1964), but as an illustration, the method for knee flexion and extension is as follows:

In a prone position on a box or bench with knees at the end of the bench and lower legs extending beyond the end of the bench, with arms at the sides of the bench and hands grasping the edges of the bench, the instrument should be fastened to the cuticle of the subject's either ankle. The foot should be moved upwards and backwards in an arc to a position as near to the buttocks as possible, and the dial locked. Then the foot should be moved forwards and downwards until the leg is forcibly extended, and the pointer locked. Finally the subject should relax and the reading taken.

Test-retest reliability is reported in the range 0.91-0.92. Table 4.1 gives a series of values from the literature from three studies of flexibility in boys.

Table 4.1 Comparison of the Means (Degrees) and Standard Deviations of Three Studies of Flexibility and Joint Motion in Boys, With Each Other and With Two Accepted Standards

Joint Measured	VAPG	AAOS	Leighton (1957 & 1964) Ages 6-18 (n=500)	Boone & Azens (1979) Ages 1-19 (n=53)	Sigerseth (1973) Ages 10-18 (n=520)
Shoulder: Flexion/ extension	225	211	238±13	236±12	245±7
Shoulder: Abduction/adduction	180	170	171±10	185±4	179±7
Shoulder: Rotation	180	160	183±12	178±12	175±5
Elbow: Flexion/extension	145	146	151±8	146±5	146±3
Radioulnar: Supination/pronation	165	155	181±12	160±8	177±14
Wrist: Flexion/extension	150	144	136±7	154±12	140±17
Wrist: Radioulnar deviation	65	52	87±8	58±8	83±6

(continued)

Table 4.1 *(continued)*

Joint Measured	VAPG	AAOS	Leighton (1957 & 1964) Ages 6-18 (n=500)	Boone & Azens (1979) Ages 1-19 (n=53)	Sigerseth (1973) Ages 10-18 (n=520)
Hip: Flexion/extension	135	141	75±15	131±6	
Hip: Abduction/adduction	85	79	54±6	80±13	56±3
Hip: Rotation	90	90	90±16	101±12	84±16
Knee: Flexion/extension	140	134	147±12	143±5	141±4
Ankle: Flexion/extension	65	66	65±5	71±11	65±9
Ankle: Inversion/eversion	60	51	45±2	60±9	46±2

VAPG: Veterans Administration Physicians Guide: Disability, Evaluation, Examination (1963), from Moore (1978).
AAOS: American Academy of Orthopaedic Surgeons (1972).

Isokinetic Dynamometers

A third method of measuring motion visible at a single joint is isokinetic dynamometry such as is performed with the Cybex II Isokinetic Dynamometer (Lumex Inc., Ronkonkoma, NY). Studies by Wiktorsson-Moller et al. (1983) and Bonci, Hensal, and Torg (1986) have used the Cybex to evaluate range of motion in the lower extremity and at the glenohumeral joint, respectively.

Specialist Devices for Measuring Range of Motion at a Single Specific Joint

Specialist devices for measuring specific joint ranges of motion have been developed due to the limitations of universal goniometers as well as of the methods of the American Academy of Orthopaedic Surgeons. Troup, Hood, and Chapman (1967) raised the problem of assessing the separate ranges of motion of the lumbar spine and hips and criticized the American Academy of Orthopaedic Surgeons' measuring technique, which initiates a movement of the hips without stabilization of the pelvis and thus the lumbar spine. The authors undertook a photographic study of lumbar posture in seven different positions, assessing reliability by a radiographic study of seven patients. Errors arose in the photographic method due to movement of the skin from the flexed to extended positions. The author noted that the radiographic methods were both prone to error and hazardous. Citing the inherent risks of radiographs and the expense of photographs, the authors developed a goniometer mounted on a base to measure straight leg raising, hip flexion, and lumbar extension. Reliability coefficients between 0.78 for hip flexion and 0.88 for femoral trunk angle flexion were recorded.

Loebl Inclinometer

Loebl (1967) developed an inclinometer to measure spinal posture and range of motion. He measured each subject in three different postures. The method takes approximately 5 min. On five weekly measuring sessions, the average variation was $14°$, with daily and hourly measurement reducing the variation to $4°$. As Loebl noted, the back is a notoriously difficult set of joints to measure. Errors arose from the reading of the inclinometer and the marking of the spinous processes, in addition to the varying flexibilities and cooperation of the subjects.

Hyperextensometer and Hand Goniometer

Further goniometers have been developed to measure joint motion in the hand. Brodie et al. (1982) used a hyperextensometer developed by Jobbins, Bird, and Wright (1979) to measure movement at the metacarpophalangeal joint of the index finger with a reliability of 0.92.

Hasselkus et al. (1981) developed a two-axis goniometer to measure metacarpophalangeal laxity; reliability varied between 0.89 and 0.98. Hamilton and Lachenbuch (1969) compared three methods of measuring finger joint angle including a pendulum, a dorsal, and a universal goniometer. The three methods showed equal reliability. The authors also concluded that there was significant variance at the $p < 0.01$ level between operators.

Miscellaneous Methods of Measuring Range of Motion at a Single Joint

Photographs, radiographs, rulers, outline tracings, and mathematical calculations are used in addition to goniometers to measure movements visible at a single joint.

Tanigawa (1972) developed a method of calculating the angle of straight leg raising in order to compare proprioceptive neuromuscular facilitation and passive mobilization stretching techniques. It involved the calculation of the sine of a right-angled triangle.

Photographs have been used in a number of studies. Wilson and Stasch (1945) used double-exposure photographs to record the measurement of joint motion. As stated earlier, Troup, Hood, and Chapman (1967) calculated the movement of lumbar spine and hips and produced reliabilities of 0.91.

Radiographs have been used to measure a variety of joints; for example, Clayson et al. (1966) evaluated the movement of the hip and lumbar vertebrae in normal young women, while Harris and Joseph (1949) used radiographs to measure the extension of the metacarpophalangeal and interphalangeal joints of the thumb, with reliabilities of 2.5°.

Photographic methods are particularly expensive and unsuitable for screening large populations, while radiographs are both hazardous and expensive. Their use is therefore unsuitable for clinical evaluation and for the physical educator.

Israel (1959) used a flexible ruler to reproduce spinal contour, marking the position of bony landmarks and drawing tangents to the curve at those points. Attempts to use a similar technique in the laboratory were abandoned due to inaccuracies of ruler alignment to the spine. Finally, several authors including Nutter and Appleton (1919), Rosen (1922), and Cureton (1941) have used outline tracings as permanent records of a subject's flexibility.

Composite Joint Measurement Techniques

Composite joint measures included in physical fitness batteries provide a less accurate indication of joint flexibility. Yet they have ecological relevance and have much merit in an epidemiological context.

Back and Hamstring Tests

Two popular tests are the standing reach test first developed by Weber and Kraus (1949) and a second similar method referred to as the sit and reach test developed by Wells and Dillon (1952). Very high test-retest coefficients are quoted for these tests, for example, 0.70 for elementary school children and 0.97 for college women for the Kraus/Weber test and 0.98 for college women for the Wells and Dillon sit and reach test.

The sit and reach tests and their numerous variations involve bending to touch the toes with legs straight in either a standing or long sitting position. Differences between adaptations of the test usually concern the length of scale and more importantly instructions to subjects. In some studies a bobbing action is permitted, while in others a single slow movement to full range of motion is required. An examination of the nomenclature surrounding flexibility would tend to suggest these two tests may be measuring different components of flexibility.

The purpose of the sit and reach test is to measure the flexibility of the hamstrings and lower back. It is used for both males and females ranging in age from 6 years to maturity. The subject sits on the floor with legs straight. For the test, the subject's arms are extended forward with the hands placed on top of each other. The subject reaches directly forward, palms down (elbows extended, wrists pronated, and meta-carpophalangeal and interphalangeal joint extended) along the measuring scale on the top panel of the standard sit and reach board box (see figure 4.1). It is advisable for the test to be repeated.

The test is easy to administer in the field and is inexpensive. Trained practitioners are not needed. A weakness of the sit and reach test is that the performance may be influenced by the length or width of the body segments. For example, an individual who has short legs relative to the trunk would have a definite advantage in the sit and reach test. It may not be a valid test for lower back flexibility in teenage girls (Jackson and Baker 1986).

The sit and reach test has acceptable face validity, and test-retest reliability ranges from 0.70 to 0.98. The score is the distance in centimeters from the "zero" point. The zero point is at 20 cm from the start of the scale, so that reaching the toes would gain a score of 20 cm. Positive values occur when the hand is taken past the zero limit. The score taken is the best of two to four repetitions.

Gender-specific means are available for the sit and reach test, as shown in figure 4.2 (Smith and Miller 1985). Percentile norms can be obtained from the American

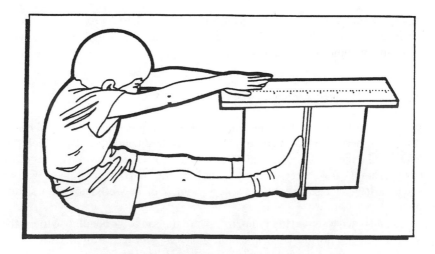

Figure 4.1 Performing the back and hamstring test using a measuring scale.

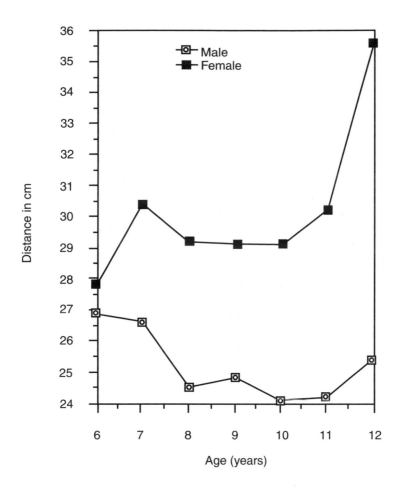

Figure 4.2 Gender-specific means for sit and reach test.

Data from Smith and Miller 1985.

Alliance for Health, Physical Education, Recreation and Dance (AAHPERD) Fitness Test Manual (1984) for both boys and girls aged 5-17 years, or from Kemper et al. (1983) for both boys and girls aged 12-17.

Several groups of researchers have chosen to concentrate on the popular sit and reach or stand and reach tests and the relationship to body segment length. Mathews, Shaw, and Woods (1959) found no significant relationship between hip joint and length of body segments. On the other hand, "A significant relationship was found between sit and reach flexibility and excess of trunk and arm length over leg length" by Laubach and McConville (1966, 241). The problem of segment length can be overcome by using single-joint measures, as described earlier.

Shoulder and Wrist Elevation Test

The purpose of testing for shoulder and wrist elevation is to measure the development of shoulder and wrist flexibility. Since it is difficult to elevate the shoulders in this test without extending the wrists, the movements of these two joints are combined for the score.

The subject assumes a prone (facedown) position with the arms straight and grasps a broomstick or meter rule with hands about shoulder-width apart. The subject then raises the stick upward as high as possible while keeping the chin on the floor and elbows straight. When the stick is raised to its highest point, the position should be maintained for 3 s and a tester notes the distance from the midpoint of the stick to the floor, to the nearest centimeter. The subject's arm length, from the acromion process to the tip of the middle finger, is measured to the nearest centimeter. The best lift from three trials is subtracted from the subject's arm length to give the score.

Goniometry and Kyphometry

Use of the goniometer and the kyphometer is common with children in clinical assessment of flexibility. Details of purpose, use, procedures, validity, reliability, and typical values can be found in chapters 3 and 4 of *A Reference Manual for Human Performance Measurement in the Field of Physical Education and Sports Science* (Brodie 1995). As these methods are less commonly used in field testing for flexibility, they will not be discussed further.

Fleishman's Flexibility Tests

The effect of speed on range of motion has received inadequate coverage in the literature. Only two devices are commonly used to measure range of motion in a kinetic state, the isokinetic dynamometer and electrogoniometer.

Fleishman (1963) used six tests in a factor analytic study to measure "extent and dynamic" flexibility. The tests for extent flexibility included an abdominal stretch in which the subjects bent backward, their hips secured to a fence; a toe-touching test in which subjects had knees straight while standing on a bench; and a twist and touch test in which subjects, with right arm outstretched, twisted as far as possible to the right touching a scale on the wall. Three dynamic flexibility tests were also included: the squat-twist-and-touch; bend-twist-and-touch; and lateral bend. The squat-twist-and-touch test required subjects to go through as many cycles of squat, twist, and touch movements as possible in 30 s. The bend-twist-and-touch test required the subject to perform a cycle of flexing, extending, and rotating the spine (in alternative directions) as many times as possible in 20 s. The lateral bend test required speed in laterally flexing the spine. The score was the number of left/right cycles in 20 s.

Fleishman proposed a battery of 10 tests to measure nine factors. Two reliabilities were reported: a reliability of 0.90 for the twist and touch test and of 0.92 for the bend-twist-and-touch. Harris (1969) obtained reliability estimates for 5 of Fleishman's flexibility tests; the results were for toe touch 0.97; for twist and touch 0.95; for squat-twist-and-touch 0.86; for bend-twist-and-touch 0.93; and for lateral bend 0.93.

To conduct a critical appraisal of Fleishman's work it is necessary to define flexibility using the definition "the maximal existing range of motion in a given joint or joints." It is clear that Fleishman's tests do not test flexibility but rather, as he himself stated, "The ability to make repeated rapid flexing movements in which the resilience of the muscles in recovering from strain or distortion is critical" (Fleishman, quoted in Campbell and Tucker 1966, 100).

Fleishman called this quality dynamic flexibility: it is recognized that within the operational definition given earlier, flexibility is a questionable term because at no stage is full range of motion necessarily achieved. However, the two tests do appear commonly in the literature and so are described in more detail in the paragraphs to follow.

Test of Extent Flexibility

The subject stands with the nonpreferred side to a wall, an arm's length away, feet together. The subject keeps his/her feet in place and twists around as far as possible to touch the wall with the preferred hand. A horizontal scale is extended on either side of a line drawn perpendicular to a line on the floor in front of the toes, and is marked from 0 to 90 cm (0-30 in.). The score is the farthest point reached on the scale and held for 2 s (see figure 4.3).

Test of Dynamic Flexibility

The subject stands with his/her back to the wall but far enough away to be able to bend forward without hitting the wall. Feet are shoulder-width apart. An X is placed on the wall in midshoulder position and another on the floor between the feet. On the signal "Go" the subject bends forward, touching the X on the floor, and straightens up, twisting to touch the X behind with both hands (see figure 4.4). This represents one cycle. The cycles are repeated and the score is the number of cycles in 20 s. The subject alternates the side of rotation with each cycle.

Both of these tests were subjected to rigorous validity and reliability tests and were selected when they fulfilled the criteria adequately. The twist and touch had a reliability of r = 0.90; the bend-twist-and-touch, of r = 0.92.

Flexibility Test Batteries

Other authors have identified flexibility as an important component of physical fitness. Perhaps noting its specific nature, and also realizing the limitations under which many practitioners work, with neither the time nor the money to use expensive technical equipment, experimenters have developed a series of field tests in a

Pediatric Anaerobic Performance

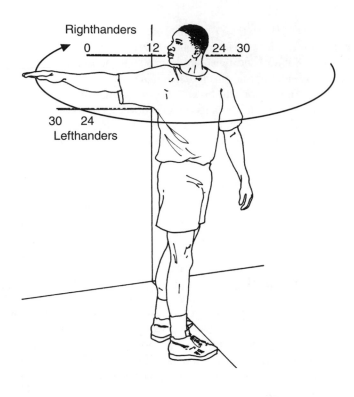

Figure 4.3 The twist-and-touch test for extent flexibility.

Data from Fleishman 1963.

flexibility battery. One such author, Cureton (1941), developed four flexibility tests, of trunk flexion, trunk extension, shoulder flexibility, and ankle flexibility, with reliabilities of 0.95, 0.71, 0.85, and 0.92, respectively. Cureton's work has been the subject of revision and reanalysis by authors such as McCloy and Young (1954) and Harris (1969).

Authors such as Daniels and Worthingham (1977) and Nicholas (1970) have published flexibility tests very much aimed at a specific coaching situation, the objective of the test being to attain an indication of the subject's flexibility weaknesses. Pass/fail tests such as Daniels and Worthingham's are satisfactory in terms of time and are much superior to a single test, but they fail to provide accurate information for rehabilitation or scientific study.

The AAHPERD health-related fitness test is commonly used to compare flexibility standards using the sit and reach test as in a recent study of 8000 Maine schoolchildren (Lehnhard et al. 1992). The criticism of this approach by Plowman (1992) is that the use of criteria-referenced standards is exclusively derived from normative data and expert opinion. This applied equally to a study by Mosher, Carre, and

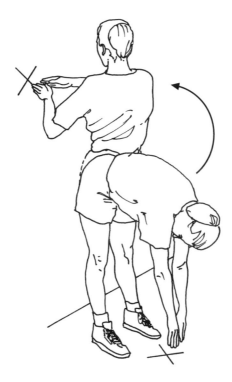

Figure 4.4 The bend-twist-and-touch test for dynamic flexibility.

Data from Fleishman 1963.

Schutz (1982) in which the results on flexibility for 3000 children were below the acceptable range set by the provincial evaluation panels. It is proposed that as these values bear no relationship to desirable and absolute levels of health, the values would be better linked to some specific status that does represent appropriate health standards.

Carter-Wilkinson Method

Medical experimenters such as Carter and Wilkinson (1964) have developed a number of tests of flexibility to assess the relationship between joint laxity and pathological conditions such as Ehlers-Danlos syndrome. The procedure of Carter and Wilkinson (1964) was later modified by Beighton, Solomon, and Soskolne (1973) and is a measure of generalized joint laxity.

In the scoring system (Brodie et al. 1982), one point is allotted for the ability to perform each of the following maneuvers: passive dorsiflexion of the little fingers beyond 90° (one point for each hand); passive opposition of the thumbs to the flexor aspects of the forearm (one point for each side); hyperextension of the elbow beyond 10° (one point for each elbow); hyperextension of the knees beyond 10° (one point for each knee); and forward flexion of the trunk with the knees extended so the palms of the hands rest flat on the floor (one point). A maximum of nine points denotes the most extreme laxity. The reproducibility of the measurement is high ($r = 0.93$, $p < 0.001$). Persistent generalized joint laxity was diagnosed if three out of five tests were positive. Brodie et al. found that 7% of normal children had persistent generalized joint laxity.

Brodie et al. (1982) used Carter and Wilkinson's method on a bilateral basis and a nine-point scoring system for comparison with a hyperextensometer and the method of the American Academy of Orthopaedic Surgeons (1965). It was found to be satisfactory as a method of distinguishing between mobile and hypermobile populations.

Choosing the Most Suitable Method of Measuring Range of Motion

The most suitable method of assessing joint range of motion, given sufficient time (at least 30 min per subject) for a full examination, is either the SFTR method of Russe and Gerhardt (1971) or the method of the American Academy of Orthopaedic Surgeons (1965). The limitations of certain joint movements may necessitate the use of specialist instruments such as the Loebl inclinometer for certain joint movements.

The Leighton flexometer is another instrument that is highly reliable and must be recommended; it has been used extensively by physical educators. However, it is not quite as adaptable as the universal goniometer and its cost may be prohibitive. Another device, the isokinetic dynamometer, is a piece of extremely expensive and highly technical instrumentation; it is unlikely to become a common device in either rehabilitation centers or fitness clinics, and its use will be restricted to scientific study. Finally, electrogoniometers and their adaptations have immense potential in the measuring of kinetic flexibility and as yet have received insufficient consideration in the literature. A simple, cheap adaptation of the Elgon would be ideal for clinical practice.

More popular methods of measuring flexibility make use of simpler procedures, cheaper materials, and limited time. Flexibility tests such as Cureton's are the best alternative to single-joint measures because they involve the use of scoring scales. Pass/fail tests give the coach an indication of flexibility weaknesses and may highlight the need for a flexibility program. They are insufficiently sensitive, however, for a scientific study or in rehabilitation programs. Medical flexibility tests such as Carter and Wilkinson's tests allow subjects to be broadly categorized into hypermobile and hypomobile populations.

Single tests of flexibility as part of a physical fitness battery are the least satisfactory methods. These procedures lack validity in that flexibility has been shown to be joint specific. Popular back and hamstring tests cannot therefore be recommended except in cases in which time permits only an indication of flexibility to be gained. They have the one advantage that they measure an important aspect of flexibility often associated with lower back pain.

Recent Research on Pediatric Flexibility

Although the foregoing includes much research on measurement techniques and methods employed, the following section provides further information on selected topics such as injury, illnesses, and special groups.

Injuries

Injury rate is always a concern when participation levels increase. Any comprehensive rehabilitation requires the reacquisition of strength, endurance, and flexibility. All reconditioning after injury must ensure that flexibility is given a high priority to achieve full recovery to the preinjury level (Thompson, Hersham, and Nicholas 1990). Special programs, even based around a 1-day sports medicine program and organized by coaches, have been shown to decrease the level of injuries (Willman et al. 1990). An explanation is that the children become aware of the importance of flexibility and other fitness components in training. There is increasing evidence that the prevention of sports injuries is associated with giving more time to fitness training, including flexibility, than to training sessions designed to develop specific skills required for the sport (ACSM 1993).

Illnesses

There are a range of illnesses in which changes in flexibility are associated with the process of the disease. Low back pain was studied by Salminen et al. (1992) from a population of over 1500 children. The authors showed that those with continual low back pain were associated with a decrease in lumbar extension and straight leg raising, an increase in lumbar flexion, and a decrease in endurance strength. The pupils reporting sciatica had decreased lumbar flexion and side-bending compared to those without sciatica.

An examination of almost 5000 Dutch children, aged 11 years, for scoliosis, kyphosis, and deviant lateral aspect, showed that 7% of the boys and 11% of the girls had an abnormal forward bending test (Hazebroek-Kampschreur et al. 1992). A separate study on idiopathic scoliosis (McCall and Bronson 1992) showed that children with lumbar curves greater than 45°and associated with a low flexibility index were significantly more likely to develop postoperative progression of the uninstrumented lumbar curve resulting in spinal decompensation. This questions the current methods of establishing the criteria for selective thoracic fusion. Polio is a disease now rarely seen in the West, but in the Indian subcontinent it can cause severe reduction in flexibility. The most common deformities associated with residual poliomyelitis are flexion-abduction contracture of the hip, flexion contracture of the knee, and vulgus deformity of the foot (Sharma et al. 1991). Flexion contractures are also a feature of the feet and hips of children who have osteogenesis imperfecta (Binder, Conway, and Gerber 1993). The degree of flexion deformity is a characteristic of the functional status of such children, especially of how ambulatory they can be, with or without leg braces. Flexibility was shown to improve significantly in children with rheumatoid arthritis (Bacon et al. 1991) who undertook aquatic exercises. This was especially the case for external and internal hip rotation.

In conditions like muscular dystrophy, cerebral palsy, and even below-knee amputation, the center of mass is critical in gait patterns. Gait is often a process of regulating the forward loss of balance that is a consequence of a greater forward flexion of the trunk compared with that of able-bodied children (Engsberg, Tedford, and Harder 1992). Children with Down syndrome, on the other hand, appeared to have greater low back and hamstring flexibility than age-matched children without disabilities (Dichter et al. 1993). This information, in association with below-average scores in lung function, aerobic capacity, and abdominal strength, suggests potential areas for physiotherapy intervention. Intervention involving flexibility was also used in a training program for children with high blood pressure (Brandon and Fillingim 1990). It was shown that the risk profiles of these children could be improved as a result of such training. Even with children who had had surgically corrected congenital heart disease, exercise classes improved flexibility by 25% in the lower body. The training also improved neck flexion, hip and oblique rotation, hamstring and low back stretch, and heel cord stretch. Such exercises will enable these children to achieve a more normal lifestyle (Koch et al. 1988).

Cerebral Palsy

Children with cerebral palsy are of special concern in terms of flexibility because their contractures often require surgery, a feature of most inflexible children. Decreased trunk and hip flexion during the stance phase of the gait cycle was observed when a posterior walker was used by such children in place of an anterior walker. This enabled the children to walk more normally and with increased stability (Greiner, Czernircki, and Deitz 1993). Upper-body exercises involving flexion and extension work have been used by children with cerebral palsy to improve muscular endurance. As this occurred (O'Connell, Barnhart, and Parks 1992), the correlation with wheelchair propulsion increased, showing the specific contribution that muscular endurance could make to mobility. A number of studies (Ounpun et al. 1993; Nene,

Evans, and Patrick 1993; Katz, Rosenthal, and Yosipovitch 1992) have examined changes in flexibility in children with cerebral palsy following surgery. Rectus femoris transfer and rectus femoris release were reported by Ounpun et al. (1993) in 105 and 31 children, respectively. It was found that when preoperative knee range of motion was greater than 80% of normal, no significant changes in knee motion occurred in either form of surgery. In children with less than 80% of normal knee flexion preoperatively, rectus femoris transfer resulted in a maintained knee flexion in the swing phase. The children who underwent distal rectus femoris release or no procedure showed a significant decrease in knee flexion postoperatively. Intrapelvic intramuscular psoas tenotomy (Nene, Evans, and Patrick 1993) resulted in an improvement of hip flexion deformity without any loss of muscle power. Fractional lengthening resolved fixed knee flexion deformity, and the knee flexion arc was improved from 28° to 45° by distal transfer of the rectus femoris. Hamstring contracture is a limiting factor in children with cerebral palsy, and the popliteal angle when the hip was held at 90° of flexion was used to measure hamstring tightness. A value of greater than 50° is an indication, in children aged 1-10 years, of abnormal hamstring tightness (Katz, Rosenthal, and Yosipovitch 1992). While most surgery occurs in the lower limbs because of their importance in gait, elbow, wrist, and finger flexion can also be improved dramatically by appropriate surgery (Koman et al. 1990). Muscle and tendon lengthening are the most common procedures, but the best results for correcting wrist flexion deformities have been through the transfer of the flexor carpi ulnaris to the exterior digitorum communis.

Asthma and Obesity

Flexibility improvement is commonly seen as a by-product of other more general training. This occurred, for example, in asthmatic children who were involved in judo training while keeping exercise-induced bronchospasm to a minimum (Huhnerbein, Achtzehn, and Kriegel 1993). In another study on children with asthma (Strunk et al. 1988), flexibility was found to be normal in comparison with that of healthy children. Obese children have also been studied widely with reference to flexibility. It has been shown that although children with obesity perceive endurance activities negatively, they perceive flexibility-coordination activities more positively than do slim children. As obese children take part in exercise programs and lifestyle modifications (Cohen, McMillan, and Samuelson 1991), they do not change in flexibility when other health-related fitness measures do alter significantly for the better. This was confirmed by another study (Suzuki and Tatsumi 1993) in which an obese group of children were compared with normal-weight controls. Flexibility was one of the measures that did not differentiate between the two groups either initially or after intervention. Even a comparison of the gait of obese versus normal-weight prepubertal children showed differences that suggested increased flexion in the normal children (Hills and Parker 1991) for both hip and knee joints.

Training and Pediatric Flexibility

Training for specific sports can also show flexibility variations in children, although in many cases differences with matched subjects are nonsignificant. A study by Bloomfield et al. (1984), for example, showed no differences in the flexibility of swimmers between competitors and noncompetitors. There was, however, a difference between swimmers and gymnasts (Haywood, Clark, and Mayhew 1986) in ankle and trunk flexibilities, which probably reflected the involvement of different body areas in the two sports. Flexibility in both sports was maintained over the 7-12-year age range. Specific strength training was shown by Sewall and Micheli (1986) to improve flexibility by 4.5% in prepubescent children, but the control group also improved by 3.6% over the 9-week training period.

In 6 months of tae kwon do training, flexibility increased significantly in children aged 5-6 years (Cho and Choe 1988), and also with soccer training (Das and Bannerjee 1992). In the latter case, the majority of the flexibility benefit occurred within the first 8 weeks of training. It has been recognized in baseball that flexibility training is essential to maintain the biomechanical balance of the shoulder and prevent damage (Pappas, Zawicki, and Goldberg 1991). Similarly in running it is recognized that the child's inherent flexibility is insufficient to prevent injury and that special exercises need to be incorporated into the training program (Apple 1985).

Nonspecific physical activities were shown not to benefit flexibility in a study by Bischoff and Lewis (1987). Children participating in a movement education program had less flexibility at ages 11-12 than the control group, and remediation was advised. In contrast, a group of children who participated in a 12-week program of sports at a mean age of 11.4 years showed a significant improvement in flexibility with an average gain of almost 4 cm in the sit and reach test (Naughton and Carlson 1991).

Occasionally one observes coaches, especially in sports such as gymnastics in which flexibility is paramount, applying *forced* dynamic flexibility. An example of this is seen when a coach uses his/her own body weight to extend the joint beyond the limit achieved by the individual undertaking a static stretch. To increase flexibility the muscle must be overloaded beyond its normal range, but the best person to judge this is the athlete, not the coach. If the stretch is taken to the point of tightness, resistance to the stretch or even some discomfort may be acceptable. However, stretching to the point of pain is likely to be damaging. The guidelines provided by Prentice (1994, 44-45) give excellent precautions for stretching.

Sex Differences

Differences in gender have long been recognized in relation to flexibility in adults, due largely to hormonal differences, but in children the results are less consistent. At puberty, girls are more flexible than boys (Kemper 1986), and although boys increase their scores in most motor performance tests as they age, girls show scarcely any changes (Kemper 1985). Andrew (1981) showed that 7-year-old New Zealand girls were superior to boys in flexibility tests, and this was confirmed by Thomas (1992) in tests of hamstring flexibility with 5-9-year-old children. At older ages (Docherty and Bell 1985) such as 12-15 years, girls were superior to boys in tests of trunk flexion/extension and trunk extension. However, in shoulder flexion/extension and arm extension, there were significant decreases with age from 6 to 15 years. In South African children (Goslin and Burden 1986), the same gender difference was observed in senior high school pupils, with no observable difference between the racial groups. The earlier study by Docherty and Bell (1985) showed an increase of trunk extension with age, and when anthropometric measures of linearity were correlated with flexibility, a high and consistent relationship was established. Others, such as Pissanos, Moore, and Reeve (1983), have used body composition with age and sex to predict flexibility. Age was the most significant variable in the prediction, and in a separate study (Leelarthaepin and Chesworth 1983), age was also the strongest predictor, followed by height and weight for boys and height alone for girls.

Directions for Future Research

Any future research needs to be based on clearer and more consistent definitions within the area of flexibility. Some of the terminology in use is still confusing, especially when adjectives like "static," "kinetic," "dynamic," and "extent" are used in association with flexibility or range of motion.

The literature on flexibility and physical performance, either in sport or in the laboratory setting, is still inconclusive. Much more rigorous, randomized controlled trials need to be undertaken to provide evidence for the efficacy of flexibility. The benefits of specific flexibility procedures such as PNF need to be assessed by similar experimental methods. This especially applies to the long-term outcomes, as the short-term benefits are clearly positive. Alternative flexibility strategies may produce very different results when considered over a matter of hours as opposed to days or weeks.

The influence of improved flexibility on injuries needs to be studied using longitudinal approaches. Most of the current work has been cross-sectional and is therefore of limited value.

Possibly the most valuable direction for future research is to use modern technologies such as magnetic resonance imaging to examine soft tissue changes as a result of flexibility increases. This will provide a clearer indication of the underlying anatomical variations and thus provide evidence for training methodologies.

Summary

The literature on flexibility can be confusing because of the range of terminology in use. A high level of flexibility is generally considered to be of benefit in sporting performance. In many sports, appropriate flexibility can be advantageous in reducing certain types of injury. Warm-up is of value for most physical activities. Flexibility is joint specific. Flexibility can be limited by fat, bone, skin, ligaments, connective tissue, muscles, and tendons. A variety of stretching methods are used, including ballistic, static, and PNF techniques; of these, PNF appears to be the most effective. Measurement of flexibility includes the use of goniometry, flexometers, dynamometers, inclinometers, radiographs, photographs, and field tests. The sit and reach test is a popular field test for back and hamstring flexibility. Other field tests include tests of extent flexibility and dynamic flexibility and test batteries such as the Carter-Wilkinson and the American Academy of Orthopaedic Surgeons test. Injuries, illnesses, disease, and training all influence flexibility, especially in children. Growth changes are apparent for flexibility in both sexes. The future direction of research is for longitudinal studies, randomized controlled trials, and the use of new imaging modalities.

References

American Academy of Orthopaedic Surgeons. 1965. *Method of measuring and recording,* 1-87. American Academy of Orthopaedic Surgeons.

American Alliance for Health, Physical Education and Recreation. 1958. *Youth Fitness Test manual.* Washington, DC: American Alliance for Health, Physical Education and Recreation.

American Alliance for Health, Physical Education, Recreation and Dance. 1980. *AAHPERD Health Related Physical Fitness Test manual.* Washington, DC: American Alliance for Health, Physical Education and Recreation.

American Alliance for Health, Physical Education, Recreation and Dance. 1984. *AAHPERD Health Related Physical Fitness Test manual.* Washington, DC: American Alliance for Health.

American Alliance for Health, Physical Education, Recreation and Dance. 1992. *AAHPERD Health Related Physical Fitness Test manual,* Washington, DC: American Alliance for Health, Physical Education and Recreation.

Andrew, R. 1981. Children's recreational patterns and opportunities in Karori. In *Women and recreation. Papers and reports from the conference on Women and Recreation,* ed. A. Welch, 364-370, Wellington, New Zealand.

Apple, D.F. 1985. Adolescent runners. *Clin. Sports Med.* 4(4): 641-655.

Bacon, M.C., Nicholson, C., Binder, H., and White, P.H. 1991. Juvenile rheumatoid arthritis: aquatic exercise and lower-extremity function. *Arthr. Care Res.* 4(2): 102-105.

Beaulieu, J.E. 1981. Developing a stretching programme. *Physician Sports Med.* 9(11): 59-65.

Beighton, P.H., Solomon, L., and Soskolne, C.L. 1973. Articular mobility in an African population. *Ann. Rheumatol. Dis.* 32: 413-418.

Bell, R.D., and Hoshizaki, T.B. 1981. Relationships of age and sex with range of motion of seventeen joint actions in humans. *Can. J. Appl. Sports Sci.* 6: 202-206.

Binder, H., Conway, A., and Gerber, L.H. 1993. Rehabilitation approaches to children with osteogenesis imperfecta: a ten year experience. *Arch. Phys. Med. Rehabil.* 74(4): 386-390.

Bischoff, J.A., and Lewis, K.A. 1987. A cross-sectional study of fitness levels in a movement education program. *Res. Q. Exerc. Sport* 58(4): 348-354.

Bloomfield, J., Blanksby, B.A., Beard, D.F., Ackland, T.R., and Elliott, B.C. 1984. Biological characteristics of young swimmers, tennis players and non-competitors. *Br. J. Sports Med.* 18(2): 97-103.

Bonci, C.M., Hensal, F.J., and Torg, T.S. 1986. A preliminary study on the measurement of static and dynamic motion at the glenohumeral joint. *Am. J. Sports Med.* 14(4): 12-17.

Brandon, L.J., and Fillingim, J. 1990. Health fitness training responses of normotensive children. *Am. J. Health Promot.* 5(1): 30-35.

Brodie, D.A. 1995. *A reference manual for human performance measurement in the field of physical education and sports science.* New York: Edwin Mellen Press.

Brodie, D.A., Bird, H.A., and Wright, V. 1982. Joint laxity in selected athletic populations. *Med. Sci. Sports Exerc.* 14(3): 190-193.

Burke, D., Hagbarth, K-E., and Lofstedt, L. 1978. Muscle spindle activity in man during shortening and lengthening contractions. *J. Physiol.* 277: 131-142.

Campbell, W.R., and Tucker, N.M. 1966. *An introduction to tests and measurement in physical education.* London: Bell and Sons.

Carter, C., and Wilkinson, J. 1964. Persistent joint laxity and congenital dislocation of the hip. *J. Bone Joint Surg.* 46B(1): 40-45.

Carter, C.A. 1978. Supplying: the myth of mobility exercising. *Track Technique Annual* 73: 2329-2331.

Cave, E.F., and Roberts, S.M. 1936. A method for measuring and recording joint function. *J. Bone Joint Surg.* 34: 455-465.

Cho, J.W., and Choe, M.A. 1988. A study on the effect of taekwondo training on the physical performance in preschool children. *WTF—Taekwondo* 8(4): 34-39.

Clark, H.H. 1975. Joint and body range of movement. *Phys. Fitness Res. Dig.* 5: 16-18.

Cohen, C.J., McMillan, C.S., and Samuelson, D.R. 1991. Long-term effects of a lifestyle modification exercise program on the fitness of sedentary, obese children. *J. Sports Med. Phys. Fitness* 31(2): 183-188.

Corbin, C.B., and Noble, L. 1980. Flexibility. *J. Phys. Ed. Recr.* 23-44, 57-60.

Cureton, T.K. 1933. Observation and tests of swimming at the 1932 Olympic Games. *J. Phys. Ed.* 30: 125-130.

Cureton, T.K. 1941. Flexibility as an aspect of physical fitness. *Suppl. Res. Q.* 12(5): 381-390.

Daniels, L., and Worthingtham, C. 1977. *Therapeutic exercise for body alignment and function.* 2nd ed. Philadelphia: Saunders.

Das, S.S., and Banerjee, A.K. 1992. Variation in duration of training period on the performance variables of young soccer players. *NIS Scientific Journal* 15(3): 116-121.

De Vries, H.A. 1986. Physiology of flexibility. *Physiology of exercise for physical education and athletics*, 462-471.

Dichter, C.G., Darbee, J.C., Effgen, S.K., and Palisano, R.J. 1993. Assessment of pulmonary function and physical fitness in children with Downs Syndrome. *Pediatr. Phys. Ther.* 5(1): 3-8.

Docherty, D., and Bell, R.D. 1985. The relationship between flexibility and linearity measures in boys and girls 6-15 years of age. *J. Hum. Mov. Stud.* 11(5): 279-288.

Ekstrand, J., Wiktorsson, M., Oberg, B., and Gillquist, J. 1982. Lower extremity goniometric measurements: a study to determine their reliability. *Arch. Phys. Med. Rehabil.* 63: 171-175.

Engsberg, J.R., Tedford, K.G., and Harder, J.A. 1992. Center of mass location and segment angular orientation of below knee amputee and able-bodied children during walking. *Arch. Phys. Med. Rehabil.* 73(12): 1163-1168.

Eston, R.G.E., and Reilly, T., eds. 1996. *Kinanthropometry and exercise physiology laboratory manual.* London: Spon.

Fleishman, E.A. 1963. *The structure and measurement of physical fitness.* Englewood Cliffs, NJ: Prentice Hall.

Goslin, B.R., and Burden, S.B. 1986. Physical fitness of South African school children. *J. Sports Med. Phys. Fitness* 26(2): 128-136.

Greiner, B.M., Czernircki, J.M., and Deitz, J.C. 1993. Gait parameters of children with spastic diplegia: a comparison of effects of posterior and anterior walkers. *Arch. Phys. Med. Rehabil.* 74(4): 381-385.

Hamilton, G.F., and Lachenbruch, P.A. 1969. Reliability of goniometers in assessing finger joint angle. *Phys. Ther.* 49(5): 465-469.

Harris, M.L. 1969. Flexibility. *Phys. Ther.* 49(6): 591-601.

Hartley-O'Brien, S.J. 1980. Six mobilization exercises for active range of hip flexion. *Res. Q.* 51(4): 625-635.

Hasselkus, B.R., Shepakaran, K.K., House, J.C., and Plaitz, K.A. 1981. Rheumatoid arthritis: a two-axis goniometer to measure metacarpophalangeal laxity. *Arch. Phys. Med. Rehabil.* 62: 137-139.

Haywood, K.M., Clark, B.A., and Mayhew, J.L. 1986. Differential effects of age group gymnastics and swimming on body composition, strength, and flexibility. *J. Sports Med. Phys. Fitness* 26(4): 416-420.

Hazebroek-Kampschreur, A.A., Hofman, A., van Dijk, A.P., and van Linge, B. 1992. Prevalence of trunk abnormalities in eleven year old school children in Rotterdam, The Netherlands. *J. Pediatr. Orthop.* 12(4): 480-484.

Hills, A.P., and Parker, A.W. 1991. Gait characteristics of obese children. *Arch. Phys. Med. Rehabil.* 72(6): 403-407.

Holland, G.J. 1949. Physiology of flexibility: review of literature. *Kinesiol. Rev.* 49-62.

Hoshizaki, T.B., and Bell, R.D. 1984. Factor analysis of seventeen joint flexibility measures. *J. Sports Sci.* 2: 97-103.

Huhnerbein, J., Achtzehn, R., and Kriegel, V. 1993. Judo in a training group for children with asthma. *Kinderarztl-Prax.* 61(7-8): 264-268.

Humphrey, L.D. 1981. Flexibility. *J. Phys. Ed. Recr.* 52: 41-43.

Hutton, R.S., and Nelson, D.L. 1986. Stretch sensitivity of golgi tendon organs in fatigued gastrocnemius muscle. *Med. Sci. Sports Exerc.* 18(1): 69-74.

Jackson, W.A., and Baker, A.A. 1986. The relationship of the sit and reach test to criterion measures of hamstring and back flexibility in young females. *Res. Q. Exerc. Sport* 57(2): 183-186.

Jobbins, B., Bird, H.A., and Wright, V. 1979. A joint hyperextensometer for the quantification of joint laxity. *Engl. Med.* 8: 103-104.

Johns, R.J., and Wright, V. 1962. Relative importance of various tissues in joint stiffness. *J. Appl. Physiol.* 17(5): 824-828.

Katz, K., Rosenthal, A., and Yosipovitch, Z. 1992. Normal ranges of popliteal angle in children. *J. Pediatr. Orthop.* 12(2): 229-231.

Kemper, H.C.G. 1985. Youth and physical fitness. *Int. Council Sport Sci. Phys. Ed. Rev.* 8: 30-36.

Kemper, H.C.G., Dekker, H., Ootjers, G., Post, B., Ritmeester, J.W., Snel, J., Splinter, P., van Essen, S., and Verschuur, R. 1983. *Growth and health of teenagers.* The Netherlands: University of Amsterdam.

Kemper, H.G. 1986. Growth, health and fitness of teenagers in the Netherlands. *Idrett og oppvekstivilkar: Rapport fro seminar pa Bardshaug herregard, (Norway), Universitetsforlaget,* 105-122.

Koch, B.M., Galioto, F.M., Vaccaro, P., and Buckenmeyer, P.J. 1988. Flexibility and strength measures in children participating in a cardiac rehabilitation exercise program. *Physician Sports Med.* 16(2): 139-143.

Koman, L.A., Gelberman, R.H., Toby, E.B., and Poehling, G.G. 1990. Cerebral palsy: management of the upper extremity. *Clin. Orthop.* 62-74.

Laubach, L.L., and McConville, J.T. 1966. Relationships between flexibility, anthropometry and the somatotypes of college men. *Res. Q.* 37(2): 241-251.

Leelarthaepin, B., and Chesworth, E. 1983. Physical performance in a group of school children aged 10-17 years. In *Measuring fitness,* ed. R. Richards, 19-33. East Melbourne: The Menzies Foundation.

Leighton, J.R. 1957. Flexibility characteristics of four specialised skill groups of college athletes. *Arch. Phys. Med. Rehabil.* 38: 24-28.

Leighton, J.R. 1964. Flexibility characteristics of males six to ten years of age. *J. Assoc. Phys. Ment. Rehabil.* 18: 19-21.

Marshall, J.L., Johanson, N., Wickiewicz, T.L., Tischler, H.M., Koslin, B.L., Zeno, S., and Meyers, A. 1980. Joint looseness: a function of the person and the joint. *Med. Sci. Sports Exerc.* 12(3): 189-194.

Mathews, D.K., Shaw, V., and Woods, J.B. 1959. Hip flexibility of elementary school boys as related to body segments. *Res. Q.* 51(4): 197-302.

Mathews, D.K.E.L., and Fox, E. 1976. *The physiological basis of physical education and athletes.* Philadelphia: Saunders.

McCall, R.E., and Bronson, W. 1992. Criteria for selective fusion in idiopathic scoliosis using Cotrel-Dubousset instrumentation. *J. Pediatr. Orthop.* 12(4): 475-479.

McCloy, C.H., and Young, N.D. 1954. *Tests and measurements in health and physical education*, New York: Appleton-Century-Crofts.

Moore, M.L. 1949. The measurement of joint motion. *Phys. Ther.* 29(5): 195-205.

Mosher, R.E., Carre, F.A., and Schutz, R.W. 1982. Physical fitness of students in British Columbia: a criterion-referenced evaluation. *Can. J. Appl. Sports Sci.* 7(4): 249-257.

Naughton, G., and Carlson, J. 1991. Sports participation: a physiological profile of children in four sports over a 12-week season. *Pediatr. Exerc. Sci.* 3(1): 49-63.

Nene, A.V., Evans, G.A., and Patrick, J.H. 1993. Simultaneous multiple operations for spastic diplegia: outcome and functional assessment of walking in 18 patients. *Br. J. Bone Joint Surg.* 75 (3): 488-494.

Nicholas, J.A. 1970. Injuries to knee ligaments: relationship to looseness and tightness in football players. *JAMA* 212: 2236-2239.

Nutter, J., and Appleton. 1919. The standardisation of joint records. *J. Orthop. Surg.* 1: 423-428.

O'Connell, D.G., Barnhart, R., and Parks, L. 1992. Muscular endurance and wheelchair propulsion in children with cerebral palsy or myelomeningocele. *Arch. Phys. Med. Rehabil.* 73(8): 709-711.

Ounpun, S., Muik, E., Davis, R.B. III, Gage, J.R., and DeLuca, P.A. 1993. Rectus femoris surgery in children with cerebral palsy. Part II: A comparison between the effect of transfer and release of the distal rectus femoris on knee motion. *J. Pediatr. Orthop.* 13(3): 331-335.

Pappas, A.M., Zawicki, R.M., and Goldberg, B. 1991. Baseball: too much on a young pitcher's shoulders? *Physician Sports Med.* 19(3): 107-110, 112-114, 117.

Pissanos, B.W., Moore, J.B., and Reeve, T.G. 1983. Age, sex and body composition as predictors of children's performance on basic motor abilities and health-related fitness items. *Percept. Mot. Skills* 56(1): 71-77.

Plowman, S.A. 1992. Criterion referenced standards for neuromuscular physical fitness tests: an analysis. *Pediatr. Exerc. Sci.* 4(1): 9-10.

Prentice, W.E. 1994. *Rehabilitation techniques in sports medicine.* 2nd ed. St. Louis: Mosby.

Rasch, P.J., and Burke, R.K. 1978. *Kinesiology and applied anatomy: the science of human movement.* 6th ed. Philadelphia: Lea & Febiger.

Rosen, N.G. 1922. A simplified method of measuring amplitude of motion in joints. *J. Bone Joint Surg.* 20: 570-579.

Russe, O.A., and Gerhardt, J.J. 1971. *International SFTR method of measuring and recording joint motion.* Bern: Hans Huber.

Salminen, J.J., Maki, P., Oksanen, A., and Pentti, J. 1992. Spinal mobility and trunk muscle strength in 15 year old school children. *Spine* 17(4): 405-411.

Sapega, A.A., Quedenfeld, T.C., Moyer, R.A., and Butler, R.A. 1982. Biophysical factors in range-of-motion exercise. *Physician Sports Med.* 9(12): 57-65.

Schultz, P. 1979. Flexibility: day of the static stretch. *Physician Sports Med.* 11(6): 130-135.

Sewall, L., and Micheli, L.J. 1986. Strength training for children. *J. Pediatr. Orthop.* 6(2): 143-146.

Sharma, J.C., Gupta, S.P., Sankhala, S.S., and Mehta, N. 1991. Residual poliomyelitis of lower limb pattern and deformities. *Indian J. Pediatr.* 58(2): 233-238.

Shyne, K., and Dominguez, H. 1982. To stretch or not to stretch? *Physician Sports Med.* 10(9): 137-140.

Smith, J.F., and Miller, C.V. 1985. The effect of head position on sit and reach performance. *Res. Q.* 56(1): 84-85.

Strunk, R.C., Rubin, D., Kelly, L., Sherman, B., and Fukuhara, J. 1988. Determination of fitness in children with asthma. Use of standardized tests for functional endurance, body fat composition, flexibility and abdominal strength. *Am. J. Dis. Child.* 142(9): 940-944.

Surburg, P.R. 1981. Neuromuscular facilitation techniques in sports medicine. *Physician Sports Med.* 9(9): 115-127.

Suzuki, M., and Tatsumi, M. 1993. Effect of therapeutic exercise on physical fitness in a school health program for obese children. *Nippon Koshu Eisel Zasshi* 40(1): 17-28.

Tanigawa, M.C. 1972. Comparison of the hold-relax procedure and passive mobilization on increasing muscle length. *Phys. Ther.* 52(7): 725-735.

Thomas, D.Q. 1992. Health related fitness in first through fourth grade students. *J. Appl. Sport Sci. Res.* 6(3): 165-169.

Thompson, T.L., Hersham, E.B., and Nicholas, J.A. 1990. Rehabilitation of the injured athlete. *Pediatrician* 17(4): 262-266.

Troup, J.D.G., Hood, C.A., and Chapman, A.E. 1967. Measurements of the sagittal mobility of the lumbar spine and hips. *Ann. Phys. Med.* 9(8): 308-321.

Weber, S., and Kraus, H. 1949. Passive and active stretching of muscles spring stretch and control group. *Phys. Ther. Rev.* 29: 407-410.

Wells, K.F., and Dillon, E.K. 1952. The sit and reach—a test of back and leg flexibility. *Res. Q.* 23: 115-118.

Willman, M.K., Jacobs, A.W., Mayhew, J.L., and Piper, F.C. 1990. Fitness day: a tool for measuring and ranking total body fitness among high school athletes. *J. Osteop. Sports Med.* 4(4): 3-10.

Wiktorsson-Moller, M., Oberg, B., Ekstrand, J., and Jillquist, G. 1983. Effects of warming up, massage, and stretching on range of motion and muscle strength in the lower extremity. *Am. J. Sports Med.* 11: 249-251.

Wilson, G.D., and Stasch, W.H. 1945. Photographic record of joint motion. *Arch. Phys. Med.* 26: 361-362.

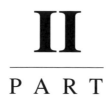

PART

Assessment of Anaerobic Performance

5

CHAPTER

The Determinants of Anaerobic Muscle Function During Growth

Anthony J. Sargeant

This chapter focuses on the following objectives:

- To provide an overview of the fundamental physiological determinants of human anaerobic power during growth with special reference to muscle fiber variability in contractile and metabolic properties
- To review how the rate and capacity of energy pathways in human muscle determine maximum performance
- To describe how the fundamental laws of muscle mechanics may determine maximum anaerobic performance
- To discuss how maximum voluntary effort may be influenced by activation level and learning
- To discuss the relationship between muscle power and muscle or body dimensions
- To describe the acute plasticity of muscle properties, including the effects of fatigue, potentiation, and temperature

The capability of human muscle to generate mechanical output for brief periods lasting for seconds rather than minutes is of fundamental importance in the daily activities of children and adults. Moreover, it is a key element determining performance level in a number of sports, in dance, and in many physically based recreational activities.

It is therefore surprising that until relatively recently this aspect of children's physical performance has received little systematic attention from the scientific community. That is not to say that its importance was not recognized by generations of physical educators who sought to include assessment of it in the many test batteries for physical ability that have been enthusiastically promoted for many decades. Unfortunately, such assessments, although of practical pedagogic value, were rarely used or suitable for objective investigation of the fundamental mechanisms governing the effect of growth and development and the trainability of this aspect of physical performance. This chapter therefore reviews some of the fundamental considerations necessary for study of the intrinsic capability of the neuro-muscular-skeletal system to generate mechanical output of short duration, primarily via anaerobic energy sources.

Energy Supply

The ultimate carrier of energy in the muscle cell is adenosine triphosphate (ATP). This releases energy when it is broken down to adenosine diphosphate (ADP) and inorganic phosphate (Pi) by the enzymatic action of myosin ATPase. The energy released is used to detach cross bridges formed between the actin and myosin filaments of muscle, thereby allowing for the subsequent power-generating phase of the cross-bridge cycle to occur (see equation 1).

$$\text{ATP} \xrightarrow{\text{myosin ATPase}} \text{ADP} + \text{Pi} + \text{energy} \tag{1}$$

Also present in the muscle fiber is another high-energy phosphate, creatine phosphate (PCr). In the presence of the enzyme creatine kinase this can be split, allowing the resynthesis of ATP from ADP (see equation 2).

$$\text{PCr} + \text{ADP} \xrightarrow{\text{creatine kinase}} \text{ATP} + \text{Cr} \tag{2}$$

In this way, PCr acts as a chemical buffer in the cell (temporally and spatially), maintaining ATP levels within the muscle fiber. If the demand for ATP exceeds the rate at which it can be supplied, then PCr will become depleted; as a consequence, the concentrations of ATP will also drop with consequent increases in the by-products of its breakdown, notably ADP, Pi, and inosine monophosphate (IMP), and the muscle will fatigue. In this context it is important to point out that the phenomenon we call muscle fatigue can be thought of as an important down-regulating mechanism reducing the energy demands of the muscle cell (and hence its mechanical output) and thus preventing a metabolic crisis in the muscle cell. In human maximal dynamic exercise lasting about 25 s, it has been calculated that PCr is almost totally depleted in most fibers (Sant'Ana Pereira, van der Laarse, and Sargeant 1996).

The energy available from the reactions represented by equations 1 and 2 can be released at very fast *rates* generating high levels of mechanical output. In contrast, however, the total amount of energy available, that is, the intrinsic *capacity*, is rather small due to the size of the stores of high-energy phosphates (ATP and PCr) present in the resting muscle cell. This pathway for energy turnover in the muscle cell has been called *anaerobic alactic* because it does not require oxygen or generate lactate.

If muscle activity is to continue for more than a few seconds, other pathways will need to be brought into play in order to resynthesize the ATP needed for muscle contraction. The first of these to be considered is anaerobic glycolysis. In the absence of oxygen, muscle glycogen is broken down in a series of enzymatically regulated steps to form lactate and release energy for the resynthesis of ATP (see equation 3). Traditionally this has been called *anaerobic lactic* energy.

$$\text{Glycogen} \longrightarrow \text{lactate} + \text{ATP} \tag{3}$$

This pathway does not require oxygen but does generate lactate, and hence an increase in the concentration of hydrogen ions $[H^+]$, which has often been associated with the phenomenon of muscle fatigue. However, it should be noted that muscle fatigue can occur in the absence of lactate and $[H^+]$ accumulation. Furthermore, recovery from muscle fatigue usually occurs with a much faster time course than does the restoration of resting levels of $[H^+]$. Thus it should be apparent that the link between $[H^+]$ accumulation in the muscle and fatigue is probably not one of simple cause and effect, but may be rather indirect and will depend upon the nature of the exercise that leads to fatigue (see Sahlin and Ren 1989; Cady et al. 1989; Sargeant and Dolan 1987). Although the maximal rate at which this anaerobic lactic pathway can supply energy for the resynthesis of ATP is only about half that of equation 2, the maximal rate has a capacity that is probably twice as large—such that significant energy turnover can be maintained for exercise of 40 to 60 s duration.

If exercise is to be sustained, oxygen must be used in aerobic metabolism to provide continuous resynthesis of ATP that matches the demand as indicated in the generalized form shown (see equation 4).

$$\text{Food (carbohydrates and fats)} + \text{oxygen} \longrightarrow CO_2 + H_2O + \text{ATP} \tag{4}$$

Although the maximal rate at which this pathway can generate energy is about half as much again as that of equation 3, it has an immense capacity, allowing submaximal exercise to continue for some hours. It should be remembered, however, that at levels close to the maximum for aerobic metabolism, exercise may be sustained for only a few minutes.

Anaerobic Versus Aerobic Contribution

The interdependence of the mechanisms that regulate and switch on the three pathways for the resynthesis of ATP is not fully understood. What is important to understand, however, is that all pathways may be operating at the same time even in short-term exercise lasting for a few seconds. Thus many measurements of anaerobic power contain a significant minority contribution from aerobic metabolism. In maximal dynamic exercise such as running or cycling, it seems likely that if the duration is less than about 2 min, the majority energy source will be anaerobic but that the contribution from the aerobic pathways will make a progressively greater contribution to the total as the duration of the exercise increases. At 2 min there will be a roughly equal contribution from aerobic and anaerobic pathways, but beyond that time the aerobic pathway will make the majority contribution to energy turnover (see figure 5.1).

The maximal power that can be delivered in exercises of different duration will decrease as duration increases. Since the energy pathways are not recruited in a mutually exclusive sequence, it is only possible to characterize the different parts of the power duration curve as "phases" in which a particular energy source may dominate—but this domination will not be to the exclusion of the other energy pathways (figure 5.2).

Rate Versus Capacity of Energy Pathways

It will be appreciated that there are formidable difficulties in making direct measurements of either the rate or the capacity of the anaerobic pathways for energy turnover in the intact human, whether child or adult. Nevertheless, Bangsbo and his colleagues (1990), using needle biopsy of muscle and arterial and venous catheter-

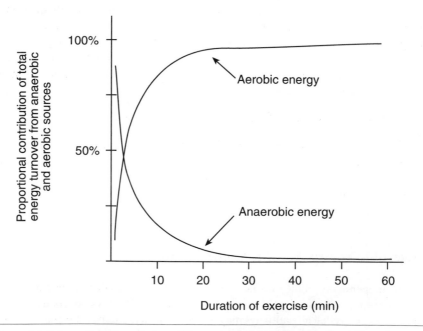

Figure 5.1 Schematic representation of the percentage contribution of aerobic and anaerobic energy to total energy turnover in relation to the duration of maximal exercise.

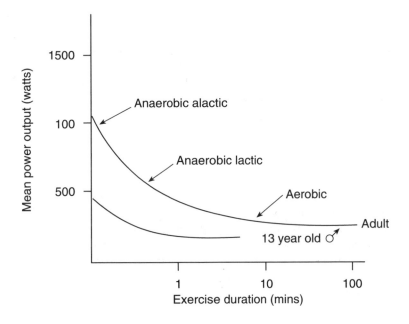

Figure 5.2 Schematic representation of maximal power output in relation to the duration of exercise.

Data from Sargeant 1989.

ization, have demonstrated that direct quantitative measurements of anaerobic energy turnover can be made during short-term dynamic exercise in adults. The multiple techniques involved are, however, highly invasive, not suitable for large-scale population studies, and not ethically justifiable in the case of children. As an alternative, indirect estimations of anaerobic metabolism have been made using calculations based on measurement of the oxygen deficit at the onset of exercise. Some caution is needed in interpreting these data, however, due to the assumptions that need to be made regarding mechanical efficiency and the energy equivalence of oxygen in high-intensity exercise (for a discussion of this point see later in this chapter; Bangsbo 1996; di Prampero 1996; and Zoladz, Rademaker, and Sargeant 1995). The use of phosphorus nuclear magnetic resonance spectroscopy (31 PNMR) offers an alternative indirect technique for investigating muscle metabolism in the intact human that is noninvasive. At the time of writing, there are no apparent health risks associated with this technique and it seems suitable for use in healthy children. As with all techniques it has limitations, and these need to recognized. One major problem relates to the type of exercise (and the muscle groups involved) that can be performed in even the largest (and therefore most expensive) bore magnets available. The time required for recording the spectra and the averaging of a number of spectra makes the technique difficult to use in looking at fast transient changes in the compounds being studied. In addition, it is difficult to take account of the continuum of metabolic and contractile properties found within the muscle fiber population, since the measurement being made is essentially a homogenate of those fibers under the measuring coil. Nevertheless, the technique does hold promise for investigating some questions regarding muscle energetics (for a recent review see Cooper and Barstow 1996).

Muscle Mechanics

Because of the problems associated with direct measurement of anaerobic energy turnover in children, attention has been focused on measuring the mechanical output attributable (predominantly) to anaerobic energy sources. In developing and applying such techniques it is important to realize that even though one may be measuring the mechanical output of whole groups of muscles operating together, the constituent muscle will still be governed by the fundamental laws of muscle mechanics.

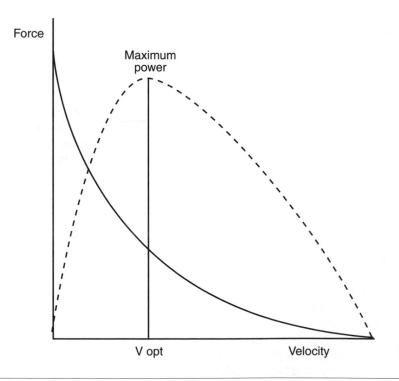

Figure 5.3 The general form of the force-velocity relationship in skeletal muscle is given by the solid line. The dashed line is the relationship of power to velocity.

Force-Velocity Relationship

The relationship between the force that a muscle can generate and its velocity of contraction is described by an inverse relationship of the general form shown in figure 5.3. The mathematical consequence of this relationship is that power (which is force times velocity) has a parabolic relationship with velocity. Maximal power is attained at an optimal velocity (V_{opt}) that in isolated animal experiments is about one-third of the maximum velocity of shortening. The implication of this for whole-body exercise is that it will be vital to know at which "velocity" the exercise is being performed and how this relates to the "global" power velocity for that specific exercise (see, e.g., Sargeant, Hoinville, and Young 1981; Sargeant 1994).

Length-Tension Relationship

The force that a muscle can generate depends upon its length as described by the length-tension relationship (figure 5.4). Active tension is related to the degree of overlap of the actin and myosin filaments, and this decreases beyond optimum length as the amount of overlap and hence potential cross-bridge sites diminishes. Passive tension is the result of the stretching of the cytoskeleton, connective tissue, and other structural elastic elements around and within the muscle fibers. Clearly great care needs to be taken to standardize the "global" muscle length in muscle strength or torque measurements, as well as the range of length excursion in measurements of muscle power. This standardization will normally be made in relation

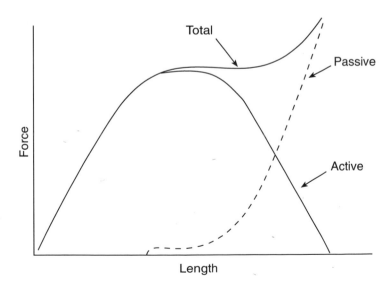

Figure 5.4 The active and passive isometric tension generated by a muscle in relation to its length.

to joint angles in the intact human rather than to muscle (sarcomere) length. Little is known of the changes that occur in the passive elastic elements during growth and development. Similarly it is not known how the active and passive components of the length-tension relationship may be related to one another and the range of use and hence joint angle.

Muscle Fiber Type Variability

The basic element of neuromuscular function is the motor unit. Each motor unit consists of a single motoneuron in the spinal cord that through its axonal branches supplies a number of muscle fibers. The number of muscle fibers that compose a motor unit may vary enormously depending on the muscle, but however many fibers there are they will be relatively homogenous with respect to their contractile and metabolic properties. This homogeneity exists because the fibers are subject to the same pattern of activation from the single controlling motoneuron. Between motor units, however, there will be considerable variability in fiber properties due to the differences in recruitment pattern according to use (for review see, e.g., Sargeant and Jones 1995). Traditionally the variability in fiber properties has been classified according to a number of systems that may be considered analogous, although it should be noted that there will be considerable variation across species and even within species among different muscles (see table 5.1).

In humans, the fiber type classification has usually been based on histochemical staining of cross sections obtained from needle biopsy. The histochemical techniques used are designed to differentiate fibers into discrete types, but this categorization, although convenient, is somewhat misleading, since it is now clear that there is a continuum in most, if not all, contractile and metabolic properties. In recent years it has become possible to show that there is a complex set of genes controlling the expression of the contractile and regulatory proteins. Of the contractile proteins it is the (iso-)form of the myosin heavy chain that is expressed that seems to be the primary determinant of the muscle fiber's maximum velocity of shortening and hence power. In human skeletal muscle this is found in three main isoforms, type I

Table 5.1　Principal Systems of Muscle Fiber Type Classification

Human muscle fibers	Contractile/metabolic	Physiological
type I	slow oxidative	ST (slow fatigue resistant)
type IIA	fast oxidative	FFR (fast fatigue resistant)
type IIX *	fast glycolytic	FFS (fast fatigue sensitive)

* Note: This type was previously designated IIB

(slow), type IIA (fast), and a third type, IIX (the fastest). Unfortunately and confusingly, this last type (so designated because of its close homology to the IIX isoform identified in other mammalian species) is associated with the human fiber type previously designated on the basis of conventional histochemistry as type IIB (see Ennion et al. 1995 for a discussion of this point).

One of the important observations made in recent years is that while the type I and type II myosin heavy-chain isoforms are not usually seen together in the same muscle fiber, many if not the majority of type II fibers have both the IIA and the faster IIX isoforms present in variable proportions. At present there is little direct evidence in humans, but it does seem probable that there is a continuum of related contractile properties and maximum power dependent on the degree of "co-expression" (Larsson and Moss 1993; Sant'Ana Pereira et al. 1995; Stienen et al. 1996). It is also probable that it is relatively easy to elicit shifts in the degree of "co-expression" by changes in the activity/activation patterns. It should be realized that such changes might have marked functional consequences but could go undetected with the use of conventional histochemistry designed to categorize fibers into discrete types. Figure 5.5 shows the possible power-velocity relationships for type I human muscle fibers and

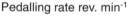

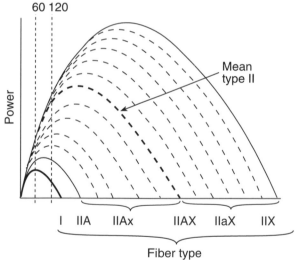

Figure 5.5 The relative power-velocity relationship of type I muscle fibers compared to that for the *mean* of type II. In fact there is probably a continuum of properties for the type II fibers dependent upon the proportion of IIA and IIX myosin heavy-chain isoforms present. This is represented by the broken lines. The uppercase letter indicates a predominance of that isoform in the coexpressing fibers. The vertical lines are suggestions for how these contraction velocities might relate to cycling at 60 and 120 rev/min (see Sargeant and Jones 1995; Sargeant 1994).

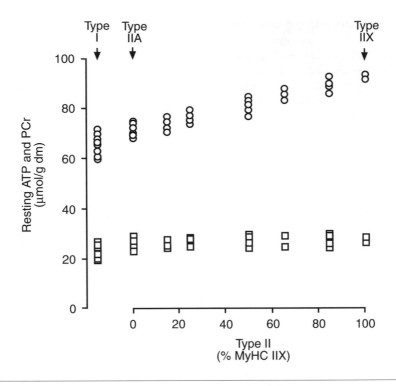

Figure 5.6 ATP (open squares) and phosphocreatine (open circles) content in resting fibers characterized according to their myosin heavy-chain composition. Each value represents one individual pool of fibers. Hybrid IIAX fibers were pooled according to the percentage of their myosin heavy-chain IIX component.

Data from Sant'Ana Pereira et al. 1996.

the *mean* for the type II fibers. The possible effects of varying proportions of the type IIA and IIX myosin heavy-chain isoforms are also shown. One of the more difficult problems has been to understand how such power-velocity relationships may be related to human movement. Our suggestion in relation to cycling exercise is indicated in figure 5.5. For a further discussion of the background to this proposal, readers are referred to Sargeant and Jones (1995) and Sargeant (1996).

Not surprisingly, there is a close link between the expression of the contractile proteins, the metabolic properties, and the concentration of substrates. For example, while the resting concentration of ATP seems to vary little between different human fibers (in contrast to those of some other mammals), phosphocreatine concentration increases systematically as the proportion of the IIX myosin heavy-chain isoform increases. Thus as the intrinsic speed of cross-bridge cycling and hence ATP breakdown increases, so does the buffering capacity provided by the phosphocreatine (see figure 5.6).

Intrinsic Isometric Strength

While the maximum velocity of contraction (V_{max}), and possibly maximum power, of human muscle fibers may vary by a factor of about 10 between type I and type IIX fibers, there is much less, if any, difference in the intrinsic isometric strength—that is, strength normalized for cross-sectional area. However, it is difficult to be certain of the true range in human muscle because of difficulties in making accurate normalized measurements in the intact human. Recent work using skinned single human fiber fragments does, however, suggest that there may be significant differences between type I, IIA, and IIX (Stienen et al. 1996).

Mechanical Efficiency

The mechanical efficiency is a measure of the amount of mechanical work that can be generated from the release of chemical energy. It has been shown in animal experiments that maximum efficiency is attained at a contraction velocity close to, but somewhat less than, that for maximum power. Unfortunately very little is known about the efficiency/contraction velocity relationships of human muscle fibers. Although there is no reason to suppose that the general relationship will differ in principle from that for other mammalian species (Lodder, de Haan, and Sargeant 1991; Rome 1993), any attempt to calculate energy turnover from the mechanical power output using an assumed mechanical efficiency is fraught with difficulty. This is especially the case since efficiency is labile depending upon the energetic status of the cell (see di Prampero 1996 for a discussion of this issue). In passing, it is also worth pointing out that the aerobic component of short-term work will also have a variable mechanical yield. This is confirmed by the observation that in incremental exercise tests the relationship between power output and oxygen uptake is not linear—despite standard text book teaching! (Zoladz, Rademaker, and Sargeant 1995; figure 5.7). In fact there is a disproportionate increase in oxygen cost for power output at levels beyond those at which blood lactate increases, and this makes calculations of energy turnover from measurements of oxygen deficit, for example, problematic (see also Bangsbo 1996).

Neuromuscular Activation and Learning

An important issue that needs to be addressed is whether in maximum voluntary exercise of short duration, subjects are able to fully activate their muscles. It is often suggested that there is a large physiological reserve of force-generating ability when maximum voluntary contractions are made. This evidence is, however, largely anecdotal and not substantiated by laboratory experiments on adults performing isometric and concentric contractions of major locomotory muscles. Such investiga-

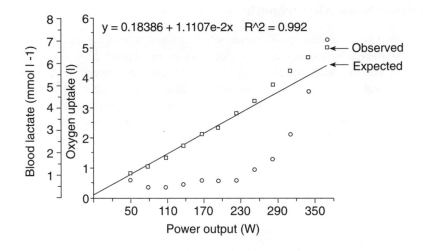

Figure 5.7 Nonlinear relationship of oxygen uptake and blood lactate to power output during progressive incremental cycle ergometer exercise ($\dot{V}O_2$ is the mean of the last minute of each 3 min incremental stage).

Data from Zoladz, Rademaker, and Sargeant 1995.

tions, using either direct electrical stimulation of the motor nerve or superimposed electrical stimulation applied transcutaneously, indicate that maximal or near-maximal (>95%) contractions can be elicited voluntarily by most subjects in most tests (see Beelen et al. 1995; James, Sacc, and Jones 1995; Gandevia et al. 1995).

These observations are, however, related to single maximal efforts or dynamic exercise of short duration involving concentric contractions in adults. They do not apply to maximum eccentric contractions, even in adults, where the forces generated are much higher than in isometric contractions and probably generate reflex inhibition. Perhaps more importantly, as the duration of the maximum voluntary effort increases, say beyond approximately 25 s, so does the likelihood that motivational factors, or possibly central fatigue mechanisms, may play a decisive role in limiting performance. Finally it should be remembered that these conclusions are drawn almost exclusively from experiments on adults, and their extrapolation to other populations, such as children or patient groups, should be treated with caution.

Another point should be taken into account in considering the maximal activation of limb muscles in children and adolescents: there is clear evidence that the maturation process of the corticospinal tract in humans continues into the second decade. Thus, for example, corticospinal conduction velocity continues to increase up to about 15 years of age. What the functional significance of the changes is—changes that occur strikingly late in human development—is not clear. They may have no significant effect, but little is known in this area, and further research is merited.

There is little doubt that the performance of even apparently simple tasks, such as lifting a bar with weights, can be dramatically improved as the subject learns the optimum pattern of muscle activation in order to generate "useful" power. There may be an added component in this "neural learning" that is the synchronizing of motor unit activation at the onset of a maximum effort so that the time to peak tension is shorter. The learning of optimal activation patterns may be especially noticeable in the performance of movements in which power needs to be translocated from proximal to distal limb segments via biarticular muscles. Care in initial training, and the inclusion of proper control groups and carefully selected criterion measurements, are clearly important in any study of anaerobic performance, but especially in training or other longitudinal studies (see Sargeant 1989, 56-58, for discussion of these points).

The Relation of Muscle Power to Muscle and Body Dimensions

The force generated by skeletal muscle is generally believed to be the consequence of the attachment of cross bridges between actin and myosin filaments. Because of the opposite directional organization of the filaments on either side of the Z line that separates one sarcomere from the next, the forces generated on either side cancel one another out as shown in figure 5.8. Thus in isometric contractions it is the number of sarcomeres acting side by side (in parallel) that determines the force that can be generated. In normal muscle this dimension might best be represented by an estimate of the physiological cross-sectional area—that is, the cross section at right angles to the fibers that compose the muscle group being studied. Unfortunately this is often a difficult measurement to make in vivo because of the complex architecture and the varying angles of the fibers of different muscles acting around a joint. A reasonable compromise may therefore be to measure the anatomical cross section of a muscle group, that is, the cross section at right angles to the limb segment.

While isometric force is independent of muscle length, power is not, since it is a product of force and velocity. Velocity is a function of the number of sarcomeres in series. The amount of shortening generated by each sarcomere adds up along the length of the fiber so that the distance moved in unit time increases with every sarcomere added (see figure 5.8). Thus measurements of muscle power should be standardized for the number of sarcomeres in series and in parallel. In practice this is probably best reflected by a measurement of muscle volume (see Sargeant 1989).

Standardization of muscle power and force for the appropriate muscle dimensions is relatively easy when isolated muscle preparations are being studied. In the intact human, accurate measurement of muscle size is more difficult but should nevertheless be attempted if the investigator wants to establish whether there are differences in the intrinsic muscle properties: between population groups, such as children and adults, or as a consequence of training or other interventions. In the past there has been uncertainty as to whether the apparently low anaerobic power of children compared

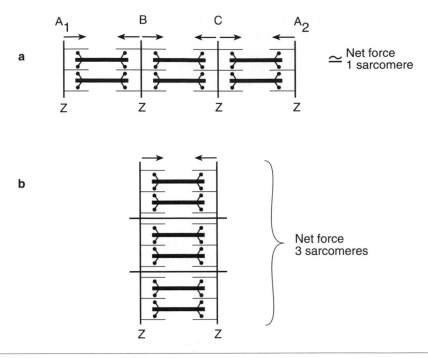

Figure 5.8 Schematic illustration to show the force generated by three sarcomeres arranged (a) in series and (b) in parallel. In (a) the forces on either side of the Z lines B and C cancel one another out; thus the net force of the system is only the forces generated at A1 and A2, that is, equivalent to that of one sarcomere. In (b) the forces generated by all three sarcomeres add up to give three times the net force delivered by (a).

Note: Conversely the distance shortened (and hence velocity) will be three times greater in system (a) compared to system (b). Thus the maximum power (i.e., force · velocity) will be the same in both systems, although it will be achieved at different optimal velocities.

to adults was a genuine phenomenon or the consequence of inappropriate or inaccurate standardization. Recent work, however, with young rat muscle, where maximal electrical stimulation can be combined with accurate measurement of the isolated muscle dimensions, shows a similar phenomenon. It seems therefore that a reduction in the appropriately normalized maximal muscle function may be a genuine and normal feature during growth (Lodder, de Haan, and Sargeant 1994).

Measurements of muscle dimensions are difficult and or very expensive in the intact human, involving, for example, magnetic resonance imaging and three-dimensional reconstruction. As a consequence, maximal power has often been expressed relative to body size, but clearly this indirect approach is inherently unsatisfactory when one is seeking to assess *intrinsic* muscle function.

The foregoing section, however, deals only with the physiological principles that need to be taken into account in normalizing short-term power in relation to the size of the active muscle mass. In situations in which the power is being generated in order to move the body, it may be relevant to express the power in relation to the forces to be overcome. In running, for example, it may be body mass; in cycling (at least on the flat), it might be frontal area. Apart from these performance-related expressions there seems to be little purpose in the current fashion of seeking to relate "anaerobic" power to some "allometric gold standard" based on body dimension, since the relationship between body dimensions and muscle size and function is so easily changed, for example, by training, immobilization, or obesity.

The Effects of Muscle Temperature and Prior Exercise

The concept of *chronic* plasticity of muscle properties is well accepted. In this, the intrinsic properties of the muscle are changed by long-term interventions such as training, immobilization, chronic stimulation, or cross innervation (in animals), or as a consequence, for example, of the aging process. Recently, Sargeant (1994) introduced the concept of "acute plasticity" to cover those short-term but often profound and quickly reversible changes consequent upon, for example, the effect of exercise itself leading to potentiation or fatigue, or the effect of temperature changes as a consequence of either the exercise itself or environmental conditions.

Muscle Fatigue

Our understanding of muscle fatigue in relation to anaerobic power and capacity relies mainly upon studies in adults (see, e.g., Sargeant and Dolan 1987; Beelen and Sargeant 1991; Greenhaff et al. 1994). An important observation made first in animal studies but subsequently confirmed in humans is that muscle fatigue may lead to a temporary transformation of the muscle toward slower properties (de Haan, Jones, and Sargeant 1989). Functionally this means that the magnitude of the measured fatigue will depend upon the contraction velocities over which it is assessed. Thus as shown in figure 5.9, a standard fatiguing exercise may lead to no significant change in leg extension power during maximum cycling exercise at slow pedal rates, but to a 25% to 30% change at faster pedal rates close to or beyond the optimum for maximum power output. It should be emphasized, however, that fatigue generated by other forms of exercise may have a different origin and can lead to different effects (for reviews see Sargeant and Kernell 1993; Gandevia et al. 1995).

Muscle Temperature

In a classic paper, Asmussen and Boje (1945) demonstrated the significant effect of increasing muscle temperature on human power output generated in an approxi-

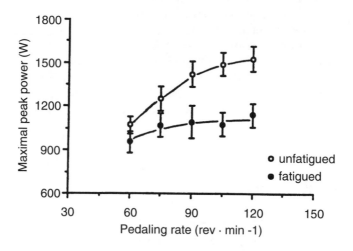

Figure 5.9 Human maximum peak power cycling at 5 different pedaling rates in fatigued and unfatigued states.

Data from Beelen and Sargeant 1991.

mately 14 s maximal sprint on a cycle ergometer. Recently that work has been extended to demonstrate that the magnitude of the temperature is velocity dependent (see figure 5.10; Sargeant 1987). This is so because the primary effect of changes in muscle temperature is to change the rate of cross-bridge detachment and hence the maximal velocity of shortening.

Temperature changes in muscle can be brought about by both exercise and changes in the ambient temperature. In relation to the latter it should be appreciated that limb muscles show a marked temperature gradient, especially in cold weather, with the more superficial layers falling by more than 5 or 6°C compared with the deeper muscle. Children have a relatively large limb surface area in relation to volume and may be more vulnerable in this respect than adults. It should be remembered that a difference of 5°C would result in a 20% to 30% difference in maximum power between superficial and deep muscle in the example given.

Ideally muscle power should be measured at a homogenous and known temperature and in a stable metabolic state (that is, from rest). However, given the difficulty and acceptability of making deep muscle temperature measurements in children, it seems more pragmatic to argue for measurements to be made under carefully standardized conditions. If a warm-up is considered desirable, this should also be incorporated into the protocol. The need for rigor in this matter cannot be overemphasized, especially with respect to longitudinal studies. A 1°C difference in the mean muscle temperature at rest might easily be produced by seasonal variations in the ambient temperature or by changes in clothing at the end compared to the beginning of the study. At optimal velocity this could produce a systematic difference of 5% in muscle power!

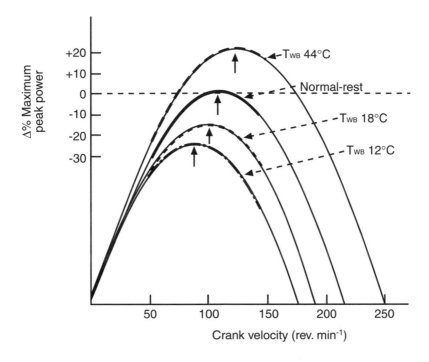

Figure 5.10 The relationship of leg extension power generated in cycling exercise to pedaling rate after immersion of the legs in water baths at different temperatures and under control conditions. The thicker sections of the lines represent the limits of the experimental data; the thinner sections are the theoretical extrapolations. Power is given in watts standardized for the upper leg muscle (plus bone) volume. Temperatures are for the water bath. The increase in the optimal velocity for maximal power with increasing temperature is indicated by the arrows.

Data from Sargeant 1987.

Directions for Future Research

A major area that has been hitherto neglected in the pediatric population is the evolution of muscle fatigue during short-term exercise. In addition, little has been done to investigate the rate of recovery from such exercise or the effect of repeated bouts of high-intensity exercise. Unfortunately an issue that cannot be separated from this, and that complicates the investigation, is the effect of muscle temperature on muscle power. High-intensity exercise will result in an increase in muscle temperature, leading to an increase in muscle power, but the same exercise might also be expected to result in a reduction in power due to fatigue processes. It has recently been shown that these two effects can occur simultaneously in the same muscle such that a real fatigue of up to 30% reduction in power can be completely masked by the increase in muscle power consequent upon an exercise-induced increase in muscle temperature (Rademaker, Zoladz, and Sargeant 1994).

Another issue that has scarcely been addressed in this population is the relationship between power generated by the contractile elements during a shortening contraction and the power that is derived from prior activity in isometric or pre-stretch contractions and has been stored in elastic structures (see, e.g., Komi 1992). It seems probable that the signals responsible for the different protein synthesis that will determine function in these two respects, although related, are independent. During growth it would not be surprising if the relationship between the two components were different from that in the adult state.

Finally, the reduced specific strength, power, and—related to this—efficiency of exercise in pediatric compared to adult populations remain to be explained. It seems probable that this will require a combination of animal (whole-muscle and single-fiber work) and human studies given the likely molecular basis of these differences.

Summary

Fundamental aspects of muscle mechanics and energetics, and the organized variability of the neuromuscular system, were reviewed in relation to children's physical performance during short-duration exercise in which anaerobic energy supply predominates. Consideration was given to factors that may modify performance, such as fatigue and changes in muscle temperature. Suggestions have been made as to important areas of future research.

References

Asmussen, E., and Boje, O. 1945. Body temperature and capacity for work. *Acta Physiol. Scand.* 10: 1-22.

Bangsbo, J. 1996. Efficiency in repeated high intensity. In *Human muscular function during dynamic exercise,* ed. P. Marconnet, B. Saltin, P. Komi, and J. Poortmans. *Med. Sport Sci.* 41, 21-31. Basel: Karger.

Bangsbo, J., Gollnick, P.D., Graham, T.E., Juel, C., Kiens, B., Mizuno, M., and Saltin, B. 1990. Anaerobic energy production and O_2 deficit-debt relationship during exhaustive exercise in man. *J. Physiol.* 422: 539-559.

Beelen, A., and Sargeant, A.J. 1991. Effect of fatigue on maximal power output at different contraction velocities in humans. *J. Appl. Physiol.: Resp. Environ. Exerc. Physiol.* 71(6): 2332-2337.

Beelen, A., Sargeant, A.J., Jones, D.A., and de Ruiter, C.J. 1995. Fatigue and recovery of voluntary and electrically elicited dynamic force in humans. *J. Physiol.* 484: 227-235.

Cady, E.B., Jones, D.A., Lynn, J., and Newham, D.J. 1989. Changes in force and intracellular metabolites during fatigue of human skeletal muscle. *J. Physiol.* 418: 311-325.

Cooper, D.M., and Barstow, T.J. 1996. Magnetic resonance imaging and spectroscopy in studying exercise in children. In *Exerc. Sports Sci. Rev.* 24, ed. J.O. Holloszy. Baltimore: Williams & Wilkins.

de Haan, A., Jones, D.A., and Sargeant, A.J. 1989. Changes in power output, velocity of shortening and relaxation rate during fatigue of rat medial gastrocnemius muscle. *Pflugers Archiv. Eur. J. Physiol.* 413: 422-428.

di Prampero, P.E. 1996. Effects of shortening velocity and oxygen consumption on efficiency of contraction in dog gastrocnemius. In *Human muscular function during dynamic exercise,* ed. P. Marconnet, B. Saltin, P. Komi, and J. Poortmans. *Med. Sport Sci.* 41, 1-9. Basel: Karger.

Ennion, S., Sant'Ana Pereira, J.A., Sargeant, A.J., Young, A., and Goldspink, G. 1995. Characterisation of human skeletal muscle fibres according to the myosin heavy chains they express. *J. Muscle Res. Cell Mot.* 16: 35-43.

Gandevia, S.C., Allen, G.M., and McKenzie, D.K. 1995. Central fatigue: critical questions, quantification and practical implications. In *Fatigue, neural and muscular mechanisms,* ed. S.C. Gandevia, R.M. Enoka, A.J. McComas, D.G. Stuart, and C.K. Thomas. *Adv. Exp. Med. Biol.* 384. New York: Plenum Press.

Gandevia, S.C., Enoka, R.M., McComas, A.J., Stuart, D.G., and Thomas, C.K., eds. 1995. *Fatigue, neural and muscular mechanisms,* ed. S.C. Gandevia, R.M. Enoka, A.J. McComas, D.G. Stuart, and C.K. Thomas. *Adv. Exp. Med. Biol.* 384. New York: Plenum Press.

Greenhaff, P.L., Nevill, M.E., Soderlund, K., Bodin, K., Boobis, L.H., and Hultman, E. 1994. The metabolic responses of human type I and type II muscle fibres during maximal treadmill sprinting. *J. Physiol.* 478: 149-165.

James, C., Sacc, P., and Jones, D.A. 1995. Loss of power during fatigue of human leg muscles. *J. Physiol.* 484: 237-246.

Komi, P.V. 1992. Stretch-shortening cycle. In *Strength and power in sport,* ed. P.V. Komi, chap. 6E. Oxford: Blackwell Scientific.

Larsson, L., and Moss, R.L. 1993. Maximum velocity of shortening in relation to myosin isoform composition in single fibres from human skeletal muscles. *J. Physiol.* 472: 595-614.

Lodder, M.A.N., de Haan, A., and Sargeant, A.J. 1991. Effect of shortening velocity on work output and energy cost during repeated contractions of the rat EDL muscle. *Eur. J. Appl. Physiol.* 62: 430-435.

Lodder, M.A.N., de Haan, A., and Sargeant, A.J. 1994. The effect of growth on efficiency and fatigue in rat EDL muscle. *Eur. J. Appl. Physiol.* 69: 429-434.

Rademaker, A., Zoladz, J.A., and Sargeant, A.J. 1994. Effect of prolonged exercise performed at different movement frequencies on maximal short-term power output in humans. *J. Physiol.* 475: 23P.

Rome, L. 1993. The design of the muscular system. In *Neuromuscular fatigue,* ed.

A.J. Sargeant and D. Kernell. Academy Series, Royal Netherlands Academy of Arts and Sciences. Amsterdam: North Holland Press.

Sahlin, K., and Ren, J.M. 1989. Relationship of contraction capacity to metabolic changes during recovery from a fatiguing contraction. *J. Appl. Physiol.* 67: 648-654.

Sant'Ana Pereira, J.A., van der Laarse, W.J., and Sargeant, A.J. 1996. Correlation between MyHC co-expression and physiological properties of human skeletal muscle fibres. *Muscle Nerve*(suppl. 4): S45.

Sant'Ana Pereira, J.A. de, Wessels, A., Nijtmans, L., Moorman, A.F.M., and Sargeant, A.J. 1995. New method for the accurate characterisation of single human skeletal muscle fibres demonstrates a relation between mATPase and MyHC expression in pure and hybrid fibres types. *J. Muscle Res. Cell Mot.* 16: 21-34.

Sant'Ana Pereira, J.A.A., Sargeant, A.J., de Haan, A., Rademaker, A.C.H.J., and van Mechelen, W. 1996. Myosin heavy chain isoform expression and high energy phosphate content of human muscle fibres at rest and post-exercise. *J. Physiol.* 496(2): 1-6.

Sargeant, A.J. 1987. Effect of muscle temperature on leg extension force and short-term power output in humans. *Eur. J. Appl. Physiol.* 56(6): 693-698.

Sargeant, A.J. 1989. Short-term muscle power in children and adolescents. In *Advances in pediatric sports sciences.* Vol. 3, *Biological issues,* ed. O. Bar-Or, chap. 2, 41-63. Champaign, IL: Human Kinetics.

Sargeant, A.J. 1994. Human power output and muscle fatigue. *Int. J. Sports Med.* 15(3): 116-121.

Sargeant, A.J. 1996. Human power output—determinants of maximum performance. In *Human muscular function during dynamic exercise,* ed. P. Marconnet, B. Saltin, P. Komi, and J. Poortmans. *Med. Sport Sci.* 41, 10-20. Basel: Karger.

Sargeant, A.J., and Dolan, P. 1986. Optimal velocity of muscle contraction for short-term (anaerobic) power output in children and adults. In *Children and exercise XII,* ed. J. Rutenfranz, R. Mocellin, and F. Klimt, 39-42. Champaign, IL: Human Kinetics.

Sargeant, A.J., and Dolan, P. 1987. Effect of prior exercise on maximal short-term power output in man. *J. Appl. Physiol.: Resp. Environ. Exerc. Physiol.* 63: 1475-1482.

Sargeant, A.J., Hoinville, E., and Young, A. 1981. Maximum leg force and power output during short-term dynamic exercise. *J. Appl. Physiol.: Resp. Environ. Exerc. Physiol.* 51(5): 1175-1182.

Sargeant, A.J., and Jones, D.A. 1995. The significance of motor unit variability in sustaining mechanical output of muscle. In *Fatigue, neural and muscular mechanisms,* ed. S. Gandevia, R.M. Enoka, A.J. McComas, D.G. Stuart, and C.K. Thomas, chap. 24. *Adv. Exp. Med. Biol.* 384, 323-338. New York: Plenum Press.

Sargeant, A.J., and Kernell, D., eds. 1993. *Neuromuscular fatigue,* 1-195. Academy Series, Royal Netherlands Academy of Arts and Sciences. Amsterdam: North Holland Press.

Stienen, G.J.M., Kiers, J.L., Bottinelli, R., and Reggiani, C. 1996. Myofibrillar ATPase activity in skinned human skeletal muscle fibres: fibre type and temperature dependence. *J. Physiol.* 493(2): 299-308.

Zoladz, J.A., Rademaker, A., and Sargeant, A.J. 1995. Oxygen uptake does not increase linearly with power output at high intensities of exercise in humans. *J. Physiol.* 488(1): 211-218.

6

CHAPTER

Assessing Accumulated Oxygen Deficit in Children

John S. Carlson
Geraldine A. Naughton

This chapter focuses on the following objectives:

- Presenting a detailed explanation of the accumulated oxygen deficit measurement
- Discussing the potential methodological issues surrounding accumulated oxygen deficit
- Examining the accumulated oxygen deficit values determined in children
- Revealing the issues pertinent to the accumulated oxygen deficit measurement in testing pediatric populations

Many of the short-term tests for anaerobic characteristics currently practiced have recently been criticized for their inability to completely exhaust the capacity of the anaerobic system (Saltin 1990; Withers et al. 1991). Most of the traditional methods for testing anaerobic characteristics in pediatric populations have focused on power output under short-term high-intensity conditions. The following discussion presents a measure for the assessment of anaerobic capacity that has application to pediatric populations. This measure is known as the accumulated oxygen deficit (AOD).

Anaerobic capacity has been described by Medbø (1991) as the total amount of adenosine triphosphate (ATP) that can be formed via the anaerobic processes/metabolism under high-intensity exercise conditions. Adenosine triphosphate resynthesis under anaerobic conditions occurs due to the breakdown of stored phosphocreatine (PCr) and from the production of lactic acid via glycolysis (breakdown of stored carbohydrate; glycogen in the muscle). Given the known limits of stores of PCr and maximal tolerance levels of lactic acid within the muscle, it would seem that measuring the total capacity of these systems would provide a valuable tool for understanding developmental considerations and limitations to anaerobic performance in pediatric populations.

Hermansen and Medbø (1984) introduced a measure of estimating maximal O_2 deficit from individual responses to steady state submaximal exercise. The authors then extrapolated this established power-O_2 relationship into supramaximal exercise intensities for the purpose of predicting energy demands under anaerobic conditions. Jon Medbø has since provided an impressive depth of research on the validity of AOD as a means of measuring maximal anaerobic capacity (Medbø 1991; Medbø et al. 1988; Medbø and Tabata 1987, 1989). Medbø et al. (1988) expressed the AOD as an amount of energy, in total liters of O_2 or in relative terms expressed in milliliters of O_2 per kilogram of body mass (ml · kg^{-1}) for the duration of the test. Green (1994) sought to clarify the definition of AOD when he expressed it as an estimation of the total amount of ATP resynthesized via anaerobic metabolism by the whole body during high-intensity exercise of short duration.

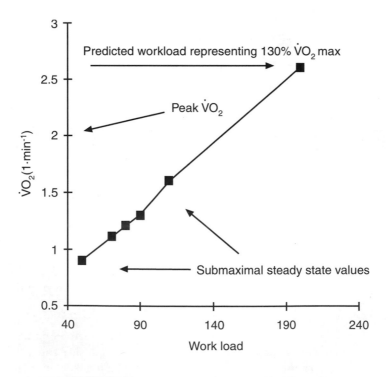

Figure 6.1 Extrapolation of submaximal steady state to supramaximal work.

Measurement of Accumulated Oxygen Deficit

Accumulated oxygen deficit is measured as the difference between the predicted (theoretical) O_2 demand and the actual O_2 uptake of a supramaximal exercise bout. The term "accumulated" refers to measurements predicted or taken over the duration of the test. The prediction is calculated by an extrapolation from the linear regression of power and O_2 within a series of submaximal O_2 uptake exercise bouts. The number of submaximal tests depends on the range of workloads at which the subject can maintain steady state. Data from the steady state tests enable the power-O_2 relationship to be established. This is calculated by a standard, least squares linear regression equation $[y = a + b(x)]$. From this information, a supramaximal workload can be obtained by rearranging the equation $y = a + b(x)$, to $x = (y - a)/b$, where $y = \dot{V}O_2$ and $x =$ workload/intensity. Figure 6.1 summarizes the statistical procedures, and figure 6.2 (p.122) provides an example of a typical calculation with pediatric data.

The measure of anaerobic capacity discussed in this chapter is independent of the rate of exercise or the amount of time taken to exhaustion during the test. For example, a test to exhaustion in 1 min will produce the same anaerobic capacity measurement as a test to exhaustion performed at a lower intensity but lasting 2 min.

Measurement of Accumulated Oxygen Deficit as a Capacity

The mode of testing and the times to exhaustion appear to be factors that influence AOD measurement in children. Figure 6.3 presents some AOD values determined from prepubertal boys using either running or cycling modes of exercising at three supramaximal intensities (110%, 130%, and 150% peak $\dot{V}O_2$) to exhaustion. An examination of the cycling AOD results across the three intensities for the males in figure 6.3 generally supports the concept that a plateau, indicative of capacity, occurred with increasing intensity. This finding complements the work of Withers et al. (1991) and Gastin (1992), who also associated the plateau effect across different test intensities with an indication of subjects reaching an exhaustive capacity within 60 and 90 s, respectively. Medbø and coworkers (1988) obtained a plateau within 120 s from supramaximal treadmill performances in adults. In the testing of younger subjects, however, the observed plateau within the responses of the males during cycling (Carlson and Naughton 1993) appeared to have occurred substantially fewer times than previously cited in adult studies (Gastin 1992; Withers et al. 1991). The male children demonstrated no significant differences in AOD values determined from three supramaximal tests representing 110%, 130%, and 150% peak $\dot{V}O_2$. Mean performance times for these intensities were 102, 68, and 47 s, respectively.

Sample calculation of the AOD from data collected on an 11 year old male tested on a constant load cycle ergometer:

"Mike" aged 11.1 years, has a mass of 37.2 kg

and his peak $\dot{V}O_2$ was 2.01 L · min^{-1}

(1) Submaximal testing

Steady state values determined from the following workloads:

Watts	$\dot{V}O_2$ L · min^{-1}
50	.091
70	1.12
80	1.23
90	1.33
110	1.62

The linear regression equation [y=a +b(x)] computed from the above data is:
$\dot{V}O_2$ (L · min^{-1}) = 0.306 + .0117 (Watts) which has a correlation coefficient r = .996

(2) Supramaximal predictions

The oxygen uptake at 130% peak $\dot{V}O_2$ is (2.01 x 1.3) = 2.61 L · min^{-1}

From the linear regression the workload representing 130% peak $\dot{V}O_2$ is calculated:

$$2.61 = 0.30 + .0115 \text{ (unknown Watt)}$$
$$\text{Watts} = [y\text{-}a] \; /b \quad = 197 \text{ Watts}$$

Sample of calculations for AOD

Mike's time to exhaustion at 197 Watts = 57.43 seconds (i.e. 0.957 min)

Total predicted oxygen demand for = 2.61 (L · min^{-1}) · .957 (min)

the exercise time Σ= 2.49 (liters)

The actual (measured) O_2 consumption for the exercise time from Douglas bag data was 1.2 (L · min^{-1}) and for the exercise time = 1.21(L·min^{-1})·.957(min)
= Σ1.07(liters)

AOD = Predicted O_2 for the exercise time - Actual O_2 for the exercise time
= 2.49 - 1.07 liters
= 1.42 liters (absolute value)
= 38.17 ml · kg^{-1} (relative value)

Figure 6.2 Sample calculation of accumulated oxygen deficit from data collected on an 11-year-old male tested on a load cycle ergometer.

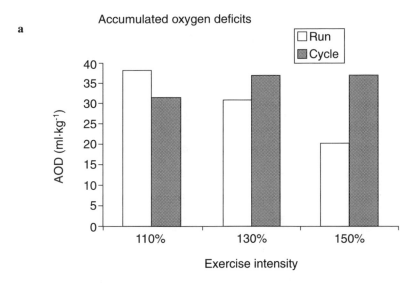

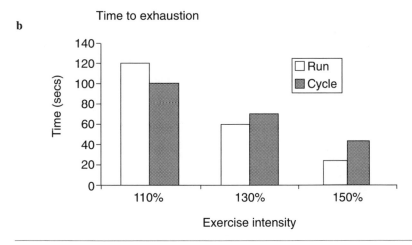

Figure 6.3 Accumulated oxygen deficits (a) and time to exhaustion (b) from three supramaximal bouts of cycling and running in preadolescent boys.

Medbø believed that for a true capacity to be obtained, the exercise period should span 120 s. Medbø et al. (1988) experienced difficulties with treadmill speeds in protocols used to predicted workloads that would exhaust the subjects in less than 2 min. It was observed that the treadmill speed may have been too intense to permit complete exhaustion of anaerobic capacities to occur in the adults studied by Medbø and his coworkers (1988). Similarly, studies with children (Carlson, Naughton, and Buttifant 1992; Naughton 1993) have been unable to demonstrate a plateau in AOD during treadmill running (figure 6.3a), and the exercise times at higher running

Table 6.1   Intraclass Correlation Coefficients (R) From Isokinetic and Constant-Load Supramaximal Cycle Ergometer Testing

Exercise mode	Sex	n	Accumulated O_2 deficit (liters)	Accumulated O_2 deficit (ml · Kg^{-1})	Exercise duration (s)
ISO	boys	7	.96	.95	.57
	girls	6	.86	.89	.88
CP	boys	9	.81	.92	.81
	girls	9	.79	.55	.74

Note: ISO = isokinetic supramaximal exercise;
        CP = constant-power supramaximal tests.

intensities were much shorter than those recorded during cycle tests to exhaustion (figure 6.3b). Similar AOD values during running and cycling were observed only in tests requiring energy outputs of 110% peak $\dot{V}O_2$. Perhaps running places a higher skill demand on younger subjects than cycling at the higher supramaximal intensities. Consequently, factors associated with difficulties in meeting the coordination and speed demands of high-intensity running may dictate premature test termination in running as compared with cycling during supramaximal efforts to exhaustion.

When investigating a protocol to measure aspects of performance or growth in the pediatric population, it is important to examine the reliability of the method. Overall, it appears that AOD is reliable (Naughton 1993). Table 6.1 demonstrates the reliability of the data from intraclass correlation coefficients (R) during AOD testing in boys and girls using constant-load and isokinetic cycle ergometers (Naughton 1993). Boys produced more reliable AOD values than girls. The observed difference in the intraclass correlation values (R) between the sexes reflected poorly on the repeatability of the girls' performances, which may be associated with factors such as motivation and skill (see table 6.1).

Aerobic and Anaerobic Contributions to Accumulated Oxygen Deficit Performances

Within the estimated total accumulated O_2 demand, measurements of accumulated O_2 uptake allow investigators to report the relative contributions of aerobic and anaerobic energy sources (i.e., the actual O_2 consumed during the test is divided by the amount predicted for the exercise time to give the percentage of aerobic contribution). Medbø and Tabata (1989) examined the relative importance of the aerobic and anaerobic processes in supramaximal tests. They emphasized that there was a substantial contribution from aerobic energy sources even in exhaustive exercise bouts of 30 s duration. Aerobic energy contributions during cycling exercise to exhaustion of 30 s, 1 min, and 2 min durations were 40%, 50%, and 65% of the total energy release (Medbø and Tabata 1989). Therefore Medbø (1991) speculated that a 50/50 split in aerobic/anaerobic contributions to exercise occurred after 1 min of intense exercise. Similarly, Withers et al. (1991) reported a 49% aerobic contribution after 60 s of work. Both of these studies indicated that relative aerobic contribution increases with exercise duration and conversely decreases with exercise intensity. Both studies also demonstrated that even in 30 s of intensive exercise, the contribution of aerobic energy sources appeared to be substantial. Within the three supramaximal workloads used to measure AOD in children, it was also shown that the percentage of aerobic contribution to energy expenditure increased significantly with increasing exercise time to exhaustion and decreased with intensity (see figure 6.4).

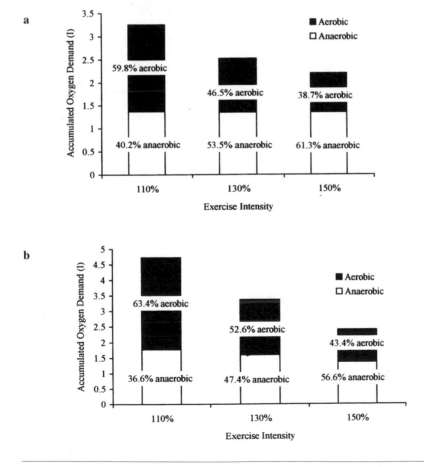

Figure 6.4 Partitioning of accumulated oxygen demand (liters) into accumulated oxygen uptake and AOD of (a) boys and (b) girls.

For example, in tests averaging 47 and 123 s of work, the aerobic contributions were 40.8% and 61.6%, respectively.

Issues Surrounding the Measurement of Accumulated Oxygen Deficit

The AOD, as a measure of anaerobic capacity, has not gained complete international acceptance. Debate surrounding this measure has been presented in recent literature (Bangsbo 1996; Medbø 1996). Many issues remain unresolved and warrant further discussion.

Accumulated Oxygen Deficit as a Measure of Capacity

Medbø et al. (1988) discussed a number of conditions that, if supported, would confirm a concomitant anaerobic capacity. One major issue centered on the need to observe some degree of leveling off, or plateauing, in AOD values determined with repeated supramaximal test conditions. Medbø et al. (1988) reported that AOD values and blood lactates continued to increase in supramaximal tests lasting up to 120 s. A plateau occurred beyond 120 s of supramaximal treadmill running, which suggested that a capacity had been reached. Pate et al. (1983) similarly reported a plateau effect in the AOD values, obtained from cycling at 110%, 120%, and 130% of maximal effort.

Gastin (1992) demonstrated that maximal AOD values could be obtained within 60 s of supramaximal exercise on a cycle ergometer. Gastin (1992) reported that after 60 s, no significant increases in AOD values occurred among tests conducted at 110% and 125% of peak O_2 uptake in a constant-power mode and an all-out protocol within isokinetic cycling. Withers et al. (1991) also achieved maximal AOD and blood lactate values within 60 s of all-out exercise on an air-braked cycle ergometer. In AOD measures with children, plateaus have been observed in AOD values for supramaximal cycling efforts in times ranging from 102 to 45 s at intensities representing work ranging from 110% to 150% of maximal aerobic power (figure 6.3).

Extrapolation From Submaximal to Supramaximal Exercise Economy

One of the biggest challenges to the validity and precision of the AOD measure is the assumption that supramaximal exercise economy is a linear function of submaximal exercise economy. Saltin (1987) suggested that the lowest mechanical efficiencies were found at the highest relative intensities. Therefore, according to Saltin (1987) the true energy costs of supramaximal exercise were likely to be underestimated. Saltin (1987) could not accept that energy costs could be extrapolated from submaximal to supramaximal conditions. He believed that supramaximal exercise conditions incurred much more O_2 than could be predicted from submaximal conditions. Saltin et al. (1972) reported 16-19% efficiency instead of 20-25% efficiency from subjects cycling close to maximal effort intensities. Given that supramaximal conditions were therefore much more inefficient than submaximal conditions, Saltin (1987) postulated that any extrapolation of supramaximal energy demands from submaximal conditions would grossly underpredict the true O_2 costs of highly intense exercise conditions. Medbø (1991) defended the criticism of possible deviations within a linear extrapolation from submaximal steady state conditions into supramaximal exercise. It must be suggested that efficiency during highly intense exercise may well be affected by functional adjustments outside the active muscle. These adjustments include energy demands from the cardiorespiratory system responding to the added work of stabilizing muscle of the upper body under highly intense conditions, as well as the thermoregulatory mechanisms adjusting to increased demands from a rise in muscle temperature (Gastin 1992; Gladden and Welch 1978; Withers et al. 1991). Catecholamine activity may also increase energy demand more under supramaximal than under submaximal exercise conditions (Galbo 1983).

Gastin (1992) hypothesized that the AOD measure could inherently account for changes in efficiency, within the process of measuring efficiencies for each incremental bout of steady state exercise. Thus, a number of data points representing the upper range of steady state data would be required to establish a power-O_2 relationship for each individual. Obtaining high-intensity steady state data would therefore be critical to the precision of the measure of AOD. Nevertheless, the ability to extrapolate from submaximal to supramaximal conditions remains open to debate (Bangsbo 1992, 1996).

Profiles of Anaerobic Capacity in Pediatric Populations

Limited data exist in the literature addressing AOD in pediatric populations. Bangsbo (1996) argued that data must be interpreted with caution when different exercise modes and populations are used in comparisons of AOD results. Table 6.2 profiles the range of AOD measures obtained from a number of pediatric groups. Testing in children has involved the use of constant-load and isokinetic cycle ergometers, as well as treadmill running (Carlson and Naughton 1993; Naughton and Carlson 1996; Carlson, Naughton, and Buttifant 1992). Table 6.2 demonstrates trends in age- and sex-related characteristics. Specifically, in the preadolescent males and females, similar AOD values are evident (Carlson and Naughton 1993). This finding is supported by several authors (Bar-Or 1983; Rowland 1990) who have indicated that prior to puberty, no physiological differences should exist that explain differ-

Table 6.2   Profile of AOD Results Across a Range of Pediatric Subjects

Developmental stage	Sex	Age	Testing device	AOD (Σ liters)	AOD (ml · kg^{-1})
Preadolescents n = 9	Male	10.6	Constant-load cycle	1.35 ±.11	36.4 ±2.1
Preadolescents n = 9	Female	10.6	Constant-load cycle	1.55 ±.10	36.7 ±1.5
Preadolescents n = 7	Male	10.8	Isokinetic cycle	1.38 ±0.1	36.7 ±2.9
Preadolescents n = 7	Female	10.7	Isokinetic cycle	1.37 ±0.1	33.1 ±2.6
Nonasthmatic preadolescents n = 10	Male	11.0	Treadmill	2.08	51.59 ±2.66
Asthmatic preadolescents n = 10	Male	10.9	Treadmill	1.77	53.23 ±4.02
Preadolescents n = 8	Male	11.1	Treadmill	1.45 ±0.23	38.7 ±5.6
Adolescent athletes n = 8	Male	14.9	Treadmill	4.38 ±0.86	68.14 ±15.3
Adolescent athletes n = 8	Female	14.5	Treadmill	3.36 ±0.28	59.98 ±4.71
Prepubertal n = 5	Male	11.8	Treadmill	1.81 ±0.54	49.8 ±8.25
Circumpubertal n = 7	Male	14.5	Treadmill	2.52 ±0.27	52.7 ±3.71

Note: Mean ± SE

ences between performances of males and females. Higher AOD values were obtained in well-trained adolescent males when compared with females of similar training backgrounds (Naughton et al. 1993). Within the acknowledged limitations of comparisons of AOD scores across studies, these data indicate that after puberty, significantly more powerful anaerobic performances may be found in males as compared to females.

Data for asthmatic and nonasthmatic preadolescent males revealed no differences for AODs between two reasonably active groups of boys (Buttifant, Carlson, and Naughton 1993; Buttifant et al. 1996). These results are contrary to findings from a previous study comparing asthmatic with nonasthmatic children that showed a lower general anaerobic fitness in the group of asthmatic children (Karila, Varray, and Préfaut 1992). Perhaps the active nature of the asthmatic group in the Buttifant, Carlson, and Naughton study (1993) provided the stimulus for comparable development of the anaerobic capacities.

Limited cross-sectional data on AOD have also been collected from children in various stages of development. These data suggest that there is a trend, somewhat reflective of age and maturation of the anaerobic system, through puberty (Stear, Carlson, and Naughton 1994). As the increase in AOD through the various stages of puberty is not linear, it may be suggested that factors other than developmental stage or age may influence anaerobic performance. Perhaps anaerobic performances are reflective of the advantages of exercise training during pubertal years.

Previously reported O_2 deficit values for children (Eriksson, Gollnick, and Saltin 1973) used only one data point to calculate O_2 deficits and assumed a similar efficiency response in all subjects. Given that efficiency is not likely to be the same in all subjects, results from Eriksson, Gollnick, and Saltin (1973) may not therefore be as accurate as the measure of AOD described in this chapter.

Methodological Issues of the Accumulated Oxygen Deficit Measurement in Pediatric Populations

Specific pediatric issues surrounding the use of the AOD must be addressed. These issues encompass many of the inherent problems associated with both maximal and submaximal effort testing with children.

Submaximal Steady State Testing

The controversy surrounding AOD becomes even more complex when children are assessed for anaerobic capacity using this measure. For example, one of the problems encountered with pediatric populations is the small range of work capacities in which to establish a series of steady state values. This is not an issue with adults, as their range of work capacity is likely to be much higher.

The work rate range is strongly linked to the size and fitness of the individual. For example, children with the smallest workload range are often unable to provide more than four to five discrete steady state performances. These steady states represent a range of between 40% and 72% of peak O_2 uptake of the subjects. Similarly on the treadmill, children have a limited span of discrete running speeds at which steady states can be determined. It is perhaps more problematic in children than in adults to obtain the greatest number of steady state values at a work rate that would not induce an O_2 drift under these submaximal conditions.

Suitability of the Protocol for Supramaximal Work Demands

Medbø et al. (1988) used a 10% incline in AOD tests on a treadmill, whereas experiments with children have documented use of a modified treadmill protocol that involved a 4% grade (Carlson, Naughton, and Buttifant 1992). Similar AOD values have been obtained from treadmill and cycle ergometer testing at 110% and 130% of maximal effort in 11-year-old boys (figure 6.3). At speeds predicted to represent 150% of peak aerobic power, however, children running on the treadmill attained significantly lower AOD values than on tests performed at less demanding supramaximal intensities. The authors believed that the comparatively smaller incline of the treadmill when used with children (4% as compared to the 10% incline selected for adults) forced the speeds at the highest intensity to be too great to allow for exhaustion of total anaerobic energy supplies. Olesen (1992) reported that AOD values of 40, 72, and 69 ml · kg^{-1} for treadmill inclines of 1%, 15%, and 20% could not solely represent the recruitment of greater muscle mass at the highest treadmill inclination. Olesen (1992) contended that when the equations from tests at a lower treadmill incline (1%) were constructed, the subsequent AOD results underpredicted true O_2 demands of the exercise in comparison with the equations used for higher gradients. Olesen (1992) attributed the underestimation of O_2 costs to differences in the role of stored elastic energy and differences in the ratio of eccentric to concentric work between performances at low and high gradients on the treadmill. The coordination and ability of the child to cope with the skills of running at very steep inclines may preclude a similar result in child-based populations. The optimal incline (%) of a treadmill during AOD testing may therefore be different in children as compared to adults. The challenge associated with this problem is therefore to investigate a series of testing modalities (e.g., treadmill inclines and speeds or cycle ergometer workloads and cadence) to determine which protocol elicits the most powerful AOD tests to "true" exhaustion. The selected mode and load settings would also need to provide the greatest number of discrete steady state points under submaximal conditions. A large number of steady state submaximal data points promotes greater precision of the measure through linear regressions. These submaximal performances must be seen as the central focus of the measure. Other major challenges that may be perceived as recommendations for future research with the AOD measure in younger populations include experimentation with modes of metabolic data collection (e.g., expired air collection in Douglas bags or breath-by-breath apparatus), the criteria for determining exhaustion during performances (e.g., volitional exhaustion or an agreed percentage decrement in cadence), and the nature and standardization of motivational techniques to obtain totally exhaustive performances in children.

Potential Advantages in Accumulated Oxygen Deficit Testing with Children

Table 6.3 summarizes several findings from the literature that may be associated with the validity of the AOD measure in children. For example, there are suggestions that the high-intensity respiratory responses of children differ from those of adults (Armon et al. 1991; Zanconato et al. 1989). The frequency of observations of O_2 drift under high-intensity steady state conditions in adults has been lower than that in children (Armon et al. 1991).

Table 6.3   Summary of the Issues of Concern With the Use of the AOD Method With Children

Issues Within the Use of the AOD Measure With Children

- Documented evidence that the child may be less susceptible to oxygen drift under relatively high steady state conditions. This characteristic is perceived as advantageous within the AOD method.
  (Armon et al. 1991)

- Inability to achieve steady state under relatively high exercise conditions on the isokinetic cycle ergometer.
  (Observations made by Carlson et al. 1992, Naughton and Carlson 1996)

- The smaller range of workloads in which steady state values could be measured, both on the treadmill and cycle ergometers in children, produced correlation coefficients on the linear regression line that were not as strong as those documented for adult populations.
  (Observations made by Carlson et al. 1992)

- Suggestion that children may be more sensitive to hypoxic conditions than adults at the onset of exercise, and move more rapidly into an aerobic preference for energy demand.
  (Springer et al. 1991)

- Inefficient ventilatory response patterns in children compared with adults.
  (Cooper et al. 1987)

- Evidence that children may respond in a different pattern from adults at the onset of highly intense exercise conditions.
  (Zanconato et al. 1991)

As previously mentioned, the precision of the prediction for accumulated O_2 demand largely depends on the maximal number of submaximal steady state points that can be provided for the linear regression. Theoretically, subjects in whom O_2 drift was not observed would be able to perform a larger number of higher-intensity tests and provide relatively more steady state values for the linear regression equation than those subjects in whom O_2 drift had been observed. Thus, according to the literature, children may have an advantage in sustaining relatively higher-intensity steady state $\dot{V}O_2$ values than adults. Additionally, Rowland et al. (1990) noted that the net mechanical efficiency of cycling in prepubertal children was not significantly different from that of adults under relative steady state conditions. Therefore, in view of the greater uncertainty of efficiency changes during running than during cycling, it appears that cycling may be a more accurate exercise mode than running for predicting supramaximal workloads from submaximal performances.

This suggests that the AOD measure may in fact be well suited to adaptation for use in children. When an isokinetic cycle ergometer was used with children, however, their performances indicated that they were unable to obtain steady state responses at high intensities. More often than not, they were unable to continue the high-intensity submaximal workloads beyond 4 min without incurring an O_2 drift. An O_2 drift was arbitrarily denoted by a greater than 5 ml $\cdot$ kg^{-1} $\cdot$ min^{-1} increase in $\dot{V}O_2$ responses between 2 consecutive minutes, after at least 3 min of exercise. Tests in which O_2 drifts occurred could not contribute to the number of data points available for the linear regression equation. Similar experiences have been encountered in pretests of submaximal exercise on cycle ergometers and treadmills. Therefore it appears that no one particular exercise mode is more favorable than others in avoiding O_2 drift. All the factors mentioned affect the AOD values and indicate the need for more child-based protocols in pediatric laboratory testing than currently exist.

Withers et al. (1991) postulated that the protocol used to measure AOD discriminated against the subject who (through training) would be able to move more quickly through the hypoxic phase at the onset of highly intense exercise than a less trained subject. This implies that the AOD of the trained individual may be falsely recorded as smaller than it could have been if true anaerobic sources had been permitted to dominate and fully deplete. There is some evidence to suggest that children also have an increased tendency to move from anaerobic to aerobic conditions rather rapidly. The findings of Poage, McCann, and Cooper (1987) and Springer, Barstow, and Cooper (1988) would suggest that factors such as increased sensitivity to hypoxic conditions, and less storage capacity for CO_2, could lead to the postulation that differences in the child's oxygen kinetics may also impair a true indication of the capacity of the anaerobic system at the onset of exercise. If children are highly sensitive to hypoxic conditions such as those occurring at the onset of very intense exercise, then assumptions about constant efficiency from extrapolations for supramaximal conditions may not be as valid in child-based populations as in adults.

Therefore, predictions of accumulated O_2 demand may be more underestimated in children than in adults. This effect, however, may well be negligible in exercise bouts of 45 s or more in supramaximal exercise designed to exhaust the anaerobic energy capacity.

Consequently there are several existing areas of contention surrounding the use of the AOD measure with pediatric populations. Some of the methodological issues may be addressed in the near future with experiments of a relatively simple design. It is, however, the validity of the assumptions underlying the method that must be perceived as the greatest challenge for pediatric work physiologists. Even if all the adult controversies were resolved, questions would remain concerning the validity of predicting supramaximal O_2 demands from submaximal performances within pediatric populations.

Directions for Future Research

As pediatric exercise science develops and increases in popularity with scientists and researchers, the need to assess the anaerobic performance capabilities of children will be greater. Future research directions involving the measurement of AOD need to concern the following questions:

- What is the relationship between AOD values obtained in different exercise modes?
- How sensitive is the AOD in detecting training adaptations in child and adolescent populations?
- Do different testing protocols influence the determination of steady state exercise values for the construction of the linear prediction equations?
- What are the developmental profiles of AOD through childhood and adolescence?

Only when all these issues have been addressed and answered will pediatric exercise researchers be totally confident in adopting the protocol.

Summary

The data on the AOD response in children are yet to be fully established in cross-sectional as well as longitudinal studies. Only limited data exist to provide a developmental profile of this anaerobic characteristic through childhood and adolescence. Clearly, more cross-sectional and longitudinal studies would substantially contribute to understanding of the responses of young children to anaerobic stimuli. Training studies have demonstrated effective increases in AOD performances of adults from differing populations (Barzdukas et al. 1991; Medbø and Burgers 1990). The degree of relative improvement to be expected from anaerobic-based training interventions remains relatively unknown in children. Therefore, it is recommended that child-based investigations of training responses in AOD performances continue in order to contribute to understanding of the anaerobic characteristics of children and adolescents.

With a consolidation of the validity of the AOD measure in pediatric populations, testing could be extended to research into the applied fields of exercise prescription and enhanced performance. The noninvasive, challenging nature of the AOD measure for determining additional anaerobic characteristics in subjects makes it a potentially viable protocol for use with children.

References

Armon, Y., Cooper, D.M., Flores, R., Zanconato, S., and Barstow, T. 1991. Oxygen uptake dynamics during high-intensity exercise in children and adults. *J. Appl. Physiol.* 70: 841-848.

Bangsbo, J. 1992. Is the O_2 deficit an accurate quantitative measure of the anaerobic energy production during intense exercise? *J. Appl. Physiol.* 73(3): 1207-1208.

Bangsbo, J. 1996. Bangsbo responds to Medbo's paper. *Can. J. Appl. Physiol.* 21: 384-388.

Bangsbo, J., Gollnick, P.D., Juel, C., Kiens, B., Mizuno, M., and Saltin, B. 1990. Anaerobic energy production and O_2 deficit-debt relationship during exhaustive exercise in humans. *J. Physiol.* 422: 539-559.

Bar-Or, O. 1983. *Pediatric sports medicine for the practitioner. From physiological principles to clinical applications.* New York. Springer-Verlag.

Barzdukas, A.P., Hollander, A.P., D'Acquisto, L.D., and Troup, J.P. 1991. Measurement of the anaerobic capacity during swimming. *Med. Sci. Sports Exerc.* (abstract) 23(4 suppl.): 546.

Buttifant, D.C., Carlson, J.S., and Naughton, G.A. 1993. The examination of the anaerobic capacity of pre-pubertal asthmatic males. *Pediatr. Exerc. Sci.* 5(4): 397.

Buttifant, D., Carlson, J.S., Naughton, G.A., and Roberts, R. 1996. Anaerobic capacity and ventilatory responses of asthmatic prepubertal males. *Pediatr. Exerc. Sci.* 8(3): 267-275.

Carlson, J.S., and Naughton, G.A. 1993. An examination of the anaerobic capacity of children using the maximal accumulated oxygen deficit. *Pediatr. Exerc. Sci.* 5(1): 60-71.

Carlson, J.S., Naughton, G.A., and Buttifant, D. 1992. Supramaximal treadmill running for the determination of the anaerobic capacity in children. *Abstracts seventh annual meeting. North American Society of Pediatric Exercise Medicine.* Miami, FL: University of Miami, School of Medicine, Department of Pediatrics.

Cooper, D.M., Kaplan, M.R., Baumgarten, L., Weiler-Ravell, D., Whipp, B.J., and Wasserman, K. 1987. Coupling of ventilation and CO_2 production during exercise in children. *Pediatr. Res.* 21(6): 568-572.

Eriksson, B.O., Gollnick, P.D., and Saltin, B. 1973. Muscle metabolism and enzyme activities after training in boys 11-13 years old. *Acta Physiol. Scand.* 87: 485-497.

Galbo, H. 1983. *Hormonal and metabolic adaptation to exercise.* Stuttgart: Georg Thieme Verlag.

Gastin, P.B. 1992. Determination of anaerobic capacity in trained and untrained cyclists. PhD diss. Victoria University of Technology, Melbourne, Australia.

Gastin, P.B. 1994. Quantification of anaerobic capacity. *Scand. J. Med. Sci. Sports* 4: 91-112.

Gladden, L.B., and Welch, H.G. 1978. Efficiency of anaerobic work. *J. Appl. Physiol.* 44(4): 564-570.

Green, S. 1994. A definition and systems view of anaerobic capacity. *Eur. J. Appl. Physiol.* 69: 168-173.

Hermansen, L., and Medbø, J.I. 1984. The relative significance of aerobic and anaerobic processes during maximal exercise of short duration. In *Physiological chemistry of training and detraining,* ed. P. Marconnet, J. Poortmans, and L. Hermansen. Basel: Karger.

Karila, C., Varray, A., and Préfaut, C. 1992. Anaerobic adaptations in the asthmatic child during exercise. In *Children and exercise XVI, Pediatric work physiology,* ed. J. Coudert and E. Van Praagh, 179-183. Paris: Masson.

Medbø, J.I. 1991. Quantification of the anaerobic energy release during exercise in man. PhD diss. University of Oslo.

Medbø, J.I. 1996. Is the accumulated oxygen deficit an adequate measure of the anaerobic capacity? *Can. J. Appl. Physiol.* 21: 370-383.

Medbø, J.I., and Burgers, S. 1990. Effect of training on the anaerobic capacity. *Med. Sci. Sports Exerc.* 22: 501-507.

Medbø, J.I., Mohn, A., Tabata, I., Bahr, R., Vaage, O., and Sejersted, O.M. 1988. Anaerobic capacity determined by maximal accumulated oxygen deficit. *J. Appl. Physiol.* 64: 50-60.

Medbø, J.I., and Tabata, I. 1987. Aerobic and anaerobic energy release during short-lasting exhausting bicycle exercise. *Acta Physiol. Scand.* (abstract) 129(3): 6A.

Medbø, J.I., and Tabata, I. 1989. Relative importance of aerobic and anaerobic energy release during short-lasting exhausting bicycle exercise. *J. Appl. Physiol.* 67: 1881-1886.

Naughton, G.A. 1993. Anaerobic characteristics of children. PhD diss. Victoria University of Technology, Melbourne, Australia.

Naughton, G.A, and Carlson, J.S. 1996. Measuring maximal accumulated oxygen deficit in children utilising isokinetic exercise conditions. *Aust. J. Sci. Med. Sport* 27(4): 83-87.

Naughton, G.A., Carlson, J.S., Buttifant, D.C., Metcalf, S.R., Selig, S.E., and Snow, R.S. 1993. Plasma lactate and ammonia responses following supramaximal anaerobic testing in trained adolescent and adult athletes. *Pediatr. Exerc. Sci.* 5(4): 450.

Naughton, G.A., Carlson, J.S., and Fairweather, I. 1992. Determining the variability of performance on Wingate anaerobic tests in children aged 6-12 years. *Int. J. Sports Med.* 13(7): 512-517.

Olesen, H.L. 1992. Accumulated oxygen deficit increases with inclination of uphill running. *J. Appl. Physiol.* 73: 1130-1134.

Pate, R.R., Goodyear, L., Dover, V., Dorociak, J., and McDaniel, J. 1983. Maximal oxygen deficit: a test of anaerobic capacity. *Med. Sci. Sports Exerc.* (abstract) 15: 121-122.

Poage, J., McCann, E.R., and Cooper, D.M. 1987. Ventilatory response to exercise in obese children. *Am. Rev. Resp. Dis.* (abstract) 137: A23.

Rowland, T.W. 1990. *Exercise and children's health.* Champaign, IL. Human Kinetics.

Rowland, T.W., Staab, J.S., Unnithan, V.B., Rambusch, J.M., and Siconolfi, S.F. 1990. Mechanical efficiency during cycling in prepubertal and adult males. *Int. J. Sports Med.* 11(6): 452-455.

Saltin, B. 1987. The physiological and biochemical basis of aerobic and anaerobic capacities in man; effects of training and range of adaptation. In *An update on sports medicine: proceedings from the second Scandinavian conference in sports medicine,* ed. S. Maehlum, S. Nilsson, and P. Renstrom.

Saltin, B., Gagge, A.P., Bergh, U., and Stolwijk, J.A. 1972. Body temperatures and sweating during exhaustive exercise. *J. Appl. Physiol.* 32: 635-643.

Springer, C., Barstow, T.J., and Cooper, D.M. 1988. Evidence that maturation of the peripheral chemoreceptors is not complete in childhood. *Res. Physiol.* 74: 55-64.

Stear, K., Carlson, J.S., and Naughton, G.A. 1994. Developmental characteristics of anaerobic capacity in children. *Proceedings: International Conference of Science and Medicine in Sport, Sports Medicine for Lifetime Activity,* 288-289. Queensland: Australian Sports Medicine Federation.

Withers, R.T., Sherman, W.M., Clark, D.G., Esselbach, P.C., Nolan, S.R., Mackay, M.H., and Brinkham, M. 1991. Muscle metabolism during 30, 60 and 90 s of maximal cycling on an air-braked ergometer. *Eur. J. Appl. Physiol.* 63: 354-362.

Zanconato, S., Baraldi, E., Santuz, P., Rigon, F., Vido, L., Da Dalt, L., and Zacchello, F. 1989. Gas exchange during exercise in obese children. *Eur. J. Pediatr.* 128: 614-617.

7

CHAPTER

Assessing Postexercise Lactates in Children and Adolescents

Joanne R. Welsman
Neil Armstrong

This chapter focuses on the following objectives:

- The ethical considerations that relate to blood sampling
- Methodological considerations that must be addressed
- The differences between children and adults in terms of postexercise lactates

Postexercise blood lactate is routinely sampled following an anaerobic exercise test to provide an indication of the extent to which glycolysis has been stressed. In this way, postexercise lactate sampling has been used to investigate the development of anaerobic metabolism in children and adolescents. The interpretation of postexercise lactates is, however, complicated by many factors. The first major influence derives from the methodology used to obtain the blood lactate measurement, that is, sampling and assay techniques. Such factors appear to have rarely been acknowledged, and documentation remains scarce. A review of these issues forms a major focus of this chapter and provides a foundation for consideration of the interpretation of children's and adolescents' postexercise lactates in relation to chronological and biological age. It has been well documented that children have a lower capacity for anaerobic exercise than adults, which is reflected in lower postexercise blood lactate levels. The underlying mechanisms that account for child-adult differences have not been determined conclusively, but the major hypotheses are reviewed and discussed later in this chapter.

Ethical Considerations Relating to Blood Sampling

Before considering the assessment and interpretation of postexercise lactates in young people it is important to clarify the ethical issues relating to blood sampling during routine exercise testing with minors. It has been suggested that children should take part in research only if the relevant knowledge could not be gained by research with adults (Working Party on Ethics of Research in Children 1980; Working Party on Research in Children 1991). Research that involves a child but is of no direct benefit to that child (nontherapeutic research) is not necessarily unethical if it places the child at no more than negligible risk of harm (i.e., not greater than risks of harm ordinarily encountered in daily life). Procedures involving negligible risk include observation of behavior, noninvasive physiological monitoring, developmental assessments, physical examinations, changes in diet, and *obtaining blood and urine specimens* (Working Party on Research in Children 1991). A child's participation in research, however, must not be through coercion, and it is advisable to obtain the informed consent of both the child and his/her guardians in advance of data collection.

Methodological Considerations for Measuring Postexercise Lactates

The influence of the methods used to sample and analyze the sampled blood on the actual lactate values obtained has not been well documented in the literature, even though an awareness and understanding of the extent of their impact are critical to the meaningful interpretation of young people's postexercise lactates.

Blood Sampling Sites

Blood for lactate sampling may be drawn from arteries, veins, or capillaries. Lactate levels in arterial blood from the arm closely approximate those in the venous blood draining the muscle groups that are active during leg exercise (Newton and Robinson 1965; Saltin et al. 1968). Arterial sampling, therefore, provides the closest indicator of muscle lactate levels.

Routine arterial blood sampling is clearly neither feasible nor ethical in nonclinical investigations with young subjects (Bar-Or 1984). In addition, the insertion of arterial lines is time consuming, requires advanced technical expertise, and should be carried only out under medical supervision. For these reasons some investigators have opted to sample venous blood. Insertion of indwelling venous catheters, for example into the back of the hand, is technically less difficult than the insertion of arterial lines but still permits serial blood sampling without repeated venipuncture.

Several studies have highlighted significant differences between arterial and venous lactate levels during exercise suggesting that venous blood lactate levels will not closely reflect the lactate levels in the blood draining the active muscles. During low-intensity cycle ergometry, arterial-venous differences are small, but with increasing intensity the arterial-venous lactate differences become more pronounced (Yoshida, Suda, and Takeuchi 1982; Yoshida 1984). Although arterial-venous lactate differences do not appear to have been investigated directly during supramaximal exercise, a similar or even greater discrepancy would be expected. Few studies have examined arterial-venous lactate differences during treadmill exercise, but it would appear that they are less pronounced, at least during steady state exercise (Busse, Muller, and Boning 1983; Williams, Armstrong, and Kirby 1992). However, the increasing discrepancy in lactate levels between the two sites remains as exercise becomes more intense (Williams, Armstrong, and Kirby 1992).

For technical simplicity and ease of collection, capillary blood sampling has much in its favor and is particularly suited to field situations (Van Praagh et al. 1989). Capillary sampling is also less traumatic than sampling at venous or arterial sites and is therefore recommended for use with children. The two most commonly sampled sites are the fingertip (Williams, Armstrong, and Kirby 1992; Mero et al. 1988) and the earlobe (Van Praagh et al. 1989; Falgairette et al. 1991, 1993).

Capillary blood lactate levels will accurately reflect arterial levels as long as a good blood flow is maintained at the sampling site (Williams, Armstrong, and Kirby 1992). This is not usually a problem during exercise after an adequate warm-up. At rest, or after a very short period of exercise or in cold environments, warming the hand will ensure a free flow of blood. In very young or sensitive subjects, the application of a topical anesthetic cream or spray to the sampling site may reduce anxiety.

Assay Techniques

Although several studies have been aimed at quantifying the magnitude of the differences in blood lactate levels measured at different sampling sites, few researchers have examined the influence of the assay method on the results obtained. Lactate may be determined in whole blood, lysed blood, serum, plasma, or a protein-free preparation using a variety of assays.

Previously, the most commonly used technique was an enzymatic-spectrophotometric assay (e.g., Hohorst 1965) that forms the basis for several commercially available kits (e.g., those of Sigma and Boehringer) and the DuPont ACA analyzer (Westgard, Lahmeyer, and Birnbaum 1972). Enzymatic-fluorometric assays (Lowry and Passeneau 1972; Maughan 1982) have also been popular and have been adapted for a variety of analyses (Rydevik, Nord, and Ingman 1982; Karlsson et al. 1983; Kumagai et al. 1986). The majority of research laboratories now use the modern semiautomatic analyzers that are based on an enzymatic electrochemical (amperometric) assay.

The various assay techniques require the blood to be treated in specific ways prior to assay. The spectrophotometric and fluorometric assays usually require the preparation of a protein-free filtrate: after the immediate expulsion of the blood sample into ice-cold perchloric acid ($HClO_4$) to precipitate the proteins, the sample is centrifuged and the clear supernatant assayed for lactate. Lactate determinations by this method have been described as "blood" or "whole blood" lactates in the literature (Tietz 1986); however, these values should not be confused with those from assays that measure whole, untreated blood.

For plasma lactate determinations, blood is collected into containers prepared with chemicals to inhibit further red cell glycolysis, for example sodium fluoride and potassium oxalate. Samples are then centrifuged to separate the cells from the plasma (Tietz 1986). Preservation of the blood by perchloric acid or glycolytic inhibitors is necessary to prevent a significant increase in lactate concentration as a result of both continued synthesis of lactate and leakage of lactate out of the red blood cells (Piquard et al. 1980). The extent of the increase varies with temperature and the elapsed time before assay but may be between 20% and 70% (Tietz 1986; Piquard et al. 1980), with the rate of increase apparently independent of the initial lactate concentration (Geyssant et al. 1985).

The majority of modern analyzers allow blood to be assayed immediately without chemical treatment. The enzyme electrodes are highly specific for lactate ions, and other potentially interfering substances are prevented from traversing the membrane (Tietz 1986). First developed for the rapid assessment of critical-care clinical conditions, their immediacy of assay—providing lactate determinations in a matter of seconds rather than minutes—and simplicity of use make them highly suitable for lactate determinations during exercise both in the laboratory and in the field. These analyzers can also assay plasma, serum, or lysed blood if required.

The disruption of the red blood cell membrane that occurs when perchloric acid or specific lysing agents are added to blood causes the intracellular lactate to be released into the extracellular fluid, contributing this lactate to the lactate from energy metabolism to the assay. In whole-blood assays, only the lactate in the plasma fraction of the blood is assayed (Mullen et al. 1986; Weil et al. 1986). This represents an important source of variation between lactate measurements from different assays.

Williams, Armstrong, and Kirby (1992) found no significant differences between lactate levels in lysed blood and those in whole blood, although levels in lysed blood tended to be higher than those in whole blood over the range 1.0 to 11.0 mmol $\cdot$ L^{-1}. Other studies have, however, recorded significant differences between lysed and whole blood (Friedham and Town 1989).

A further source of variation arises from the volume difference between whole blood and plasma or protein-free filtrates. In the whole blood of an individual with a normal hematocrit of around 40%, the aqueous phase represents about 88% of the total volume, and the nonaqueous phase, consisting of cells, proteins, and cellular debris, about 12%. Lactate levels measured in whole blood are therefore lower than those in plasma, serum, or deproteinized samples from which the cellular material has been removed. The main differences between the types of blood preparation that may be used for lactate assay are summarized in table 7.1.

Protein-free filtrates and lysed whole-blood assays measure "total" lactate, that is, plasma and erythrocyte lactate. Plasma assays may or may not measure total lactate according to treatment. Whole-blood assays measure lactate only in the plasma compartment. In addition, volume differences exist between plasma and protein-free filtrates and whole or lysed blood. Plasma lactate levels have been shown to be some 7% higher than those in protein-precipitated samples (Tietz 1986), although other authors have noted good agreement between the two assays (Westgard, Lahmeyer, and Birnbaum 1972). Williams, Armstrong, and Kirby (1992) demonstrated a 30% difference between plasma and whole-blood lactates assayed using the same analyzer.

In the majority of cases, values obtained from whole blood are markedly lower than those from protein-free samples (Mullen et al. 1986; Weaver and Vadgama 1986; Weil et al. 1986; Friedheim and Town 1989), although the degree of under-

Table 7.1   Types of Blood Preparation Used for Lactate Assay

Whole blood	The majority of modern semiautomatic analyzers assay whole blood. Capillary blood is collected into a heparinized container to prevent clotting and is assayed within a few minutes without further treatment.
Plasma	Blood is collected as above and centrifuged to separate the plasma from the cellular solids. Lactate is then measured in the plasma.
Serum	Serum is formed when blood is allowed to clot. The sample is centrifuged to separate the serum from the solids and is then assayed for lactate.
Lysed blood	The sample is treated with chemicals to break open (lyse) the red blood cells releasing the cellular lactate. The blood is not separated before assay.
Protein-free preparation	The sample is chemically treated to lyse the red blood cells and break down blood proteins. The blood is then centrifuged and the clear liquid portion assayed for lactate.

estimation varies. Friedheim and Town (1989) noted that during submaximal exercise, whole-blood lactate levels were 63.7% lower than those in protein-free samples while at maximal levels the difference was reduced to 20.4%.

It is evident from this discussion that postexercise blood lactates are specific to the assay used and that values determined using different methods are not directly comparable. Furthermore, Williams, Armstrong, and Kirby (1992) demonstrated a consistent discrepancy between two makes of analyzer despite the fact that both were enzymatic, whole-blood assays.

The interpretation and comparison of young people's postexercise lactates must include consideration of the lactate sampling and assay procedures used. The majority of published papers clearly specify aspects of methodology such as the exercise protocol used and the site and technique of blood sampling. The assay is rarely so well defined, despite its potential as a major source of variation between studies.

Timing of Postexercise Sampling

After an anaerobic test lasting 30-60 s, blood lactate levels progressively rise as lactate diffuses from muscle into blood. Thus maximal blood lactate levels are not reached until 5-8 min postexercise in adults (Crielaard and Franchimont 1985), although there is considerable variation between individuals. In children, the peak blood lactate following supramaximal exercise has been shown to occur at 2-3 min postexercise (Van Praagh et al. 1989; Van Praagh et al. 1990; Chia, Armstrong, and Childs 1997). It is not always practical or desirable to obtain serial blood samples from young subjects to identify individual peak lactates; therefore standardizing sampling to 3 min postexercise may be appropriate. The duration of the supramaximal effort will also influence the postexercise lactate obtained. A test lasting 60 s will produce higher postexercise lactates than a 30 s effort, reflecting the longer period of glycolytic stress (see table 7.2).

Child-Adult Differences in Postexercise Lactates

It has frequently been demonstrated that children and adolescents respond to all intensities of exercise with lower blood lactates than adults. Several lines of evidence have been examined in order to identify the factors that contribute to child-adult differences in postexercise lactates, but a definitive explanation remans elusive. Methodological differences and a scarcity of either cross-sectional or longitudinal data make it impossible to identify accurately the rate and timing of the progression of children's postexercise lactates toward values typical of adults.

Table 7.2   Blood Lactates Following Supramaximal Cycle Ergometry in Children and Adolescents

Study	Sex	Age (y)	n	Test duration (s)	Time of sample (min post-ex)	Site[1]	Assay[2]	Mean (SD) blood lactate (mmol · L[-1])
Van Praagh et al. 1989	M	7.4 (0.3)	19	30	From 1 to 5	E	1	7.0 (3.2)
Falgairette et al. 1991	M	7.7 (0.4)	36	30	2	E	1	6.2 (2.1)
Falgairette et al. 1991	M	9.3 (0.7)	27	30	2	E	1	5.1 (1.8)
Armstrong & Welsman (unpublished)	F	9.9 (0.3)	17	30	3	F	1	5.2 (1.4)
Falgairette et al. 1993	M	11.3 (1.0)	26	30	2	E	1	8.0 (1.8)
Falgairette et al. 1991	M	11.6 (0.5)	34	30	2	E	1	7.7 (2.1)
Armstrong et al. 1997	M	12.2 (0.4)	100	30	3	F	1	6.2 (1.6)
Armstrong et al. 1997	F	12.2 0.4)	100	30	3	F	1	6.0 (1.3)
Van Praagh et al. 1990	F	12.8 (0.4)	12	30	3	E	1	9.0 (1.8)
Van Praagh et al. 1990	M	12.9 (0.5)	15	30	From 1 to 7	E	1	10.0 (1.6)
Falgairette et al. 1991	M	13.1 (0.4)	29	30	2	E	1	8.4 (2.1)
Chia et al. 1997	M	9.7 (0.3)	25	30	From 30 s to 3	F	1	3.6
Chia et al. 1997	F	9.7 (0.3)	25	30	From 30 s to 3	F	1	4.9
Armstrong & Welsman (unpublished)	M	13.2 (0.4)	78	30	3	F	1	6.2 (1.7)

(continued)

Table 7.2 *(continued)*

Study	Sex	Age (y)	n	Test duration (s)	Time of sample (min post-ex)	Site[1]	Assay[2]	Mean (SD) blood lactate (mmol · L⁻¹)
Armstrong & Welsman (unpublished)	F	13.1 (0.4)	67	30	3	F	1	6.1 (1.8)
Armstrong & Welsman (unpublished)	M	14.1 (0.3)	16	30	3	F	1	7.3 (1.3)
Crielaard et al. 1986	M	12.3 (0.5)	12	47.2[3]	7	?	2	7.2 (1.1)
Falgairette et al. 1991	M	14.4 (0.4)	18	30	2	E	1	7.8 (1.6)
Mero et al. 1989	M	11.6 (0.9)	17	60	5	F	2	9.8 (2.5)
Mero 1988	M	12.0 (1.0)	19	60	5	F	2	13.1 (2.6)
Crielaard et al. 1986	M	14.2 (0.4)	13	55.9[3]	7	?	2	9.3 (1.7)
Mero et al. 1989	M	14.6 (0.9)	17	60	5	F	2	13.9 (1.7)
Crielaard et al. 1986	M	16.3 (0.6)	12	76.8[3]	7	?	2	11.2 (1.4)

[1]Site: E = earlobe, F = fingertip.

[2]Assay: 1 = whole-blood assay, 2= protein-free assay.

[3]This value represents the mean time to exhaustion.

Muscle Metabolic Profile and Postexercise Lactates

The lactate measured in blood reflects all those processes by which lactate is produced and eliminated (Brooks 1985). Consequently, postexercise blood lactates provide only a qualitative indication of the degree of stress placed on anaerobic metabolism by a bout of exercise, not a precise measure of glycolytic energy generation. It cannot be assumed, therefore, that children's lower postexercise blood lactates simply result from lower intramuscular lactate production.

The ethical restrictions surrounding the use with children of the invasive techniques necessary to study the intramuscular environment have limited the data available to accurately describe child-adult differences in muscle metabolism. However, there is evidence to suggest that muscle stores of glycogen are lower in children than in adults and increase with age (Eriksson and Saltin 1974; Karlsson et al. 1972). Rates of glycogen utilization also appear markedly lower in children and adolescents and are reflected in significantly lower muscle lactate levels. Mean muscle lactates of 8.8 mmol · kg^{-1} in 11- to 13-year-olds at peak $\dot{V}O_2$ (Eriksson, Karlsson, and Saltin 1971) compare with 15.0 mmol ·kg^{-1} at 15 years and 17.0 mmol · kg^{-1} in adults (Karlsson et al. 1972).

Eriksson and colleagues attributed children's lower lactates to lower activity of the glycolytic rate-limiting enzyme, phosphofructokinase (PFK), having observed activity levels some 30-50% lower in 11-year-old boys (Eriksson, Karlsson, and Saltin 1971) than in adults (Gollnick et al. 1972). Although providing some unique insights into the development of muscle metabolism, Eriksson himself acknowledged the limitations of his studies, which were based on small, select, single-sex samples, stating that "the results must be interpreted with caution and no general conclusions may be drawn" (Eriksson and Saltin 1974). Despite this, a lower PFK activity continues to be the most frequently cited explanation for children's lower blood lactates (Wirth et al. 1978; Mero 1988; Crielaard et al. 1986).

An examination of more recent data suggests that the cause of young people's lower lactates is more complex than this, although once again, different analytical procedures used to measure muscle enzymes preclude the formulation of a complete and satisfactory explanation. The hypothesis of lower PFK levels has been supported (Fournier et al. 1982), but other investigators have failed to observe significant or consistent child-adult differences in the maximal activities of a variety of glycolytic enzymes including PFK (Haralambie 1982; Berg, Kim, and Keul 1986).

Although lactate is a direct by-product of the glycolytic pathway, it may be misguided to focus on the functional capacity of a single energy system in the search for an explanation for young people's lower lactate responses. Adenosine triphosphate for muscular contraction is generated from a complex interplay of both anaerobic and oxidative pathways depending upon the intensity and duration of exercise. While the evidence pointing to inferior glycolytic enzyme activity is equivocal, there appears to be a general consensus that the activity of aerobic enzymes in children's muscle is significantly higher than in adult muscle (Eriksson, Gollnick, and Saltin 1973; Haralambie 1982; Berg, Kim, and Keul 1986). An examination of the ratio between key enzymes of the aerobic and anaerobic energy pathways suggests that children are preferentially equipped for aerobic energy generation (Haralambie 1982).

Oxygen On-Transients and Postexercise Lactates

Another explanation for young people's lower postexercise lactates that has been popular is a faster adjustment of the cardiopulmonary system to exercise, enabling oxygen to be available rapidly for energy generation and thus reducing the contribution from glycolysis. At exercise intensities approaching or exceeding peak $\dot{V}O_2$, there is evidence to suggest that children attain a higher percentage peak $\dot{V}O_2$ during the first 30 s of exercise than adults (Macek and Vavra 1977; Macek and Vavra 1980) and have a faster $t^1/_2$ $\dot{V}O_2$ than adults (Sady 1981; Macek et al. 1984) with correspondingly lower blood lactate levels (Macek et al. 1984).

Few studies have quantified the relative contribution of the aerobic system to energy generation during supramaximal exercise. Estimates for the aerobic contribution to a 30 s supramaximal test in adults have been from 13% (Inbar, Dotan, and Bar-Or 1976) to 28% (Seresse et al. 1988). Van Praagh et al. (1991) reported a significant decline in the aerobic contribution (by 64%) to a modified Wingate anaerobic test between the ages of 9.5 and 15 years. Over the group as a whole, the children attained 60-70% $\dot{V}O_2$ max during the 30 s test. In our laboratory, using breath-by-breath expired gas analysis, we have calculated the aerobic component of a 30 s supramaximal cycling test, assuming a 25% mechanical efficiency, to be 33% and 36% in 10-year-old girls and boys, respectively. Calculations based on a 15% efficiency reduced these values to 20% and 21% (Armstrong and Welsman 1997). Chia, Armstrong, and Childs (1997) reported aerobic components of 17.7% and 44.3% for mechanical efficiencies of 13% and 30%, respectively, for a similar test. This will inevitably reduce lactate accumulation and thus contribute to lower postexercise lactates. With such a high aerobic contribution it may be questioned whether children's lower postexercise lactates reflect a "true" metabolic difference between children and adults. It may be that the tests traditionally used to assess anaerobic performance do not accurately isolate and stress anaerobic metabolism in youngsters. An evaluation of the validity of the recognized anaerobic tests is urgently required and represents a fruitful area for research (Armstrong and Welsman 1997).

Postexercise Lactates and Chronological Age

The evidence for age-related changes in lactate responses to submaximal and maximal postexercise lactates is conflicting, with studies showing both significant changes between childhood and adolescence (Åstrand 1952; Tanaka and Shindo 1985; Cumming, Hastman, and McCort 1985) and no significant change between the ages of 11 and 16 years (Williams and Armstrong 1991; Sjödin and Svedenhag 1992).

The database on post-supramaximal exercise blood lactates is small, and few published studies have included sufficient cross-sectional or longitudinal data for this problem to be clarified. Data from females are notably lacking. The results presented in table 7.2 are arranged by chronological age and duration of test to give some indication of age-related changes. However, it is impossible to infer a true pattern of change with increasing age because of the many methodological differences among the various studies. Even within those studies using a 30 s supramaximal effort and whole-blood capillary sampling, postexercise lactate values are not directly comparable due to differences in the braking forces applied.

The study by Falgairette et al. (1991) is perhaps the most comprehensive, indicating age-related changes following a 30 s supramaximal effort in 9- to 14-year-old boys. Although significant differences were noted between the youngest and oldest groups, the data do not suggest a consistent progression in postexercise lactates across the age range. Further studies using consistent methodology with a wide age range of young people are required to clarify the emergence of lactate metabolism with age.

Postexercise Lactates and Maturation

Examining the development of young people's exercise responses by chronological age alone gives an incomplete and potentially inaccurate representation of the underlying metabolic changes. Because children grow and mature at very different rates, individuals of the same age may vary considerably in their actual biological age. Interpretation of young people's exercise responses should, therefore, include consideration of maturity stage.

Since Eriksson and colleagues (Eriksson, Karlsson, and Saltin 1971) indicated a relationship between sexual maturation (testicular volume) and lactate metabolism there has been a long-standing hypothesis that the evolution of glycolytic capacity is somehow dependent upon the hormonal changes occurring during maturation. Eriksson's work has often been cited as evidence for this hypothesis (Bar-Or 1984; Paterson, Cunningham, and Bumstead 1986; Fellmann et al. 1988) despite the fact that he reported an "almost significant" correlation ($p > 0.05$) observed in eight 13- to 15-year-old boys.

Results from animal studies that have indicated relationships between testosterone levels and the maturation of glycolytic capacity in skeletal muscle (Krotkiewski, Kral, and Karlsson 1980; Dux et al. 1979; Dux, Dux, and Guba 1982) reinforce the view that testosterone and glycolysis are causally linked, but research evidence from children and adolescents is equivocal. Several studies have noted significant relationships between postexercise lactates and testosterone levels in boys (Mero 1988; Mero et al. 1988; Fellman et al. 1988; Falgairette et al. 1990, 1991) with correlation coefficients typically around $r = 0.40$. However, although the study by Mero has been cited as supporting a maturational dependency of glycolytic capacity, all the subjects were classified as prepubertal with testosterone levels lower than would be expected to induce changes in muscle mass or metabolism. Indeed, Falgairette et al. (1991) noted significant increases in anaerobic performance and postexercise lactate between the ages of 6 and 12 years despite no increase in testosterone levels.

In other studies the significance of the relationship between lactate and testosterone may be questioned, as the influences of growth have not been adequately controlled for with the use of testosterone as the maturity indicator. Testosterone levels are highly correlated with stature and mass and therefore they should be partialled out of investigations of the relationships between testosterone and anaerobic performance or glycolytic capacity. In a recent analysis that separated the influ-

ence of body size on postpeak ˙VO$_2$ lactates from the independent influence of testosterone, no significant relationship between lactate and testosterone remained
(Welsman, Armstrong, and Kirby 1994). Similarly, we have noted no significant
relationship (p>0.05) between salivary testosterone level and post-Wingate test blood
lactate in a sample of 52 boys who were 12-13 years old (Armstrong, Welsman, and
Kirby 1997).

Further evidence exists to refute the postulated link between maturation and lactate metabolism. Paterson and Cunningham (1985) found no significant differences
in postexercise blood lactates in children of the same age classified as early or late
maturers, despite a 2-year differential in biological age as determined by skeletal
maturity. Similarly, using Tanner's indexes to indicate maturity, no significant changes
from early to late puberty have been observed in blood lactates after maximal
treadmill exercise in 11- to 16-year-olds (Williams and Armstrong 1991) or after the
Wingate Anaerobic Test in 12-year-olds (Armstrong, Welsman, and Kirby 1997).
The data presented in table 7.3 support these findings with no significant differences
in post-Wingate test blood lactates by stage of maturity, although adult values remain higher than those observed in 13- to 14-year-olds classified as Tanner stage 5.

**Table 7.3   Blood Lactates Following a 30 s Supramaximal Cycle Test by
Maturity (Data From Armstrong, Welsman, and Kirby 1997)**

Maturity group		Males			Females	
	n	Age (yr)	Lactate (mmol · L^{-1})	n	Age (yr)	Lactate (mmol·L^{-1})
Group 1	30	12.0 (0.4)	5.9 (1.6)	17	12.1 (0.3)	5.9 (1.5)
Group 2	34	12.2 (0.4)	6.2 (1.6)	22	12.0 (0.3)	6.3 (1.2)
Group 3	19	12.2 (0.3)	5.9 (1.3)	25	12.0 (0.4)	5.6 (1.1)
Group 4	7	12.8 (0.4)	6.8 (1.3)	15	12.6 (0.4)	6.4 (1.7)

Note: Male-female differences are not significant.

Directions for Future Research

Although it is well documented that children demonstrate lower post-supramaximal
exercise lactates than adults, inconsistent methodologies prevent the precise identification of patterns of change in relation to either chronological or biological age.
Further research using consistent methodology in large groups of subjects is required. Data from girls, as mentioned earlier, are notably lacking.

A muscle metabolic profile that is qualitatively different from that of adults, faster oxygen on-transients, and low levels of anabolic hormones have been hypothesized to account for children's lower lactates; but these explanations remain speculative, as limited data exist to provide conclusive supporting evidence, and further research is required.

The high aerobic component of the Wingate test with children indicates that the test, in its conventional form, does not adequately stress glycolysis—providing a nonphysiological explanation for children's lower lactates. Further research is required to refine supramaximal tests to quantify the aerobic contribution so that child-adult differences may be examined more accurately.

Summary

Methodological factors such as the site of sampling, assay method, and timing of postexercise sampling will significantly influence the measured blood lactate level. Full and detailed methodologies must be included when one reports blood lactate data. Young people's postexercise blood lactates must be interpreted in relation to the methodology employed.

Postexercise blood lactates in children and adolescents are invariably demonstrated to be lower than those of adults after a similar bout of exercise. Several hypotheses have been proposed to explain this difference, but a definitive answer has proved elusive. There are insufficient data to attribute young people's lower lactates simply to a lower activity of PFK, but there are clear indications that their muscle metabolic profile is geared toward aerobic rather than anaerobic energy generation.

A faster adjustment of the cardiopulmonary system at the onset of exercise will reduce reliance upon lactate-producing glycolysis. Again, evidence is limited, but it would appear that traditional anaerobic tests, such as the Wingate test, do not sufficiently stress glycolysis or produce a high aerobic component in young people.

The evidence suggesting a causal link between the ability to generate lactate during exercise and sexual maturation is weak. Further research is required with children, adolescents, and young adults to elucidate further the development of the production of muscle lactate and subsequent accumulation of blood lactate.

References

Armstrong, N., and Welsman, J. 1997. *Young people and physical activity.* Oxford: University Press.

Armstrong, N., Welsman, J.R., and Kirby, B.J. 1997. Performance on the Wingate Anaerobic Test and maturation. *Pediatr. Exerc. Sci. 9.*

Åstrand, P.O. 1952. *Experimental studies of physical working capacity in relation to sex and age.* Copenhagen: Munksgaard.

Bar-Or, O. 1984. The growth and development of children's physiologic and perceptional responses to exercise. In *Children and sport,* ed. J. Ilmarinen and I. Välimäki, 3-17. Berlin: Springer-Verlag.

Berg, A., Kim, S.S., and Keul, J. 1986. Skeletal muscle enzyme activities in healthy young subjects. *Int. J. Sports Med.* 7: 236-239.

Brooks, G.A. 1985. Anaerobic threshold: review of the concept and directions for future research. *Med. Sci. Sports Exerc.* 17: 22-31.

Busse, M.W., Muller, M., and Boning, D. 1983. A method of continuous treadmill testing. International Congress on Sports and Health, Maastricht, The Netherlands. *Int. J. Sports Med.* (abstract suppl.): 2.

Chia, M., Armstrong, N., and Childs, D. 1997. The assessment of children's anaerobic performance using modifications of the Wingate Anaerobic Test. *Pediatr. Exerc. Sci.* 9: 80-89.

Crielaard, J.M., and Franchimont, P. 1985. La mesure de la capacité anaérobie lactique: mise au point actuelle. *Med. Sport* 59: 150-152.

Crielaard, J.M., Piront, B., Franchimont, P., Pirnay, F., and Petit, J.M. 1986. Evolution de la capacite anaérobie lactique au cours de la croissance. *Med. Sport* 60.

Cumming, G.R., Hastman, L., and McCort, J. 1985. Treadmill endurance times, blood lactate, and exercise blood pressures in normal children. In *Children and exercise XI,* ed. R.A. Binkhorst, H.C.G. Kemper, and W.H.M. Saris, 140-150. Champaign, IL: Human Kinetics.

Dux, L., Dux, E., and Guba, F. 1982. Further data on the androgenic dependency of the skeletal musculature: the effect of prepubertal castration of the structural development of the skeletal muscles. *Horm. Metab. Res.* 14: 191-194.

Dux, L., Dux, E., Mazareau, H., and Guba, F. 1979. A non-neural regulatory effect on the metabolic differentiation of the skeletal muscle. Effect of castration and testosterone administration on the skeletal muscles of the rat. *Comp. Biochem. Physiol.* 64A: 177-183.

Eriksson, B.O., Gollnick, P.D., and Saltin, B. 1973. Muscle metabolism and enzyme activities after training in boys 11-13 years old. *Acta Physiol. Scand.* 87: 485-497.

Eriksson, B.O., Karlsson, J., and Saltin, B. 1971. Muscle metabolites during exercise in pubertal boys. *Acta Paediatr. Scand.* 217(suppl.): 154-157.

Eriksson, B.O., and Saltin, B. 1974. Muscle metabolism during exercise in boys aged 11-16 years compared to adults. *Acta Paediatr. Belg.* 28(suppl.): 257-265.

Falgairette, G., Bedu, M., Fellmann, N., Van Praagh, E., and Coudert, J. 1991. Bio-energetic profile in 144 boys aged from 6 to 15 years with special reference to sexual maturation. *Eur. J. Appl. Physiol.* 62: 151-156.

Falgairette, G., Bedu, M., Fellmann, N., Van Praagh, E., Jarrige, J.F., and Coudert, J. 1990. Modifications of aerobic and anaerobic metabolisms in active boys during puberty. In *Children and exercise,* ed. G. Beunen, J. Ghesquiere, T. Reybrouck, and A.L. Claessens, 42-49. Stuttgart: Enke.

Falgairette, G., Duché, P., Bedu, M., Fellman, N., and Coudert, J. 1993. Bioenergetic characteristics in prepubertal swimmers: comparison with active and nonactive boys. *Int. J. Sports Med.* 14: 444-448.

Fellmann, N., Bedu, M., Spielvogel, H., Falgairette, G., Van Praagh, E., Jarrige, J., and Coudert, J. 1988. Anaerobic metabolism during pubertal development at high altitude. *J. Appl. Physiol.* 64: 1382-1386.

Fournier, M.J., Ricci, J., Taylor, A.W., Ferguson, R.J., Montpetit, R.R., and Chaitman, B.R. 1982. Skeletal muscle adaptation in adolescent boys: sprint and endurance training and detraining. *Med. Sci. Sports Exerc.* 14: 453-456.

Friedheim, L.C., and Town, G.P. 1989. Blood lactate methodologies compared. *Med. Sci. Sports Exerc.* 21(suppl.): S21.

Geyssant, A., Dormois, D., Barthelemy, J.C., and Lacour, J.R. 1985. Lactate determination with the lactate analyser LA 640: a critical study. *Scand. J. Clin. Lab. Invest.* 2: 145-149.

Gollnick, P.D., Armstrong, R.B., Saubert, C.W., Piehl, K., and Saltin, B. 1972. Enzyme activity and fibre composition in skeletal muscle of untrained and trained men. *J. Appl. Physiol.* 33: 312-319.

Haralambie, G. 1982. Enzyme activities in skeletal muscle of 13-15 years old adolescents. *Bull. Eur. Physiopath. Resp.* 18: 65-74.

Hohorst, H.J. 1965. L-(+) Lactate determination with lactic dehydrogenase and DPN. In *Methods of enzymatic analysis,* ed. H.V. Bergmeyer, 226-270. 2nd ed. New York: Academic Press.

Inbar, O., Dotan, R., and Bar-Or, O. 1976. Aerobic and anaerobic components of a thirty second supramaximal cycling test. *Med. Sci. Sports* 8: 51.

Karlsson, J., Jacobs, I., Sjödin, B., Tesch, P., Kaiser, P., Sahl, O., and Karlberg, B. 1983. Semi-automatic blood lactate assay: experiences from an exercise laboratory. *Int. J. Sports Med.* 4: 52-55.

Karlsson, J., Nordesjo, L.O., Jorfeldt, L., and Saltin, B. 1972. Muscle lactate, ATP, and CP levels during exercise after physical training in man. *J. Appl. Physiol.* 33: 199-203.

Krotkiewski, M., Kral, J.G., and Karlsson, J. 1980. Effects of castration and testosterone substitution on body composition and muscle metabolism in rats. *Acta Physiol. Scand.* 109: 233-237.

Kumagai, S., Hiral, Y., Hasegawa, T., Tokudome, S., Tomokuni, K., and Nishizumi, H. 1986. Enzymatic determination of blood lactate by flow injection analysis. *Ann. Physiol. Anthrop.* 5: 97-100.

Lowry, O.H., and Passeneau, J.V. 1972. *A flexible system of enzymatic analysis.* New York: Academic Press.

Macek, M., and Vavra, J. 1977. Relation between aerobic and anaerobic energy supply during maximal exercise in boys. In *Frontiers of activity and child health,* ed. H. Lavallée and R.J. Shephard, 157-159. Quebec: Editions du Pelican.

Macek, M., and Vavra, J. 1980. The adjustment of oxygen uptake at the onset of exercise: a comparison between prepubertal boys and young adults. *Int. J. Sports Med.* 1: 75-77.

Macek, M., Vavra, J., Benesova, H., and Radvansky, J. 1984. The adjustment of oxygen uptake at the onset of exercise: relation to age and to workload. In *Children and sport,* ed. J. Ilmarinen and I. Välimäki, 129-134. Berlin: Springer-Verlag.

Maughan, R.J. 1982. A simple rapid method for the determination of glucose, lactate, pyruvate, alanine, 3-hydroxybutyrate and acetoacetate on a single 20μl blood sample. *Clin. Chim. Acta* 122: 231-240.

Mero, A. 1988. Blood lactate production and recovery from anaerobic exercise in trained and untrained boys. *Eur. J. Appl. Physiol.* 57: 660-666.

Mero, A., Kauhanen, H., Peltola, E., and Vuorimaa, T. 1988. Changes in endurance, strength and speed capacity of different prepubescent athletic groups during one year of training. *J. Hum. Mov. Stud.* 14: 219-239.

Mullen, W.H., Churchouse, F.H., Keedy, F.H., and Vadgama, P.M. 1986. Enzyme electrode for the measurement of lactate in undiluted blood. *Clin. Chim. Acta* 157: 191-198.

Newton, J.L., and Robinson, S. 1965. The distribution of blood lactate and pyruvate during work and recovery. *Fed. Proc.* 24: 590.

Paterson, D.H., and Cunningham, D.A. 1985. Development of anaerobic capacity in early and late maturing boys. In *Children and exercise XI,* ed. R.A. Binkhorst, H.C.G. Kemper, and W.H.M. Saris, 119-128. Champaign, IL: Human Kinetics.

Paterson, D.H., Cunningham, D.A., and Bumstead, L.A. 1986. Recovery O_2 and blood lactic acid: longitudinal analysis in boys aged 11-15 years. *Eur. J. Appl. Physiol.* 55: 93-99.

Piquard, F., Schaefer, A., Dellenback, P., and Haberey, P. 1980. Rapid bedside estimation of plasma and whole blood lactic acid. *Intens. Care Med.* 7: 35-38.

Rydevik, U., Nord, L., and Ingman, F. 1982. Automatic lactate determination by flow injection analysis. *Int. J. Sports Med.* 3: 47-49.

Sady, S.P. 1981. Transient O_2 uptake and heart rate responses at the onset of relative endurance exercise in prepubertal boys and adult men. *Int. J. Sports Med.* 2: 240-244.

Saltin, B., Blomqvist, G., Mitchell, J.H., Johnson, R.L., Jr., Wildenthal, K., and Chapman, C. 1968. Response to exercise after bedrest and after training. *Circulation* 38(suppl. 5).

Seresse, O., Lortie, G., Bouchard, C., and Boulay, M.R. 1988. Estimation of the contribution of the various energy systems during maximal work of short duration. *Int. J. Sports Med.* 9: 456-460.

Sjödin, B., and Svedenhag, J. 1992. Oxygen uptake during running as related to body mass in circumpubertal boys: a longitudinal study. *Eur. J. Appl. Physiol.* 65: 150-157.

Tanaka, H., and Shindo, M. 1985. Running velocity at blood lactate threshold of boys aged 6-15 years compared with untrained and trained young males. *Int. J. Sports Med.* 6: 90-94.

Tietz, N.W. 1986. *Textbook of clinical chemistry.* Philadelphia: Saunders.

Van Praagh, E., Bedu, M., Falgairette, G., Fellmann, N., and Coudert, J. 1991.

Oxygen uptake during a 30s supramaximal exercise in 7-15 year old boys. In *Children and exercise: pediatric work physiology XV,* ed. R. Frenkl and I. Szmodis, 281-287. Budapest: National Institute for Health Promotion.

Van Praagh, E., Falgairette, G., Bedu, M., Fellmann, N., and Coudert, J. 1989. Laboratory and field tests in 7-year-old boys. In *Children and exercise XIII,* ed. S. Oseid and K.H. Carlsen, 11-17. Champaign, IL: Human Kinetics.

Van Praagh, E., Fellmann, N., Bedu, M., Falgairette, G., and Coudert, J. 1990. Gender difference in the relationship of anaerobic power output to body composition in children. *Pediatr. Exerc. Sci.* 2: 336-348.

Weaver, M.R., and Vadgama, P.M. 1986. An O_2 based enzyme electrode for whole blood lactate measurement under continuous flow conditions. *Clin. Chim. Acta* 155: 295-308.

Weil, M.H., Leavy, J.A., Rackow, E.C., and Halfman, C.J. 1986. Validation of a semi-automated technique for measuring lactate in whole blood. *Clin. Chem.* 32: 2175-2177.

Welsman, J.R., Armstrong, N., and Kirby, B.J. 1994. Serum testosterone is not related to peak $\dot{V}O_2$ and submaximal lactate responses in 12- to 16-year-old males. *Pediatr. Exerc. Sci.* 6: 2120-2127.

Westgard, J.O., Lahmeyer, B.L., and Birnbaum, M.L. 1972. Use of the DuPont "Automatic Clinical Analyser" in direct determination of lactic acid in plasma stabilised with sodium fluoride. *Clin. Chem.* 18: 1334-1338.

Williams, J.R., and Armstrong, N. 1991. The influence of age and sexual maturation on children's blood lactate responses to exercise. *Pediatr. Exerc. Sci.* 3: 111-120.

Williams, J.R., Armstrong, N., and Kirby, B.J. 1992. The influence of the site of sampling and assay medium upon the interpretation of blood lactate responses to exercise. *J. Sports Sci.* 10: 95-107.

Wirth, A., Trager, E., Scheele, K., Mayer, D., Diehm, K., Reisch, K., and Weicker, K. 1978. Cardiopulmonary adjustment and metabolic response to maximal and submaximal physical exercise of boys and girls at different stages of maturity. *Eur. J. Appl. Physiol.* 39: 229-240.

Working Party on Ethics of Research in Children. 1980. Guidelines to aid ethical committees considering research involving children. *Br. Med. J.* 280: 229-231.

Working Party on Research in Children. 1991. *The ethical conduct of research in children.* London: Medical Research Council.

Yoshida, T. 1984. Effect of exercise duration during incremental exercise on the determination of anaerobic threshold and the onset of blood lactate accumulation. *Eur. J. Appl. Physiol.* 53: 196-199.

Yoshida, T., Suda, Y., and Takeuchi, N. 1982. Endurance training regimen based upon arterial blood lactate: effects on anaerobic threshold. *Eur. J. Appl. Physiol.* 49: 223-230.

8

CHAPTER

Measuring Maximal Short-Term Power Output During Growth

Emmanuel Van Praagh
Nanci M. França

This chapter focuses on the following objectives:

- Discussing the critical issues and controversies relating to anaerobic power
- Presenting testing guidelines for anaerobic power
- Discussing power diagnosis and athletic performance in children
- Evaluating which among the testing procedures should be used to assess maximal short-term power output

Testing of prolonged maximal power output (VO_2max) in children has been extensively studied (see Krahenbuhl, Skinner, and Kohrt 1985 for general review), but comparatively little attention has been given to high-intensity exercise lasting only a few seconds. This is surprising considering that this type of activity often occurs in daily tasks and leisure or sporting events. Studying daily physical activity in prepubertal children, Cooper (1995) reported that the children were more often engaged in short bursts of intense exercise than in long-term activities. The average duration of these high-intensity activities was only 6 s, and the average interval between the short bursts of activity was about 20 s. This typical activity seems to be a more "natural" pattern during growth than extensively longer exercise bouts. The growth-related differences in the adaptive response to short-term high-intensity exercise might be related to the maturation of muscle metabolic pathways, but no definitive mechanism has been established. Neither has much research been done on the correlation between short-term power measures and athletic performance. This is, however, essential in "multiple sprint sports" (Williams 1987) such as ice hockey, racket sports, jumping events, basketball, and other popular participation sports. Moreover, the use of such indicators seems to be central to talent identification. The lack of noninvasive methods for studying energy metabolism is a real drawback in child studies. New technologies (e.g., phosphorus nuclear magnetic resonance spectroscopy [^{31}P NMR]) will provide clearer information in the near future, but these tools are, of course, not available for current routine assessment. As a reasonable alternative, valid and specific power tests must be elaborated in order to evaluate short-term power capabilities during childhood and adolescence.

Anaerobic Power: Critical Issues and Controversies

Power assessment during growth is a difficult task because of the fledging status of research within the area and our limited understanding of the mechanisms that underpin pediatric anaerobic performance.

What Is the Physiological Significance?

Exercise physiologists have concentrated their research more on fuel intake (O_2 consumption) than on the resulting mechanical power output (Wilkie 1960). This statement also seems relevant in developmental exercise physiology when the purpose is to quantify the anaerobic energy yield in short-term exercise. Recently, Zanconato et al. (1993) and Kuno et al. (1995), both using ^{31}P NMR spectroscopy, reported that children aged 7-10 years and adolescents aged 12-15 years, respectively, had a lower glycolytic ability during exercise than adults. One of the limitations of these important studies is that only arm or leg exercise could be investigated. The amount of energy obtained by anaerobic processes during whole-body exercise cannot yet be measured directly. No relevant quantitative measurement techniques for anaerobic energy yield from adenosine triphosphate or glycolysis are available, probably because of the nonlinear relationship between the anaerobic energy expenditure and time (Saltin 1990). Attempts have been made in adults (Medbø et al. 1988) as well as in children (Carlson and Naughton 1992) to estimate muscle anaerobic adenosine triphosphate production using the accumulated O_2 deficit method. However, the validity of the VO_2-power regression to predict energy demand during high-intensity exercise is still a matter of debate (Green et al. 1996).

Defining the Key Terms

In performing "anaerobic" tests, it is assumed that the energy yield is derived from anaerobic pathways (5'-adenosine triphosphate [ATP], phosphocreatine degradation, and glycolysis). Margaria, Cerretelli, and Mangili (1964) proposed that phosphocreatine degradation was the immediate and only substrate for ATP resynthesis during the early stages (<10 s) of short-term high-intensity exercise. However, in adults, Saltin et al. (1971) reported a significant [La-] increase after 10 s supramaximal exercise (110% $\dot{V}O_2$max). This observation was also confirmed by the study of Mercier, Mercier, and Préfaut (1991), who found a significant venous blood lactate increase during 6 s force-velocity cycling sprints in young trained male adults. Direct measurements of "anaerobic capacity" or the maximum amount of ATP that can be supplied by the anaerobic energy pathways is still a matter for research, while the precise amount cannot actually be quantified. Furthermore, anaerobic capacity should not be confused with power, as this mechanical parameter is defined as a certain amount of energy (work) done per time unit ($J \cdot S^{-1}$ or watts).

Since the substrate utilization cannot be accurately measured during whole-body ultrashort-term exercise (100-200 ms), it is more appropriate to measure the mechanical energy yield. Ferretti et al. (1987) were able to monitor instantaneous force-velocity during a vertical jump lasting only 4 ms. They assumed that this activity was possible only via the muscle (ATP) and could therefore be considered as an estimate of the maximal ATP in vivo splitting rate. One main problem, among others, in anaerobic testing procedures is the accurate quantification of work done in a very short time. Before publication of the Margaria protocol (Margaria, Aghemo, and Rovelli 1966), most, if not all, short-term tests measured work (e.g., vertical jump), time (e.g., 30-50 m dash) or distance (e.g., softball throw) but not mechanical power. One must keep in mind that

- anaerobic tests are highly specific to the muscle group being evaluated, and
- anaerobic performance of a muscle group depends highly on the force and the velocity of its contraction.

Therefore a distinction must be made between the more general maximal short-term power tests and the more specific maximal short-term athletic power tests.

Maximal Short-Term Power

Mechanical energy yielded during overall exercises (running, cycling, jumping) of very short duration (4 ms to 40 s) will be termed maximal short-term power in this chapter (MSTP). The aim is to assess the subject's ability to yield the highest power possible during "natural" daily activity patterns. The MSTP tests also assess basic muscular characteristics (e.g., leg or arm power). The measurements are done by classic ergometry and dynamometry (cycle ergometer, static or dynamic dynamometers, treadmill ergometer). The energy requirement for external short-term performance can be calculated indirectly, depending on the specific ergometer used.

Maximal Short-Term Athletic Power

Mechanical energy yielded during specific sport patterns (high jump, "dunks," sprint starts, ball throwing, ball kicking, weight or power lifting) will be termed maximal short-term athletic power in this chapter (MSTAP). The purpose is to evaluate the ability of the young athlete to develop power in a specific training or competitive situation. Many sports require a person to produce high power in order to perform successfully. While this power is often exhibited in the sport movements themselves, its measurement is more restricted in laboratory and field situations (e.g., kicking velocity in young soccer players, throwing velocity in young athletes, seated shot put in adolescent wrestlers).

Testing of Anaerobic Power

Whether performance tests are done in a laboratory or in field settings, they must respect research criteria such as validity, reliability, and objectivity. The scientific value of physical fitness testing has been frequently debated. Field tests are less accurate than those performed in research laboratories. However, even if several independent variables (i.e., environmental variables) are better controlled in a laboratory, the child's motivation for field tests is probably higher than in the "colder" environment of a laboratory. Nevertheless, in both situations, the choice of a test must correspond to various test criteria, or test characteristics. *Validity* of a test indicates the degree to which the test or instrument measures what it is supposed to measure. In deciding whether or not to use a test, the user should check that the test has established validity. The test description should clearly indicate the type of validity (e.g., concurrent validity or predictive validity). *Reliability* pertains to the consistency or repeatability of a test. A test cannot be considered valid if it is not reliable. A test may be valid and reliable for one group of subjects but not for another (e.g., reliable for adults but not for children). Moreover, a test may be quite valid and reliable when given in a careful and systematic manner but totally unreliable and hence invalid in the hands of an incompetent tester. *Objectivity* of a test concerns whether the test measures consistently when given by two different testers. Statistical techniques, like correlation or test-retest procedures, are used to judge the construct (internal) validity and reliability of tests. However, *feasibility* (practical aspects) in pediatric testing must be taken into account: requirements for equipment, ease and cost of administration, time of administration, suitability for the intended age category and/or ability level, suitability for research purposes, and norms available. The reader is directed to Abernethy, Wilson, and Logan (1995) and Docherty (1996) for more detailed information.

Maximal Short-Term Power Assessment: Modalities and Protocols

The power produced during muscular shortening depends on both force and velocity factors; therefore force and speed of movement must be matched (Hill 1938). Maximal muscular power is thus obtained at optimal values of force and velocity (see figure 8.1). The relationship between force, velocity, and power can be more or less accurately assessed with various protocols such as *force-velocity tests*—monoarticular dynamometry (Wilkie 1950; Perrine and Edgerton 1978) and polyarticular cycle ergometry (Vandewalle et al. 1987; Sargeant, Hoinville, and Young 1981); *stair running* (Margaria, Aghemo, and Rovelli 1966); *vertical jump tests* (Davies and Rennie 1968); and *nonmotorized treadmill running tests* (Lakomy 1984; Van Praagh et al. 1993). For recent reviews concerning this topic in pediatric populations, see also Bar-Or 1996, Rowland 1996, and Van Praagh 1996.

Monoarticular Force-Velocity Tests

Movement across a single joint (e.g., elbow or knee) can be measured with devices that control the force (dynamic) or the velocity (isokinetic) of the movement. In

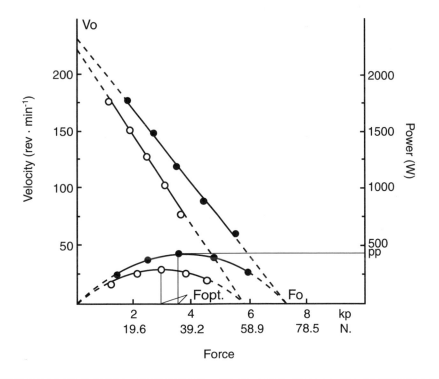

Figure 8.1 Force-velocity and force-power relationships in 12-year-old girls (o) and boys (•).

Data from Van Praagh et al. 1990.

adults, the first measurements were done via an isokinetic ergometer with monoarticular ballistic exercises such as elbow flexion or extension (Ralston et al. 1949; Wilkie 1950). (For a review, see Vandewalle et al. 1987.) This technique has several drawbacks. First, isokinetic dynamometer recordings are rarely generated under true constant angular velocity (Murray and Harrison 1986). Secondly, torque is measured throughout a range of motion at different limb velocities; in addition, Sargeant (1989) reported the difficulty of voluntarily accelerating a limb to optimal velocity for peak power output. Thirdly, there is a need to standardize the torque-velocity relationship. Some authors have reported measured torque in slow ($30° \cdot s^{-1}$) and/or fast ($300° \cdot s^{-1}$) movements. Finally, because isokinetic dynamometers are designed for adults, modification of the equipment is required to test children. Few data are available for children. Weltman et al. (1986) reported torque scores throughout the entire range of motion between the dominant and the nondominant sides in prepubertal boys. The reliability coefficients ranged from $r = 0.60$ to $r = 0.90$. Saavedra et al. (1991) reported excellent reliability and validity for repeated knee extensions and flexions in 9- to 19-year-old girls and boys. (For further discussion of this topic, see Baltzopolous and Kellis in this volume.) The maximal power measured during monoarticular exercises is clearly lower than half the maximal power measured during polyarticular exercise (Avis, Hoving, and Toussaint 1985). This is partly explained by the additional power produced by the other joints that act simultaneously during polyarticular exercise (e.g., jumping, running, kicking).

Jump Tests

The following is a discussion of two jump tests that have been used to assess leg power.

Standing Vertical Jump. The first scientific investigation of leg power, done by the French exercise physiologist E.J. Marey (Marey and Demenÿ 1885), recorded force (pneumatic force platform) and displacement during a vertical jump. (See description of the equipment in Van Praagh 1996, 605). Sargent (1921) developed the vertical jump (VJ) test to measure maximal leg power in adults. Subjects are required to jump vertically as high as they can. At the peak of the jump, the examinee marks the measuring board with chalk. The subject's ability to exert leg power is derived from the height of the jump. The best average value of the three jumps is generally taken as the test score. The VJ has been accepted as a valid measure of leg power, and various VJ protocols have been derived from the Sargent test (e.g., jump and reach test, Abalakow test; for review see Kirby 1991). The objectivity and reliability coefficients are high. Reliability coefficients of 0.91 to 0.93 suggest high intraindividual consistency (Glencross 1966).

No test-retest reliability has been reported in pediatric populations. The validity of the test, compared with the sum of four power events in track and field, is rather low ($r = 0.78$, Safrit 1990). The test does not involve high motor ability and can be easily learned by children. Norms are available (Baumgartner and Jackson 1991).

A major weakness is the lack of standardization in test administration. For instance, a countermovement increases the VJ performance by about 10% (Bosco, Luhtanen, and Komi 1983), probably because of the more relevant participation of muscle elasticity. Moreover, a more rapid elevation of the arms also improves the height of a VJ. The Lewis nomogram test has been designed to be used concomitantly with the Sargent Jump. One must remember that the Sargent Jump has the dimension of work (force · distance). The aim of the Lewis nomogram is to add "velocity" to the body mass and the vertical distance performed. This kind of artificial manipulation cannot be taken into consideration for research purposes. In addition, Harman et al. (1991) conducted a validation study on male adults and concluded that the Lewis formula does not provide an accurate estimate of muscle leg power.

Sophisticated instrumentation (force platform plus computer analysis) allows the recording of the ground reaction forces and of acceleration of the body's center of mass. Peak power output is calculated from the product of instantaneous force exerted by the subject on the force platform and the acceleration of the body's center of mass. Use of the force platform technique improves the validity of the test. In a study of children, Davies and Young (1984) found a high correlation ($r = 0.92$) between the height of a VJ and the data obtained on the force platform. Recently, Ferretti et al. (1994) measured maximal leg power in children aged 8 to 13 (see table 8.1) using the method described by Davies and Rennie (1968). However, the jump started from a squatting position in order to minimize countermovements (see figure 8.2). The velocity was obtained by time integration of the instantaneous acceleration, which is equal to the ratio of force to subject's mass.

In 1983, Bosco, Luhtanen, and Komi presented a VJ test that measured the muscular power of the leg extensors. The authors criticized the Margaria and Wingate

Table 8.1   Representative Values of Jump Power and Jump Height Performance in Girls and Boys

Age (yrs)	Sex	Ergometer	Power (W)	Power (W · kg⁻¹)	Height (cm)	v max (ms)	Ref.
11	G and B	Force plate	711	18.1	-	200	Davies & Young 1984
8 to 13	G and B	Force plate	1103	31.6	-	4	Ferretti et al. 1994
7 to 17	B	Squat	-	-	20 to 32	280-320	Bosco 1991
8 to 13	G	Jump			16 to 23		

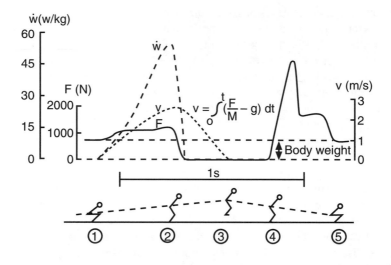

Figure 8.2 Time courses of instantaneous force (F, solid line), velocity (v, dotted line), and power (w, dashed line) during a maximal vertical jump on a force platform.

Adapted from Ferretti et al. 1987.

tests in that they did not make it possible to evaluate any functional-morphological characteristics of particular importance for the development of leg explosive power, such as the elastic property of the muscle. The test consists of jumping vertically from a static squatting position with a knee angle of 90°. Subjects keeps their hands on their hips throughout the entire jump. Each jump is recorded on a magnetic tape, and a vertical force-time curve produced by each jump is analyzed by computer (Komi and Bosco 1978). For field purposes, it is easy to monitor leg power using a digital timer and a contact mat (Bosco and Komi 1980). It was assumed that the stretch-shortening cycle that occurs during this type of jump allowed the stored elastic energy to be utilized during positive work and thus increased the vertical performance. In athletes, the test showed a high correlation ($r = 0.86$) when leg muscle power, expressed as a percentage of fast-twitch fibers, was related to the power calculated from the squat jump. Reliability coefficients ranged between $r = 0.90$ and $r = 0.95$.

Standing Broad Jump. Because of its easy execution and administration, the standing broad jump (SBJ) test is often used instead of the VJ as a measure of leg muscle power. The problem with all field-based assessments is that the tests do not reflect a single factor (leg power, in this case) but also learning, coordination, and maturation. The test appears to be objective as well as reliable, but the validity is questionable. Coefficients of 0.79 between SBJ and VJ assume that either SBJ or VJ can be used as a criterion measure for the other. Docherty (1996) asserts that no studies have examined the specific issue of validity for either test. The test is feasible for girls and boys from 6 years on (Council of Europe 1988). Normative data are available for both age and sex groups (American Alliance for Health, Physical Education and Recreation 1975).

Running Tests

The tests that follow have been implemented to measure running velocity.

Field Tests. *30-50 Sprints*. Historically in the United States and in Europe, as well as in most other countries, physical educators and coaches have used a 30-50 m dash as a measure of running velocity. The test is easy to administer and can be done indoors or outdoors, and pediatric populations can be assessed in a short time. This simple test enables one to categorize subjects as "slow," "medium slow," or "rapid." However, it cannot be considered a "real" power test, according to Wilkie (1950), as the force component is not measured. Generally, logical (face) validity is accepted for this test (Johnson and Nelson, 1986). In the author's laboratory, we compared the peak power ($W \cdot kg^{-1}$) measured by the cycle force-velocity test with a 30 m dash in a group of 7- and 12-year-old girls and boys. All in all, the correlation was rather high ($r = 0.80$, $p < 0.001$), but it was significantly lower when only the girls' results were analyzed (Van Praagh et al. 1990). The higher fat mass in girls may partially explain their handicap in running velocity at that age. Reliability coefficients of 0.66 to 0.94 (only for boys) have been reported. Learning effects for this test seem to have not been investigated.

30 s Shuttle Run. In this test, the child runs to and fro (20 m for each lap). The average velocity is calculated from the distance covered in 30 s. Nonsignificant differences in peak blood lactate could be observed between the 30 s Wingate and the 30 s shuttle run test, suggesting that the field test was a rather strenuous effort for 12-year-old girls and boys (Van Praagh et al. 1990; Falgairette et al. 1994). The reproducibility of this test has not yet been investigated.

Laboratory Tests. There are four main laboratory tests used to measure running velocity and short-term power output in children and adolescents. The representative values for running power in girls and boys are presented in table 8.2.

1. *Sprinting upstairs.* Margaria, Aghemo, and Rovelli (1966) were the first to measure short-term power during upstairs running (first quantitative power test in children). Untrained girls and boys 10 to 15 years old were investigated. The authors measured the vertical component of the maximum constant speed by having subjects run up a staircase for 4-5 s. Body mass (kg) of the subject represented the external force. To measure the power output, the time recorded was about 400-500 ms. For additional information, see recent reviews (Bar-Or 1996; Van Praagh 1996).

Table 8.2   Representative Values of Running Power in Girls and Boys

Age (years)	Sex	Ergometer	Power (W)	Power (W · kg⁻¹)	Ref.
4 to 7 Longitudinal	G and B	Staircase	17.8	1.1	Amano et al. 1983
			50.4	2.8	
			98.9	4.7	
			178.3	7.6	
10	G and B	Staircase	294	9.8	Margaria et al. 1966
8 to 14 Longitudinal	G and B	Nonmotorized treadmill	161 to 434	5.5 to 8.4	Fargeas et al. 1993

Statistically significant ($p < 0.05$) sex differences were found in absolute maximal anaerobic power between males and females at ages 11 and 15 years. No significant sex differences were observed when maximal anaerobic power was expressed relative to body mass. It was concluded that psychomotor, biomechanical, and/or biochemical changes that occur in children of these ages contribute to fairly linear increases in absolute maximal anaerobic power up to approximately age 13. After that age the values for boys continue to increase, while those for girls level off (Davies, Barnes, and Godfrey 1972). Despite the statements made by Margaria, Aghemo, and Rovelli (1966), the test's results may be influenced by factors like skill of climbing at maximal velocity and leg length, stride pattern, and body mass. In young children, because of risk of injury in taking two steps at a time, the administrator might consider the 30 m dash, discussed earlier, as an alternative. The intraindividual variation of the test is rather large (about 15%) compared with cycle or force platform measurements (around 4% and 7%, respectively; Davies and Young 1984).

2. *Acceleration in sprint running.* The effects of various training regimes on anaerobic power and the possible transfer of training among the different types were examined by Nielsen et al. (1980). A total of 249 girls, ages 7-19, took part in the training experiments. Subject made a standing start and ran 10 m as fast as possible. Running velocity was measured by means of three adjustable photocell systems placed at hip height. Accelerations were calculated using the time recordings from the cells placed at 0.2 and 4 m from the starting line. In this study, the actual contraction times were very short (200-300 ms) in both the VJ and fast stepping during the sprint start. In girls, but not in pubescent boys (Asmussen 1973), the acceleration in sprint running was independent of height; this is in contrast to what occurs with VJ performance, which increases with

height. All types of training improved performance except in acceleration.

3. *Motorized treadmill running.* In a longitudinal study, Paterson and Cunningham (1985) measured 19 boys over 5 years (mean age 10.8 to 14.9 years). Subjects performed a treadmill run designed to estimate "anaerobic capacity." The boys ran at a 20% grade at speeds ranging from 7.8 km · h^{-1} (in 10-11-year-olds) to 11.9 km · h^{-1} (in 14-15-year-olds). Treadmill time to exhaustion (which ranged from 80 to 100 s according to the different age groups), postexercise blood lactate levels, and O_2 debt served as "anaerobic capacity" indexes. One drawback of this method is that it can measure only the "anaerobic" endurance performance. Only speed is recorded; the force component cannot be measured, and thus power cannot be calculated. The reliability coefficients of the test ranged from $r = 0.76$ at age 10 to $r = 0.84$ at age 15.

4. *Nonmotorized horizontal treadmill running.* Several methods have been used to study the mechanics of running. Force plates have been applied since the early 20th century ("trottoir dynamographique" of Amar 1920) to study ground reaction forces. Film or video analysis is convenient for recording displacements. In adults, attempts have been made to measure maximal velocity and power output during maximal short-term running on a nonmotorized treadmill (Lakomy 1987). The same methodology was used in our laboratory to examine short-term power output (< 10 s) in untrained and trained children (Van Praagh et al. 1993). Fargeas (1993) studied the longitudinal running and cycling power of 38 girls and boys aged 8-14. The subject develops maximal velocity while connected to a belt at the waist. The belt, which is attached to a horizontal bar, is connected to a potentiometer (vertical displacement) and strain gauges (horizontal traction force). A constant-torque motor installed in the rear wheel of the treadmill is not used to drive the treadmill but to compensate for belt friction or to simulate various loads. Signals from the potentiometer, the transducer, and the treadmill (belt speed) allow one to calculate the mechanical power (potential + kinetic power).

This test seems promising for the measurement of an individual's running muscle power. Performing on a cycle ergometer is ideal for the cyclist but has less practical value for runners or participants in game sports (Saltin 1990). In adults, Lakomy (1987) reported reliability coefficients of $r = 0.93$. Fargeas et al. (1993) studied the validity of the test in comparing it with the force-velocity test ($r = 0.94$). Cycling power performed during the force-velocity test was found to be significantly higher ($p < 0.001$) than running power on the treadmill. Moreover, no learning effects were observed during the force-velocity test, but a significant learning effect ($p < 0.05$) was observed (test-retest) during running on the treadmill.

Cycling Tests

External leg (or arm) power can be assessed on a cycle ergometer by measuring the velocity of cycling (v) for a given braking force (N). This method is used by the popular Wingate test (WAnT). Power can also be measured by determining the relationship between force and velocity, as is done in the force-velocity test.

Arm Cycling.   As early as 1883, Speck (Germany) used a hand cranking device to measure anaerobic arm performances in adults. Few data are available for children. Blimkie et al. (1988) reported anaerobic peak and mean power of arms in girls and boys 14 to 19 years of age. Peak power and local muscle endurance determined during arm cranking (Wingate protocol) increased for boys but not for girls during the adolescent period. Recently, Nindl et al. (1995) measured upper-body anaerobic power in male and female adolescent athletes. The WAnT was administered to assess peak and average power. Peak arm power normalized for body mass, fat free mass, and cross-sectional area was significantly higher in boys than in girls.

Leg Cycling.   In April 1897, Elysée Bouny (France) described the first mechanically braked cycle ergometer. This equipment was able to measure simultaneously the variations of the cranking force and the velocity of the legs (see table 8.3 for the results of leg cycling power tests in children) and thus to measure cranking power. At about the same time, Atwater and Benedict (1897) used a cycle ergometer, electrically braked by a small dynamo generator, in a caloric chamber to measure energy used during exercise. In adults, sprint tests on cycle ergometers have been performed since 1913 (Benedict and Cathcart, n.d.).

The following are four such tests:

1. *30 s Wingate test.* Cumming (1973) was the first to investigate short-term power on a cycle ergometer in 12- to 17-year-old children (the 30 s cycling test). This supramaximal test was presented for the first time during the Fourth International Symposium on Pediatric Work Physiology held in Israel. The absolute braking force to overcome was 4 to 4.5 kg (39.2 to 44.1 N) for girls and boys, respectively. This test was later developed by the researchers of the Wingate Institute (Bar-Or 1987, 1996; Inbar, Bar-Or, and Skinner n.d.). The subject pedals on a cycle ergometer at a maximal velocity against a constant braking force for 30 s; the constant braking force has been predetermined to produce mechanical power equivalent to two to three times the metabolic power obtained during $\dot{V}O_2$ max test. Peak power reflects the ability of the leg muscles to produce short-term mechanical power, whereas mean power or total work represents the local muscle endurance of the legs. For further information concerning the WAnT protocol, the reader can consult recent reviews (Van Praagh 1996; Rowland 1996). The Wingate test has been examined more extensively than any other anaerobic performance test for several pediatric populations (abled, disabled, trained) and found to be highly valid and reliable. Test-retest reliability coefficients ranged from 0.89 to 0.97 (Bar-Or 1987; Tirosh, Rosenbaum, and Bar-Or 1990). Representative values in children are available (Bar-Or 1996).

Table 8.3   Representative Values of Leg Cycling Power in Girls and Boys

Age (years)	Sex	Ergometer	Power (W)	Power ($W \cdot kg^{-1}$)	Ref.
7	B	Frictional	146	5.8	Van Praagh 1990
12	B	Frictional	280	-	Bar-Or 1978
12	G B	Frictional	310 415	7.4 9.7	Van Praagh 1990
11	G and B	Isokinetic	1283	32.7	Davies & Young 1984

2. *20 s isokinetic cycling test.* To obtain "true" maximal power output, it is essential to match the external load to the capability of the active muscles so that they operate at their optimal velocity. Since the velocity in constant-force anaerobic tests is progressively reduced due to muscle fatigue, these conditions are hard to fulfill. To overcome this shortcoming, Sargeant, Hoinville, and Young (1981) developed an isokinetic cycle ergometer that maintains velocity at a constant level throughout the test. The level of peak force is inversely and linearly related to crank velocity over the range studied. In children, the intraindividual variation of the peak force was found to be < 6% (Sargeant, Dolan, and Thorne 1984).

3. *Sprint cycling tests.* The first cycle ergometer tests used either standard braking forces (Katch, Weltman, and Traeger 1976) or forces related to body mass (Ayalon, Inbar, and Bar-Or 1974). However, according to Wilkie's rationale (maximal power = optimal forces · optimal velocities), one cannot accurately measure maximal power with standard braking force (whether related to body mass or not). Therefore, Maréchal et al. (1979) and Pirnay and Crielaard (1979) developed a cycle sprint test. The subject performed several all-out sprints (5 to 7 s) on a Monark cycle ergometer. Increased loads (from 3 to 7 kp) were applied. After each short sprint (n = 5) the subject recovered for 3 min. The authors investigated 11-year-old boys (average peak power: 7.6 W · kg^{-1}) and 19-year-old male adults (10.1 W· kg^{-1}). The highest value of peak power was assumed to correspond to peak power. This test was the precursor of the actual force-velocity test (FVT).

4. *5-10 s force-velocity cycling test.* In adults, Pérès, Vandewalle, and Monod (1981) on a friction-loaded ergometer, and Sargeant, Hoinville, and Young (1981) on an isokinetic cycle ergometer, observed that cycling velocity decreased linearly as a function of increasing loads. In contrast to the situation in the in vitro studies, in which the relationship between force and velocity is exponential (Fenn and Marsh 1935) or hyperbolic (Hill 1938), in polyarticular cycling exercises, linear force-velocity and parabolic force-power relationships have generally been obtained in adults (Vandewalle et al. 1987), as in children (Van Praagh et al. 1989). Recently, Bar-Or (1996) reviewed the advantages of the FVT. However, the 30 min total time required (five sprints interspersed with 3 min recovery) for completion is great. In the author's laboratory, a high correlation ($r = 0.93$, $p < 0.001$) was found between peak power measured in young boys during the FVT and that obtained with the WAnT, suggesting that both tests measure the same factor (Van Praagh et al. 1990). C. Williams (unpublished data) examined the test-retest reliability of the FVT performed by 9-year-old boys. A significant correlation ($r = 0.80$, $p < 0.05$) was found for peak power. Correlations between other dependent variables, however, ranged from $r = 0.58$ to $r = 0.86$. The coefficient of variation of peak power was about 12%.

Testing of Athletic Power (MSTAP)

Athletic power refers to the forces or torques generated during sport activities. Their assessment can be used for talent identification, to observe the effects of training programs, and to evaluate the relative significance of power to particular athletic performances (Abernethy, Wilson, and Logan 1995).

Throwing Tests

Throwing power has traditionally been measured in field conditions with throwing tests such as ball-throwing or medicine ball put tests (see Kirby 1991). In such "power" tests, it is assumed that the best distance attained reflects anaerobic arm power.

In 1988, Viitasalo developed a new test to measure throwing velocity of balls with different masses. In this test the subject threw balls of the same diameter, but of different masses (from 0.3 to 4.0 kg), through a photocell gate to a $0.4 \cdot 0.4$ m contact mat hanging on a wall. The throws were randomly performed from a standing position with both hands held over the head while the feet were kept parallel. Flight time and distance between the photocell gate and the contact mat were used to calculate the velocity of the ball. Mass-velocity relationships could be established and could allow power discriminations as a function of age and sport practice (see figure 8.3). The test was found to be reliable for 10- to 12-year-old subjects, and the reliability of the test increased with age. Moreover, the throwing test had rather high correlations with the respective traditional field tests.

The seated shot put (SSP) test has been proposed in recent years to assess upper-body power in field testing (Gillespie and Keenum 1987). The SSP test was administered by having subjects sit on the floor with their backs against a support. The knees were flexed at a right angle, and the feet applied firm pressure backward. A 4.5 kg indoor shot was grasped with both hands and pushed from the center of the chest. The score was the achievement of maximum distance. Validity correlations between a constant-load bench press power test and the SSP ranged between r = 0.57 (Gillespie and Keenum 1987) and r = 0.73 (Mayhew et al., unpublished data) in young adults. However, the SPP test was only moderately related to upper-body power in adolescent wrestlers (Mayhew, Bemben, and Rohrs 1992).

Kicking Tests

Studies on pediatric populations practicing sports that are popular worldwide, such as soccer, rugby, or American football, have mostly focused on learning technical skills and motor abilities. Some research has been done on assessment of the power of specific muscles involved during maximal in-step kicking, for example. Observations have been made especially with respect to the relationship between isokinetic testing and maximal ball-kicking velocity (Cabri et al. 1988; Mognoni et al. 1994). Seventeen-year-old soccer players were asked to perform three maximal in-step kicks with a run-up of two steps. To calculate the ball velocity, the two sounds generated by the impact of the ball against the foot and against the square barrier

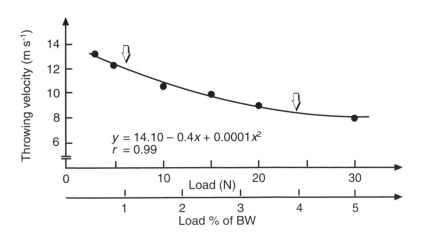

Figure 8.3 Throwing velocity of a 14-year-old boy for six different loads. Arrows indicate velocity values of 1% and 40% body mass.

Adapted from Viitasalo et al. 1992.

were recorded on a tape recorder. The highest attained velocity was used for analysis. Players chose the limb they considered to be the dominant one. The authors concluded that for both knee extensor and hip flexor muscles, isokinetic torques are poor predictors of ball-kicking velocity. The latter variable is nevertheless considered one of the main factors that determine global performances in all ball-kicking events.

Hopping Tests

The power output measured during running or jumping events not only estimates the power of the chemomechanical conversion, but also gives information regarding the mechanical energy stored in the elastic elements of the muscles involved (Cavagna, Saibene, and Margaria 1965). Although this topic is extremely interesting in relation to the habitual activity of the child (various motor tasks on playgrounds) or during specific youth training sessions (e.g., bouncing or hopping drills in track and field training), very few research reports are available. In 9-year-old boys, Moritani et al. (1989) investigated neural and biomechanical variables during fast and maximal hopping tasks on a force platform. The hopping exercises represent a cyclical motor task, with repeated stretch-shortening cycles of the leg extensor muscles. The children were asked to hop on both legs, with either the fastest possible frequency (FAST) or the maximal height in each jump (MAX). Each trial lasted about 10-15 s. The order of the trials was randomized. A rest interval of 1-2 min was allowed between trials. The mechanical power (normalized to body mass) was significantly higher for adults than for boys during maximal hopping (26 W · kg^{-1} vs. 15.4 W · kg^{-1}, p < 0.01). However, as shown in figure 8.4, during fast hopping the boys

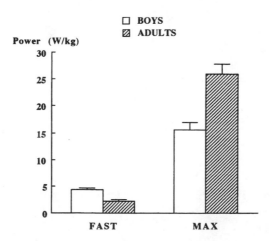

Figure 8.4 Mechanical power (normalized to body mass) during fast and maximal hopping in boys and adults.

Adapted from Moritani et al. 1989.

generated significantly higher power than the adults (4.3 W · kg⁻¹ vs. 2.3 W · kg⁻¹, p < 0.01). During MAX hopping, when the adults and boys were compared there was a significantly larger potentiation of leg muscle activity in the adults, particularly in the eccentric phase. However, there were striking similarities between boys and adults with respect to the potentiation of muscle activity during the concentric phase. Therefore, selective neural control of the leg muscles involved appears to be manifested in prepubertal boys. Conversely, the utilization of stored elastic energy and stretch reflex potentiation is age dependent.

Vertical Rebound Tests

The squat jump allows accurate and consistent testing of leg power. However, increasing demands in limits to training and more knowledge of muscle mechanics, when added together, have permitted the development of other very specific athletic power tests.

With the countermovement jump (CMJ) test (with added masses), Viitasalo et al. (1992) examined a voluntary sample of more than 300 male adolescent athletes ranging in age from 9 to 16 years and representing six sports events. After a warm-up, each subject performed three to five maximal CMJs with each of four different barbell loads. For the smallest children, the loads were 2, 50, 100, and 150 N, while the older children had to overcome loads of 2, 100, 200, and 400 N. Jumping height (the height of rise of the body's center of gravity = hCG) was calculated using the flight time (t) of the jump and the following formula:

$$hCG = \frac{t^2 - g}{8} \text{, where } g = 9.81 \text{ m·s}^{-2}$$

The flight time was measured using a digital timer and a contact mat (Bosco 1980). In a previous study (Viitasalo 1988), the coefficients of variation between determinations of the test in its present form decreased with age from 13% at 10 years of age to 6% at 16 years. It is noteworthy that the quantity of training had no effect on vertical jumping height. Conversely, subjects who trained more achieved better throwing results. One possible explanation for this finding is that much of the training concentrated especially on the lower limbs. The test may be considered reliable for young males age 12 and older. Moreover, it shows significantly high correlations with traditional jumping field tests. However, the authors did not give any information concerning possible injuries, especially during maturation.

In the drop jump, the subject drops from heights of 0.2 to 0.8 m onto a force platform with a subsequent upward jump. The young athlete is to keep his/her hands on hips throughout the entire jump. The tolerance to progressive dropping height increases from childhood up to the age of 20-25 years (Bosco and Komi 1980). It is therefore strongly recommended that the young athlete be protected against high stretch loads, especially when ossification processes have not been totally achieved.

In repeated rebound jumps, Bosco, Luhtanen, and Komi (1983) proposed a 5 to 15 s VJ test in order to measure mechanical leg power (W · kg⁻¹). In children aged 5 to 10, a 5 s test is sufficient. In adolescents (11 to 16 years), the duration can be increased to 10-15 s. It was shown (Bosco 1992) that the 5-15 RRJ test is very relevant and sensitive to neuromuscular adaptations induced by training in relation to individual characteristics and the specific sport activity practiced (more specifically, all jump activities: basketball, volleyball, high jump, ice hockey, alpine skiing, sprinting). The purpose is to assess mean leg power or total work of a subject during a series of VJs on a force platform or a contact mat. The child stands on the contact mat and begins performing as many VJs as possible in 5 or 60 s. The performance is derived by plugging the total flight time and total number of jumps into a formula (Bosco, Luhtanen, and Komi 1983). A high degree of logical validity was found in athletic populations (basketball or volleyball players), but the test lacks validity as a general power test. Even if it is suitable for males from age 16 years on, the reliability needs to be established for pediatric populations.

Power Diagnosis and Athletic Performance

There is little published material correlating anaerobic power indexes with athletic performance. This is surprising, as such information allows us to understand whether short-term power output has any relationship to an athletic event.

Anaerobic Scope

World records indicate the highest outputs of which human beings are capable. Unfortunately, scientists are not yet able to measure effective muscular power output during competitions. Wilkie (1960) argued that the theoretical limit of power output for an Olympic champion specialized in short events (sprinter, jumper, thrower) should be around 6 hp (>4400 W). For a typical individual (70 kg of body mass), this value represents a theoretical relative power output of around 60 W · kg⁻¹. Recently, Grassi et al. (1991) reported figures for 20-year-old power athletes who were able to achieve more than 6500 W during a VJ. Again for a typical subject, this means an actual value of about 90 W · kg⁻¹. The power scale (see table 8.4) shows an increase from approximately 150 W at age 7 to 6500 W for a highly trained 20-year-old power athlete (40-fold increase). However, when corrected for body mass, the maximal anaerobic power (about 30 W · kg⁻¹) of the typical child is approximately 30% of power athlete values. These data agree with observations done in 1984 by Davies and Young. This also indicates that anaerobic performance not only is age and sex related, but also depends on exercise duration, the muscle group involved, and the ergometer (inertia of the device) used.

Table 8.4   Anaerobic Scope in Children as a Function of Age, Sex, and Type of Exercise

Sex/age	Activity (ergometer)	Duration (s)	Power (W)	Power (W · kg⁻¹)	Ref.
B/7 yr	Cycling (frictional)	>10	146	5.8	Van Praagh et al. 1990
G&B/8 yr	Running (nonmotorized treadmill)	<10	197	6.8	Fargeas et al. 1993
B/12	Cycling (frictional)	5	280	-	Bar-Or 1978
G/12 yr	Cycling (frictional)	5-8	310	7.4	Van Praagh et al. 1990
G&B/10-15 yr	Running upstairs	4-5	400	10.0	Margaria et al. 1966
B/12 yr	Cycling (frictional)	5-8	415	9.7	Van Praagh et al. 1990
G&B/11 yr	Vert jumping (force platform)	.02	711	18.1	Davies & Young 1984
B/8-13 yr	Vert jumping (force platform)	<0.01	1103	31.6	Ferretti et al. 1994
G&B/11 yr	Cycling (isokinetic)	Single revolution (0.02)	1283	32.7	Davies & Young 1984
Power Athlete/20 yr	Vert jumping	<0.01	>6500	90.0	Grassi et al. 1991

Talent Identification

The issue to be addressed here is whether results on anaerobic power tests predict athletic performance. The following discussion will attempt to flesh this out.

Prediction of Athletic Performance

In 1968, di Prampero et al. (1970) investigated 116 male athletes (age range 16-38) during the Olympic Games in Mexico City. Maximal anaerobic power was measured during upstairs running according to the method of Margaria (Margaria, Aghemo, and Rovelli 1966). Mean absolute values of 4500-5000 W were observed in pentathletes and sprinters. However, in relative terms (W · kg^{-1} body mass) this test did not discriminate between long distance runners and middle distance runners or sprinters. These results are disappointing, but also reveal that performance predictions from tests batteries are not necessarily relevant. In the case of meaningful correlations, it is possible to determine whether differences in power discriminate between individuals or whether power indexes can be used to predict future performance (Abernethy, Wilson, and Logan 1995). Therefore, the limited number of scientific papers correlating power indexes with athletic performance during growth is somewhat surprising.

Åstrand (1992) reported a study done on the five best Swedish male tennis players (Carlson and Engström 1986). The subjects had been all-around participants in sports before the age of 14 and had started to specialize in tennis at age 14. They were compared with a group of players who had specialized earlier in tennis, trained more, matured earlier, and had better performances at ages 12-14. A conclusion that could be drawn from this study is that performance at age 12-14 was not a good predictor of future elite achievements.

Most investigations concerned with prediction have been conducted on heterogeneous rather than homogenous populations. For recent review, see Matsudo (1996). The following five tests have addressed issues of prediction:

1. *Isokinetic monoarticular test.* Berg, Miller, and Stephens (1986) concluded that sprint ability of 12-year-old boys was not related to knee torque production at 30° · s^{-1} and 300° · s^{-1}.

2. *30 s leg cycling (WAnT).* Cumming (1973) reported that the 30 s leg cycling test proved to be a disappointing predictor of track and field events. Short-term cycling power proved to be a significant predictor (r = 0.55) only for the 100 yd run and for the long jump (r = 0.69) in 15-year-old boys. Bar-Or (1987) reviewed a few studies in which performance in the Wingate test was correlated with performance in sprint running, sprint swimming, short-term ice skating, and vertical jumping. Correlations ranged from r = 0.32 to r = 0.90. Bar-Or concluded that the correlation between the power indexes and performance tasks is quite high, but not high enough to warrant use of the Wingate test as a predictor of athletic performances.

3. *Force-velocity running test.* In her longitudinal study on pubescent female and male athletes, Fargeas (1993) concluded that the FVT could not predict specific performance in young elite tennis players.

4. *VJ test.* In 16-year-old male volleyball players, Bosco (1992) observed a significant correlation between Bosco's CMJ test and a 60 m running perfor-

mance (s) (r = −.75, p < .001). Considering that performance of a fast run depends to a large extent on muscle elasticity, assessment of elastic potential during short-term weight-bearing activities has real practical application in many sports.

5. *Short-term running test.* Seiler et al. (1990) investigated anaerobic power in 41 American football players. Typically, football programs include only the 40 yd dash, VJ, and SBJ in their performance evaluations. Therefore, a more complete battery of tests, purported to measure anaerobic power, included VJ (Lewis formula), standing long jump, standing five-jump test, 40 yd dash with 5 yd increment, the WAnT, and the Margaria stair test. Multiple comparisons showed that while backs and linebackers were similar in power output (W · kg⁻¹) and performance scores, linemen exhibited significantly lower relative power output. Common variance between average velocity after 5 yd and average velocity in a running-start 35 yd dash was only 0.41. Considering that the quality of initial acceleration is critical in American football, it was suggested that the commonly used 40 yd dash is a poor predictor of initial acceleration and therefore not specific to the demands of most positions on a collegiate football team.

Comparing the Best Performances of Children to Adult World Records

Best performances obtained during track and field competitions are valid with respect to the individual's potential and are mostly highly reliable (e.g., control of wind speed, accurate distances). This is, of course, also the case in other individual sports (swimming, cycling, etc.), but more difficult to assess in game sports.

Maximal Athletic Performance During Growth.   As an example of maximal anaerobic performances we report the performances obtained by 9- to 18-year-old girls and boys during the United States Junior Olympic Championships in table 8.5a and b. Figures 8.5 and 8.6 show a remarkable regular growth curve in all short-term performances between ages 10 and 18 in both sexes.

Child-Adult Comparisons.   As an example of comparison between children and adults, we studied 10-year-old U.S. champions and world record athletes (mean age 22 years). Table 8.6a and b, shows an increase of about 25% in sprint performances between the 10-year-old gifted athletes and the 22-year-old world record holders (100-400 m). This observation is in line with the work done by Rowland and Cunningham (unpublished data).

In a 5-year longitudinal study of 10 boys and 8 girls, Rowland and Cunningham found a progressive improvement in 50 yd dash performance in both sexes. Improvement in sprint performances over the 5 years was 14.2% in boys and 10.5% in girls. Thus the prediction that high-performance sprinting will improve by about 25% in 10 years in both sexes seems a rather reasonable one. However, the child-adult difference in jumping performances is strikingly more important (between

Table 8.5a   Track and Field Performances of 9- to 18- Year-Old American Girls

Girls	9-10	11-12	13-14	15-16	17-18
100 m (s)	14.04	13.16	12.11	11.96	12.18
200 m (s)	28.17	26.57	24.70	24.41	24.64
400 m (s)	63.61	58.35	56.73	56.86	56.12
High jump (m)	1.40	1.51	1.62	1.67	1.72
Long jump (m)	4.13	4.78	5.31	5.66	5.73

Table 8.5b   Track and Field Performances of 9- to 18- Year-Old American Boys

Boys	9-10	11-12	13-14	15-16	17-18
100 m (s)	13.39	12.15	11.58	10.72	10.92
200 m (s)	27.21	24.57	23.06	21.62	21.66
400 m (s)	59.15	54.77	51.97	48.59	47.37
High jump (m)	1.43	1.65	1.82	1.95	2.13
Long jump (m)	4.35	5.62	6.41	6.93	7.20

30% and 50%), suggesting that the marked increase in body dimensions and muscle mass after puberty (especially in boys) is a more determinant factor than velocity alone in these activities. Young subjects become more powerful after puberty (see figure 8.7a and b, on page 180).

Which Tests to Use?

During childhood, the power measured in a test may not necessarily correspond to the "true" maximal power because of several factors: (1) motivation and learning, (2) optimal force to attain a maximal value, (3) measurement of mean power instead of instantaneous power, (4) measurement of power at a time when muscular power is no longer maximal, (5) failure to take into account inertia of the devices (Doré et al. 1997). For review on this topic, see Vandewalle et al. 1987.

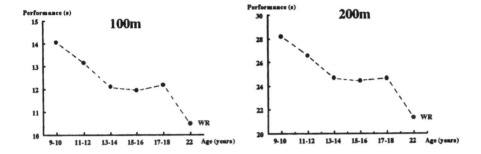

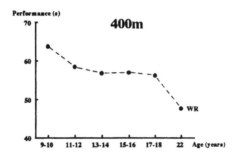

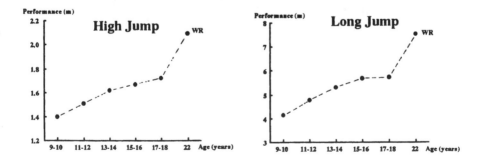

Figure 8.5 Growth curves of short-term athletic performances in girls.

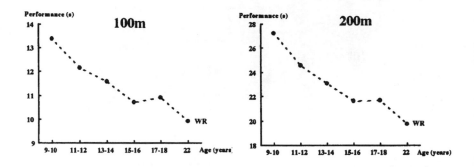

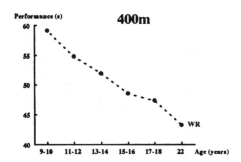

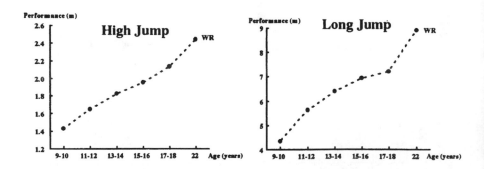

Figure 8.6 Growth curves of short-term athletic performances in boys.

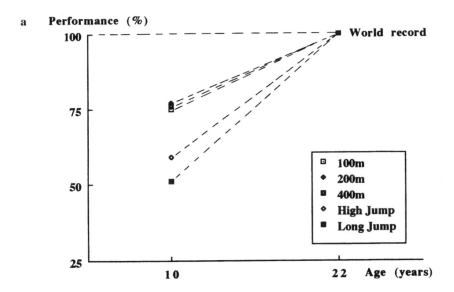

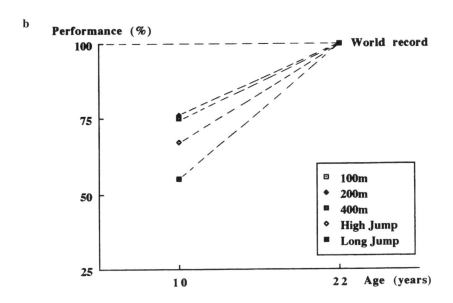

Figure 8.7 Elite child-adult comparisons: 10-year-old girls (a) and boys (b) (U.S. track and field champions) vs. 22-year-old women and men (world record holders, 1989), respectively.

Table 8.6a   Best Performances of a 10-Year-Old U.S. Champion Girl Compared with a Female World Record Holder

	10-year-old girl (1989)	22-year-old female world record holder (1989)	Performance difference (%)
100 m (s)	14.04	10.49	25
200 m (s)	28.17	21.34	24
400 m (s)	63.61	47.60	25
High jump (m)	1.40	2.09	33
Long jump (m)	4.13	7.52	45

Table 8.6b   Best Performances of a 10-Year-Old U.S. Champion Boy Compared with a Male World Record Holder

	10-year-old boy (1989)	22-year-old male world record holder (1989)	Performance difference (%)
100 m (s)	13.39	9.92	26
200 m (s)	27.21	19.72	28
400 m (s)	59.15	43.29	27
High jump (m)	1.43	2.44	41
Long jump (m)	4.35	8.90	51

Field Testing

The goal of any test is to measure the subject's highest potential. Review of the literature indicates (see the section on anaerobic scope earlier in this chapter) that among all available tests, the highest anaerobic performance during growth (> 30 $W \cdot kg^{-1}$) is attained similarly by means of an isokinetic cycle test (Davies and Young 1984) and a VJ force platform test (Ferretti et al. 1994). These maximal values measured during childhood represent approximately 30% of maximal adult values. Davies and Young (1984) reported that peak power achieved by children during isokinetic cycling was 45% higher than during vertical jumping. But, as could be demonstrated by Ferretti et al. (1987), when maximal instantaneous muscular power can be assessed on a time basis of only 0.004 s, that is, an interval 50 times shorter than during the procedure proposed by Davies and Rennie (1968) and 1000-1500 times shorter than that for the Margaria test (1960), the anaerobic performance of the child during vertical jumping is very close to the maximal values obtained during isokinetic cycling. Therefore, with respect to its simplicity and high validity and reliability, the VJ test remains a suitable field and laboratory test for leg muscle power. Unfortunately, there is a general lack of standardization in the way the VJ test is conducted. Some testers allow children to start from an upright position and do countermovements (Davies and Young 1984); they can therefore jump higher and generate more power (elastic energy utilization). Other investigators ask the child to use a squatting starting position in order to minimize the unavoidable negative work done by the legs at the onset of the jump. Difference in jump performance between the two procedures can be about 5-10% in favor of the CMJ. Although the Lewis formula and nomogram test has been used increasingly by physical educators and coaches, this formula does not provide accurate estimates of peak power output (Harman et al. 1991). With respect to the strengths and weaknesses of the various power tests used in pediatric work, as already discussed, we recommend the Bosco test (see discussion earlier in this chapter for the methodology) for practical and research purposes.

Laboratory Testing

Not only must the choice of a test address scientific measurement aspects (validity, reliability, objectivity), but the results obtained must also be carefully interpreted. The following questions must be raised: Which muscle group is to be tested (arm or leg power)? What kind of anaerobic power is to be investigated (peak power or local muscle endurance)? Is the duration of the test short enough to avoid fatigue, which irremediably reduces power? If maximum power output is to be measured, then the external load must be optimally matched with the capability of the active muscles to operate at their optimal velocity. Only the force-velocity and power-velocity relationships constructed by means of isokinetic (constant velocity) or dynamic (constant force) muscle contractions on suitable ergometers fulfill these conditions. However, these conditions cannot be met in freely accelerating or decelerating cycle or running protocols (for further discussion see Sargeant 1992). The Wingate test has been used more extensively than probably any other anaerobic performance test. However, this practical test has some methodological shortcomings. First, the WAnT, like the Margaria or the Sargent test, does not provide information on the force-velocity components of muscle power. Secondly, the optimal force selected for the WAnT is based on total body mass and therefore does not take into account the active muscle mass. Standardization for active muscle mass is particularly important in children during growth, in subjects who are obese, and in children with a neuromuscular disease. Thirdly, during the WAnT, peak power is measured by only one experimental value, whereas during the FVT at least three to five experimental plots are necessary to measure peak power. Finally, power output must be measured at a time when muscular power is still maximal. This is the case only during ballistic exercises, such as monoarticular FVTs and VJ tests. Recent advances in technology allow researchers to measure, over a few milliseconds, maximal instantaneous muscle leg power in children (Ferretti et al. 1994). Although more insights are available in muscle power testing, it should be mentioned that researchers must also take into account the specificity of human movements. Anaerobic power in young cyclists must be evaluated by a specific and accurate cycle test. In this case, the use of a valid and reliable jump test can give misleading results.

Directions for Future Research

There is a lack of published reports on anaerobic performance during childhood, which is surprising because of the importance of anaerobic performance in daily exercise and sport skills. Therefore, for future research the following suggestions are proposed:

- Because of ethical restrictions and methodological limitations, there is a need for noninvasive technologies in pediatric research. Biochemical investigations of children's muscle during exercise can now be pursued using nuclear magnetic resonance spectroscopy (Zanconato et al. 1993; Kuno et al. 1995). Unfortunately, because of bore limitations in the actual spectrometers, only partial limb measurements can be made at the present time. Whole-body spectrometers linked with ergometers will be available in the near future and will certainly provide more insight, in a nondestructive way, into the underlying mechanism of the anaerobic metabolism during short-term exercise.
- Literature reviews reveal few longitudinal studies. In developmental exercise physiology, there is a need for prospective studies.
- There is a dearth of studies on young girls. More research in this area is necessary for an understanding of anaerobic performances in relation to gender.
- In children, there has been little research on the association between power indexes and athletic performance.
- Astonishingly few studies on trainability of anaerobic power in adolescents are available, in spite of a huge increase in the participation of this age group in worldwide competitions.

However, the assessment of anaerobic muscle power during growth remains a difficult task. Limited understanding of the underlying mechanisms due to ethical considerations, the fledgling status of research within this area, and limitations of testing methodology are some of the possible reasons for the difficulties encountered.

Summary

Pediatric exercise scientists are often interested in bone structure, muscle strength or power, or cardiac output or maximal oxygen intake alone. On the other hand, coaches and physical education teachers are more involved in the development of functional capacities such as the ability to increase, for example, running (or swimming or throwing) velocity, to extend joints, or to lift body mass or weights. These athletic performances are also of interest to the exercise scientists, but the complexity of the skills necessary to perform well in these tests makes assessment difficult. Trained adults have quite specialized structural and functional characteristics. Due to the combination of selection and training, a power lifter will have a completely different shape and very different metabolic capabilities than an ultramarathon runner. It seems that during growth, the same level of specialization does not exist. Teachers often observe that a child or adolescent can be among the best sprinters in the class and at the same time be a good endurance runner and a key member of the football team. Thus one of the difficulties in the assessment of the short-term power output in a growing child is to analyze the participation and influence of the different energy pathways. To quote Wilkie (1980), "In children, exercise scientists instead of attempting to quantify anaerobic energy yield by ATP or glycolysis, are more inspired to measure the resulting mechanical power output during short-term exercise, which is the truly useful product." This statement makes the assessment of anaerobic performance more "powerful," since only the subject's maximal performance will be considered as the criterion.

Thus, during growth, the measurement of mechanical output during short-term, high-intensity exercise is a reasonable and useful alternative for elaborating innovative techniques and procedures.

Notes

Nanci M. França is supported by a fellowship awarded through the CNPq (The National Council of Scientific Development, Brasilia, Brasil).

References

Abernethy, P., Wilson, G., and Logan, P. 1995. Strength and power assessment. Issues, controversies and challenges. *Sports Med.* (New Zealand) 19: 401-417.

Amano, Y., Mizutani, S., and Hoshikawa, T. 1983. Longitudinal study of running of 58 children over a four-year period. In *Biomechanics VIII-B*, ed. H. Matsui and K. Kobayashi, 663-668. Champaign, IL: Human Kinetics.

Amar, J. 1920. *The human motor.* London: Routledge & Sons.

American Alliance for Health, Physical Education and Recreation. 1975. *Youth fitness test manual.* Washington, DC: American Alliance for Health, Physical Education and Recreation.

Asmussen, E. 1973. Growth in muscular strength and power. In *Physical activity— human growth and development,* ed. G.L. Rarick, 60-79. New York: Academic Press.

Ästrand, P.O. 1992. Children and adolescents: performance, measurements, education. In *Children and exercise XVI, Pediatric work physiology,* ed. J. Coudert and E. Van Praagh, 3-7. Paris: Masson.

Avis, F.J., Hoving, A., and Toussaint, H.M. 1985. A dynamometer for the measurement of force, velocity, work and power during an explosive leg extension. *Eur. J. Appl. Physiol.* 54: 210-215.

Ayalon, A., Inbar, O., and Bar-Or, O. 1974. Relationship among measurements of explosive strength and anaerobic power. In *International series on sport sciences.* Vol. 1, *Biomechanics IV,* ed. R.C. Nelson and C.A. Morehouse, 572-577. Baltimore: University Press.

Bar-Or, O. 1987. The Wingate Anaerobic Test, an update on methodology, reliability and validity. *Sports Med.* (New Zealand) 4: 381-394.

Bar-Or, O. 1996a. Anaerobic performance. In *Measurement in pediatric exercise science,* ed. D. Docherty, 161-182. Champaign, IL: Human Kinetics.

Bar-Or, O., ed. 1996b. *The encyclopaedia of sports medicine. The child and adolescent athlete.* International Olympic Committee. London: Blackwell Scientific.

Baumgartner, T.A., and Jackson, A.S. 1991. *Measurement for evaluation in physical education and exercise science.* Dubuque, IA: Brown.

Benedict, F.G., and Cathcart, E.P. (n.d.). *Muscular work: a metabolic study with reference to the efficiency of the human body as a machine* (report no. 187). Washington, DC: Carnegie Institute of Washington.

Berg, K., Miller, M., and Stephens, L. 1986. Determinants of 30-meter sprint time in pubescent males. *J. Sports Med.* 26: 225-231.

Blimkie, C.J.R., Roache, P., Hay, J.T., and Bar-Or, O. 1988. Anaerobic power of arms in teenage boys and girls: relationship to lean tissue. *Eur. J. Appl. Physiol.* 57: 677-683.

Bosco, C. 1992. *L'évaluation de la force par le test de Bosco (Force assessment by means of the Bosco test).* Rome: Società Stampa Sportiva.

Bosco, C., and Komi, P.V. 1980. Influence of aging on the mechanical behavior of leg extensor muscles. *Eur. J. Appl. Physiol.* 45: 209-219.

Bosco, C., Luhtanen, P., and Komi, P.V. 1983. A simple method for measurement of mechanical power in jumping. *Eur. J. Appl. Physiol.* 50: 273-282.

Cabri, J., De Proft, W., Dufour, W., and Clarys, J.P. 1988. The relation between muscular strength and kicking performance. In *Science and football,* ed. T. Reilly, A. Lees, K. Davids, and W.J. Murphy, 186-193. London: Spon.

Carlson, J.S., and Naughton, G.A. 1992. Determination of the maximal accumulated oxygen deficit in male children. In *Children and exercise XVI, Pediatric work physiology,* ed. J. Coudert and E. Van Praagh, 23-25. Paris: Masson.

Carlson, R., and Engström, L-M. 1986. *80-talets Svenska tennisunder (The*

Swedish tennis wonder during the 1980's) (report no. 7). Stockholm: College of Physical Education.

Cavagna, G.A., Saibene, P.F., and Margaria, R. 1965. Effect of negative work on the a-mount of positive work performed by an isolated muscle. *J. Appl. Physiol.* 20: 157-158.

Cooper, D.M. 1995. New horizons in pediatric exercise research. In *New horizons in pediatric exercise science,* ed. C.J.R. Blimkie and O. Bar-Or, 1-24. Champaign, IL: Human Kinetics.

Council of Europe, Committee for the Development of Sport. 1988. *European Test of Physical Fitness (Eurofit).* Rome: Edigrat Editionale Grafica.

Cumming, G.R. 1973. Correlation of athletic performance and aerobic power in 12-17-year-old children with bone age, calf muscle, total body potassium, heart volume and two indices of anaerobic power. In *Pediatric work physiology,* ed. O. Bar-Or, 109-134. Natanya, Israel: Wingate Institute.

Davies, C.T.M., Barnes, C., and Godfrey, S. 1972. Body composition and maximal exercise performance in children. *Hum. Biol.* 44: 195-214.

Davies, C.T.M., and Rennie, R. 1968. Human power output. *Nature* 217: 770.

Davies, C.T.M., Wemyss-Holden, J., and Young, K. 1984. Measurement of short term power output: comparison between cycling and jumping. *Ergonomics* 3: 285-296.

Davies, C.T.M., and Young, K. 1984. Effects of external loading on short-term power output in children and young male adults. *Eur. J. Appl. Physiol.* 52: 351-354.

di Prampero, P.E., Pinera-Limas, F., and Sassi, G. 1970. Maximal muscular power (aerobic and anaerobic) in 116 athletes performing at the XIX Olympic Games in Mexico. *Ergonomics* 6: 665-674.

Docherty, D., ed. 1996. *Measurement In pediatric exercise science.* Champaign, IL: Human Kinetics.

Doré, E., França, N.M., Bedu, M., and Van Praagh, E. 1997. The effect of flywheel inertia on short-term cycling power output in children. *Med. Sci. Sports Exerc.* 29(5): S170.

Falgairette, G., Bedu, M., Fellmann, N., Spielvogel, H., Van Praagh, E., Obert, P., and Coudert, J. 1994. Evaluation of physical fitness from field tests at high altitude in circumpubertal boys: comparison with laboratory data. *Eur. J. Appl. Physiol.* 69: 36-43.

Fargeas, M.A. 1993. Mesure de la puissance mécanique externe chez l'enfant lors d'un exercise de courte durée sur ergocycle et tapis roulant (étude longitudinale) (Measurement of short-term external mechanical power in children, performed on a cycle ergometer and a "power" treadmill). PhD diss. Université Blaise Pascal, Clermont-Ferrand, France.

Fargeas, M.A., Lauron, B., Léger, L., and Van Praagh, E. 1993. *A computerized treadmill ergometer to measure short-term power output,* 394-395. Fourteenth International Congress of Biomechanics, Paris.

Fargeas, M.A., Van Praagh, E., Léger. L., Fellmann, N., and Coudert, J. 1993. Comparison of cycling and running power outputs in trained children. *Pediatr. Exerc. Sci.* 5: 415.

Fenn, W.O., and Marsh, B.S. 1935. Muscular force at different speeds of shortening. *J. Physiol.* (London) 85: 277-297.

Ferretti, G., Gussoni, M., di Prampero, P.E., and Cerretelli, P. 1987. Effects of exercise on maximal instantaneous muscular power of humans. *J. Appl. Physiol.* 62: 2288-2294.

França, N.M., Matsudo, V.K.R., and Brandao, M.R.F. 1992. Impact of menarche on velocity and agility performance among girls at the same chronological age. In *Children and exercise XVI, Pediatric work physiology,* ed. J. Coudert and E. Van Praagh, 229-231. Paris: Masson.

Gillespie, J., and Keenum, S. 1987. A validity and reliability analysis of the seated shot put as a test of power. *J. Hum. Mov. Stud.* 13: 97-105.

Glencross, D.J. 1966. The nature of the vertical jump test and the standing broad jump. *Res. Q.* 37: 353-359.

Grassi, B., Cerretelli, P., Narici, M.V., and Marconi, C. 1991. Peak anaerobic power in master athletes. *Eur. J. Appl. Physiol.* 62: 394-399.

Green, S., Dawson, B.T., Goodman, C., and Carey, M.F. 1996. Anaerobic ATP production and accumulated O2 deficit in cyclists. *Med. Sci. Sports Exerc.* 28(3): 315-321.

Harman, E.A., Rosenstein, M.T., Frykman, P.N., et al. 1991. Estimation of human power output from vertical jump. *J. Appl. Sport Sci. Res.* 5: 116-120.

Hill, A.V. 1938. The heat of shortening and the dynamic constraints of muscle. *Proc. Roy. Soc. Br.* 126: 136-195.

Inbar, O., Bar-Or, O., and Skinner, J.S. n.d. *The Wingate Anaerobic Test: development, characteristics, and application.* Champaign, IL: Human Kinetics. In press.

Johnson, B.L., and Nelson, J.K. 1986. *Practical measurements for evaluation in physical education.* 4th ed. Edina, MN: Burgess International.

Katch, V.L., Weltman, A., and Traeger, L. 1976. All out versus steady-paced cycling strategy for maximal work output of short duration. *Res. Q.* 47: 164-168.

Kirby, R.F. 1991. *Kirby's guide for fitness and motor performance tests.* Cape Girardeau, MO: BenOak.

Komi, P.V., and Bosco, C. 1978. Utilization of stored elastic energy in men and women. *Med. Sci. Sport* 10: 261-265.

Krahenbuhl, G.S., Skinner, J.S., and Kohrt, W.M. 1985. Developmental aspects of maximal aerobic power in children. In *Exerc. Sports Sci. Rev.,* ed. R.J. Terjung, 503-538. New York: Macmillan.

Kuno, S., Takahashi, H., Fujimoto, K., et al. 1995. Muscle metabolism during exercise using phosphorus-31 nuclear magnetic resonance spectroscopy in adolescents. *Eur. J. Appl. Physiol.* 70: 301-304.

Lakomy, H.K.A. 1984. An ergometer for measuring the power generated during sprinting. *J. Physiol.* 354: 33P.

Lakomy, H.K.A. 1987. The use of a non-motorized treadmill for analysing sprint performance. *Ergonomics* 30: 627-638.

Maréchal, R., Pirnay, F., Crielaard, J.M., and Petit, J.M. 1979. *Influence de l'âge sur la puissance anaérobie (Influence of age on anaérobic power).* Paris: Economica.

Marey, E. J., and Demenÿ, G. 1885. Locomotion humaine; mécanisme du saut (Human locomotion; the jump mechanism). *Compte Rendu Séances Acad. Sci.* 489-494.

Margaria, R., Aghemo, P., and Rovelli, E. 1966. Measurement of muscular power (anaerobic) in man. *J. Appl. Physiol.* 21: 1662-1664.

Margaria, R., Cerretelli, P., and Mangili, F. 1964. Balance and kinetics of anaerobic energy release during strenuous exercise in man. *J. Appl. Physiol.* 19: 623-628.

Matsudo, V.K.R. 1996. Prediction of future athletic excellence. In *The encyclopaedia of sports medicine. The child and adolescent athlete,* ed. O. Bar-Or, 92-109. International Olympic Committee. London: Blackwell Scientific.

Mayhew, J.L., Bemben, M.G., and Rohrs, D.M. 1992. Seated shot put as a measure of upper body power in adolescent wrestlers. *Pediatr. Exerc. Sci.* 4: 78-84.

Medbø, J.I., Mohn, A.C., Tabata, I., et al. 1980. Anaerobic capacity determined by maximal accumulated oxygen deficit. *J. Appl. Physiol.* 64: 50-60.

Mercier, J., Mercier, B., and Préfaut, C. 1991. Blood lactate increase during the force velocity exercise test. *Int. J. Sports Med.* 12: 17-20.

Mognoni, P., Narici, M.V., Sirtori, M.D., and Lorenzelli, F. 1994. Isokinetic torques and kicking maximal ball velocity in young soccer players. *J. Sports Med. Phys. Fitness* 34: 357-361.

Moritani, T., Oddsson, L., Thorstensson, A., and Ästrand, P.O. 1989. Neural and biomechanical differences between men and young boys during a variety of motor tasks. *Acta Physiol. Scand.* 137: 147-155.

Murray, D.A., and Harrison, E. 1986. Constant velocity dynamometer: an appraisal using mechanical loading. *Med. Sci. Sports Exerc.* 6: 612-624.

Nielsen, B., Nielsen, K., Behrendt Hansen, M., and Asmussen, E. 1980. Training of "functional muscle strength" in girls 7-19 years old. In *Children and exercise IX,* ed. K. Bergh and B.O. Eriksson, 69-78. Baltimore: University Park Press.

Nindl, B.C., Mahar, M.T., Harman, E.A., and Patton, J.F. 1995. Lower and upper body anaerobic performance in male and female adolescent athletes. *Med. Sci. Sports Exerc.* 27: 235-241.

Paterson, D.H., and Cunningham, D.A. 1985. Development of anaerobic capacity in early and late maturing boys. In *Children and exercise XI,* ed. R.A. Binkhorst, H.C.G. Kemper, and W.H. Saris, 119-28. Champaign, IL: Human Kinetics.

Pérès, G., Vandewalle, H., and Monod, H. 1981. Aspect particulier de la relation charge-vitesse lors du pédalage sue cycloergomètre (Particular aspect of the load-velocity relationship during pedalling on the cycle ergometer). *J. Physiol.* (Paris) (abstract) 77: 10A.

Perrine, J.J., and Edgerton, V.R. 1978. Muscle force-velocity and power-velocity relationships under isokinetic loading. *Med. Sci. Sports* 10: 159-166.

Pirnay, F., and Crielaard, J.M. 1979. Mesure de la puissance anaérobie alactique (Measurement of alactic anaerobic power). *Med. Sport* 53: 13-16.

Ralston, H.J., Polissar, M.J., Inman, V.T., et al. 1949. Dynamic features of human isolated voluntary muscle in isometric and free contractions. *J. Appl. Physiol.* 1: 526-533.

Rowland, T.W. 1996. *Developmental exercise physiology.* Champaign, IL: Human Kinetics.

Saavreda, C., Lagassé, P., Bouchard, C, and Simoneau, J. 1991. Maximal anaerobic performance of the knee extensor muscles during growth. *Med. Sci. Sports Exerc.* 23: 1083-1089.

Safrit M.J. 1990. The validity and reliability of fitness tests for children. *Pediatr. Exerc. Sci.* 2: 9-28.

Saltin, B. 1990. Anaerobic capacity: past, present, and prospective. In *Biochemistry of exercise VII,* ed. Taylor, A., et al., 387-412. Champaign, IL: Human Kinetics.

Saltin, B., Gollnick, P.D., Eriksson, B.O., and Piehl, K. 1971. Metabolic and circulatory adjustments at onset of work. In *Proceedings from meeting on physiological changes at onset of work,* ed. A. Gilbert and P. Guille, 46-58. Toulouse.

Sargeant, A.J. 1989. Short-term muscle power in children and adolescents. In *Advances in pediatric sports sciences.* Vol. 3, *Biological issues,* ed. O. Bar-Or, 41-63. Champaign, IL: Human Kinetics.

Sargeant, A.J. 1992. Problems in, and approaches to, the measurement of short term power output in children and adolescents. In *Children and exercise XVI, Pediatric work physiology,* ed. J. Coudert and E. Van Praagh, 11-17. Paris: Masson.

Sargeant, A.J., Dolan, P., and Thorne, A. 1984. Isokinetic measurement of maximal leg force and anaerobic power output in children. In *Children and sport XII,* ed. J. Ilmarinen and I Välimäki, 93-98. Berlin: Springer-Verlag.

Sargeant, A.J., Hoinville, E., and Young, A. 1981. Maximum leg force and power output during short-term dynamic exercise. *J. Appl. Physiol.* 51: 1175-1182.

Sargent, D.A. 1921. The physical test of a man. *Am. Phys. Ed. Rev.* 26: 188-194.

Seiler, S., Taylor, M., Diana, R., et al. 1990. Assessing anaerobic power in collegiate football players. *J. Appl. Sport Sci. Res.* 4: 9-15.

Thorland, W.G. 1990. Muscular strength and power in elite young male runners. *Pediatr. Exerc. Sci.* 2: 73-82.

Tirosh, E., Rosenbaum, P, and Bar-Or, O. 1990. A new muscle power test in neuromuscular disease: feasibility and reliability. *Am. J. Dis. Child.* 144: 1083-1087.

USA Junior Olympic Championships. July 1989 Spokane, Washington. *Track and Field Journal.*

Vandewalle, H., Pérès, G., Heller, J., et al. 1987. Force-velocity relationship and maximal power on a cycle ergometer. *Eur. J. Appl. Physiol.* 56: 650-656.

Vandewalle, H., Pérès, G., and Monod, H. 1987. Standard anaerobic exercise tests. *Sports Med.* (New Zealand) 4: 268-289.

Van Praagh, E. 1996. Testing of anaerobic performance. In *The encyclopaedia of sports medicine. The child and adolescent athlete,* ed. O. Bar-Or, 602-616. International Olympic Committee. London: Blackwell Scientific.

Van Praagh, E., Falgairette, G., Bedu, M., et al. 1989. Laboratory and field tests in 7-year-old boys. In *Children and exercise XIII,* ed. S. Oseid and K-H. Carlsen, 11-17. Champaign, IL: Human Kinetics.

Van Praagh, E., Fargeas, M.A., Léger, L., et al. 1993. Short-term power output in children measured on a computerized treadmill ergometer. *Pediatr. Exerc. Sci.* (abstract) 5: 482.

Van Praagh, E., Fellmann, N., Bedu, M., et al. 1996. Analysis of "anaerobic fitness" in 7-and 12-year-old boys. *Pediatr. Exerc. Sci.* (abstract) 8: 92.

Van Praagh, E., Fellmann, N., Bedu, M., Falgairette, G., and Coudert, J. 1990. Gender difference in the relationship of anaerobic power output to body composition in children. *Pediatr. Exerc. Sci.* 2: 336-348.

Viitasalo, J.T. 1988. Evaluation of explosive strength for young and adult athletes. *Res. Q. Exerc. Sport* 59: 9-13.

Viitasalo, J.T., Österback, L., Alén, M., et al. 1987. Mechanical jumping power in young athletes. *Acta Physiol. Scand.* 131: 139-145.

Viitasalo, J.T., Rahkila, P., Österback, L., and Alén, M. 1992. Vertical jumping height and horizontal overhead throwing velocity in young male athletes. *J. Sports Sci.* 10: 401-413.

Weltman, A., Janney, C., Rians, C.B., and Berg, K. 1986. The effects of hydraulic resistance strength training in prepubertal males. *Med. Sci. Sports Exerc.* 18: 629-638.

Wilkie, D.R. 1950. The relation between force and velocity in human muscle. *J. Physiol.* (London) 110: 249-280.

Wilkie, D.R. 1960. Man as a source of mechanical power. *Ergonomics* 3: 1-8.

Wilkie, D.R. 1980. Equations describing power input by humans as a function of duration of exercise. *Exercise bioenergetics and gas exchange,* 25-34. Amsterdam: Elsevier/North Holland Biomedical Press.

Williams, C. 1987. Short term activity. In *Exercise: benefits, limits and adaptations,* ed. D. Macleod et al., 59-62. London: Spon.

Williams, C.A. 1995. Anaerobic performance of prepubescent and adolescent children. PhD diss. University of Exeter, UK.

Zanconato, S., Buchtal, S., Barstow, T.J., and Cooper, D.M. 1993. 31P-magnetic resonance spectroscopy of leg muscle metabolism during exercise in children and adults. *J. Appl. Physiol.* 74: 2214-2218.

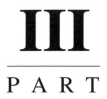

PART

Anaerobic Trainability and Training

9

CHAPTER

Strength Development and Trainability During Childhood

Cameron J.R. Blimkie
Digby G. Sale

This chapter focuses on the following objectives:

- Describing the development of human strength as a function of age, gender, and maturity
- Describing the major factors besides age, gender, and maturity that influence the expression and development of strength
- Reviewing the effects of resistance or weight training on strength development
- Describing the mechanisms underlying strength adaptations to training and detraining

Strength testing of children is performed routinely by rehabilitation therapists to assess the degree of muscle disability and to diagnose the rate of recovery from injury, by physical educators to grade student performance, by coaches to monitor effectiveness of training and to select athletes for sports teams, and by researchers to identify both the determinants and trainability of strength during childhood. Given the variety of applications of strength testing, it is important for administrators of such tests to be familiar with the normal age- and gender-associated variations in strength and the various factors that can both influence and confound interpretation of strength results.

Additionally, questions often arise from parents and coaches about the effectiveness, benefits, and risks of strength training during childhood. Both of these topics—strength development and strength trainability during childhood—have been thoroughly reviewed elsewhere (Asmussen 1973; Beunen and Malina 1988; Blimkie 1989, 1992, 1993; Cahill 1988; Froberg and Lammert 1996; Malina 1975, 1978, 1986). This review will be limited to a summary of the key concepts and findings relevant to the topics of strength development and trainability during childhood.

Strength Development During Childhood

Strength may be discussed in terms of peak force or torque development achieved under various conditions, e.g., during maximal voluntary contractions, electrically evoked twitch contractions, or electrically evoked tetanic contractions. In this chapter, discussion will be confined mostly to maximal voluntary strength measures, since these are the most abundant in the literature and are perhaps the most relevant given their utility and broad application in both clinical and athletic assessment. Discussion will also be limited to strength changes for only a selected number of muscle groups for which comprehensive published data sets were available. Lastly, since the data are derived mostly from normal, healthy, non-athletic children, statements and conclusions about strength development and trainability may not be wholly generalizable to other pediatric populations, such as young athletes or clinical groups.

Age Differences

Strength, which increases tremendously between birth and adulthood, has traditionally been described in relation to age and gender. While useful in describing general growth trends, neither provides much insight into the biological mechanisms underlying strength changes during childhood.

Strong positive correlations have been reported between chronological age and various measures of maximal voluntary strength in males during the period spanning mid-childhood and adolescence (Blimkie 1989; Carron and Bailey 1974). Weaker but nevertheless moderate positive correlations have also been reported between strength and age for girls during the prepubertal period. Correlations are generally low and sometimes negative, however, for females during the postpubertal and adolescent periods (Faust 1977). It is likely that these correlational relationships reflect the covariation of age with other perhaps more important biological and morphological determinants of strength than age itself. Nevertheless, age might exert an independent influence on strength development through the mechanism of enhanced neuromotor maturation (Asmussen 1973; Clarke and Degutis 1962).

The most abundant "strength" literature focusing on children exists in the form of maximal voluntary isometric grip strength data. The age-related development of single hand absolute grip strength is shown for boys and girls in figure 9.1. For boys, there appears to be a curvilinear increase in grip strength with advancing age from

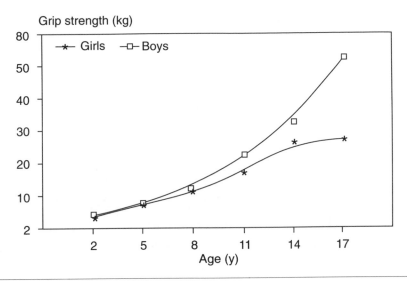

Figure 9.1 Age- and gender-associated variation in single-hand grip strength.

Data from Blimkie 1989.

early childhood until the onset of puberty. Strength increases rapidly during the pubertal period and continues to increase considerably, albeit at a slightly slower rate, during adolescence. The pattern is similar for girls until the onset of puberty at about 12 years of age. In contrast to boys, there is only a slight (barely perceptible from cross-sectional analyses) increase in the rate of strength gain in girls during puberty, and strength appears to have peaked by around the age of 15 with little further increase during adolescence. The pattern of strength development is similar for both single hand and double hand grip strength measures (Blimkie 1989).

Gender Differences

Gender-related differences in strength are evident as early as 3 years of age. Boys have consistently higher average single and double hand grip strength than girls between 3 and 18 years of age (Blimkie 1989). Gender differences are small, however, with considerable overlap between girls and boys prior to the male pubertal growth spurt. With increasing age, and from the onset of the male pubertal growth spurt, the percentage of boys who outscore girls on various strength measures increases considerably (Faust 1977; Jones 1949; Malina 1986). The sexual differentiation in strength development is most apparent when performance is expressed as a ratio of the female-male strength scores. As shown in figure 9.2, there is a dramatic decrease in the female-male absolute grip strength ratio with advancing age. Girls have about 92% of the absolute strength of boys at the age of 7, compared with less than 60% at the age of 18 years. This age-related decline is also evident for

Pediatric Anaerobic Performance

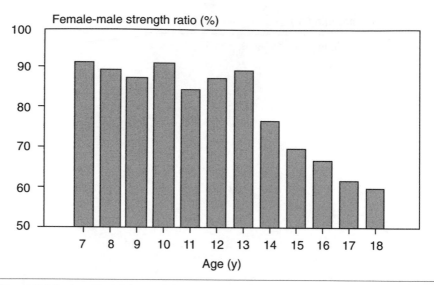

Figure 9.2 Ratio of female-to-male hand grip (both hands combined) strength in relation to age.

Data from Blimkie 1989.

female-male grip strength ratios normalized for height and weight, although the magnitude of the reduction is not as great (Blimkie 1989).

Measures of composite strength (summed measures from several muscle groups) provide an assessment of overall or general strength. The age based composite strength development curves derived from the studies by Faust (1977) and Stolz and Stolz (1951) are presented in figure 9.3. The pattern for absolute composite strength performance in both sexes is very similar to that previously described for grip strength. Females demonstrate consistently lower absolute composite strength scores than males but a fairly similar rate of increase in strength during the prepubertal years. There is an acceleration in the rate of strength gain for males during the pubertal period, with a continued but diminished rate of increase during postpuberty. For females, there is only a slight increase in the rate of strength gain during the pubertal period, and this is followed by a plateau in strength performance during the postpubertal years.

These patterns are similar to those described for other measures of composite strength for males (Carron and Bailey 1974; Clarke 1971), and females (Carron et al. 1977) at comparable ages and stages of development. It appears that the age- and gender-based developmental patterns for absolute grip strength are an accurate reflection of selected composite isometric strength development patterns for both sexes during childhood. Despite the similarity in developmental patterns, hand grip strength generally is only weakly to moderately correlated with strength of other muscle groups, especially during late adolescence (Asmussen 1973), and should not be considered as a representative measure of strength for all muscle groups during the childhood period.

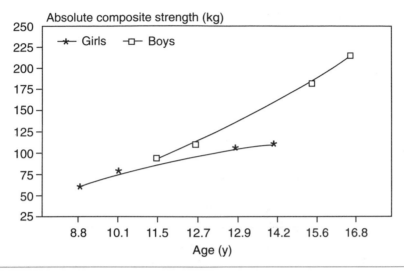

Figure 9.3 Age- and gender-associated changes in composite grip strength.

Data from Blimkie 1989.

Somatic Correlates and Determinants of Strength

Strength gains and gender differences in strength during childhood appear to be closely related to changes in somatic growth, muscle size, and neuromuscular and neuroendocrine development. Heredity and lifestyle factors such as physical activity and sports participation can also influence strength.

Body Weight

Correlations between weight and strength for both sexes range from low to moderate during the prepubertal years, then increase and peak during the pubertal growth period (with higher correlations in males than in females), and finally diminish during the postpubertal or adolescent years (Carron and Bailey 1974; Clarke 1971; Faust 1977; Jones 1949). Additionally, strong positive correlations have been reported between weight and maximal voluntary strength in males spanning the broader period from mid-childhood to late adolescence (Blimkie 1989). These findings suggest that growth related changes in body weight probably account for part of the age- and gender-associated differences in strength that are apparent during childhood.

However, as shown in figure 9.4, grip strength continues to increase throughout childhood in males and up to puberty in females, even after correcting or normalizing for body mass. A similar pattern is evident for leg extension, elbow flexion, and abdominal flexion strength (Froberg et al. 1992), as well as for composite maximal voluntary strength in boys (Blimkie 1989). This suggests that some factor or factors

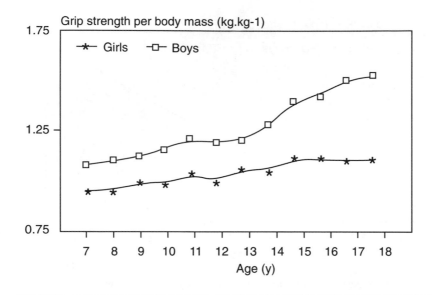

Figure 9.4 Grip strength (both hands combined) normalized for body mass in relation to age and gender.

Data from Blimkie 1989.

other than body weight are primarily responsible for the age-associated changes and gender differences in strength development during childhood.

The gender difference in relative strength (per kg body mass) before puberty is probably due in part to the higher proportion of body weight as fat in females during this period (Kemper 1986; Saris et al. 1986). The divergence in relative strength between the sexes during puberty and adolescence may also be attributed to a greater absolute and proportional increase in body fat in females (Canada Fitness Survey 1985; Kemper 1986) and to a proportionately greater increase in muscle mass in males (Malina and Bouchard 1991; Malina and Johnston 1967). Sociocultural influences, including differences between the sexes in sports and physical activity participation, may also contribute to these gender differences in relative strength and are discussed in more detail later.

Height

Correlations between height and strength are generally significant. The correlation is low to moderate in both sexes during the prepubertal years, increases to a moderate level during puberty, and diminishes to a lower and sometimes insignificant level (especially in females) during postpuberty (Carron and Bailey 1974; Clarke 1971; Faust 1977; Maglischo 1968). Strong positive correlations have also been reported between maximal voluntary strength and height in males spanning the period from prepuberty to late adolescence (Blimkie 1989). Additionally, the developmental patterns for both grip strength and composite strength normalized for height are also remarkably similar to the age based developmental pattern for absolute grip strength (Blimkie 1989). The persistence of age and gender differences in these strength measures, even after correction for height, suggests that some other factor or factors play a more important role in strength development during childhood than height itself.

Dimensionality

The effects of somatic growth on strength development have also been studied using dimensional analysis theory. By this theory, both muscle cross-sectional area and strength are predicted to increase in proportion to the change in height squared (Ht^2) during growth. Studies that have used this approach have provided mixed results. In both sexes, some strength measures (e.g., elbow flexor strength) increase fairly proportionally to height squared during the prepubertal period (Asmussen 1973; Parker et al. 1990). For other muscle groups (e.g., knee extensor strength), however, strength increases have been substantially greater than predicted by dimensional theory in both sexes prior to puberty (Parker et al. 1990) and both lower and higher than predicted in females and males, respectively, from puberty to late adolescence (Asmussen and Heeboll-Nielsen 1955; Carron and Bailey 1974; Froberg and Lammert 1996; Parker et al. 1990).

The greater than predicted increase in strength for many muscle groups suggests that other factors besides dimensional or quantitative differences contribute to the size-associated changes and gender differences in strength development during childhood. Despite assertions to the contrary (Asmussen and Heeboll-Nielsen 1955), the assumptions about geometric similarity and constancy of tissue composition during childhood, which underlie this theory, are highly questionable. While the dimensionality theory provides an interesting theoretical means by which to account for the effects of size on strength development, it is too simplistic and problematic, and it detracts from the search for more basic explanations for the age changes and gender differences in strength during childhood.

Lean Body Mass

There is little information about the relationship between development of lean body mass and strength during childhood. Forbes (1965) reported a highly significant positive correlation ($r = 0.91$) between grip strength and lean body mass in boys between 12 and 18 years of age. There are no comparable data to our knowledge describing this relationship in young females. Lean body mass is comprised mostly of muscle mass, and the relationship between lean body mass and strength is probably mediated by the influence of muscle size or mass. When composite strength (Faust 1977; Stolz and Stolz 1951) is normalized for adjusted

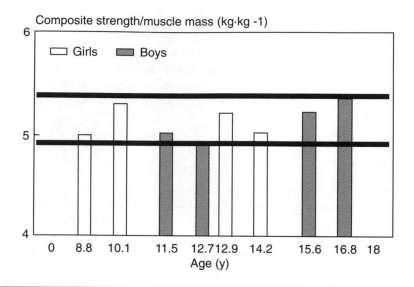

Figure 9.5 Age- and gender-associated changes in composite strength measures normalized for muscle mass.

Data for strength from Faust 1977 and Stolz and Stolz 1951; data for muscle mass from Malina and Bouchard 1991.

measures of muscle mass according to age and gender (Malina and Bouchard 1991), strength differences between the sexes and across ages virtually disappear (see figure 9.5). Normalized strength measures for both sexes fall within a very narrow band between 4.88 and 5.40 kg per kg muscle mass. This suggests that muscle mass accounts for a large proportion of the age-associated changes and gender differences in strength development during childhood.

Muscle Mass

Skeletal muscle is the tissue responsible for force generation, and theoretically one might predict a strong association between muscle mass and strength development during childhood. Muscle mass increases approximately 3.5 fold in females and 5 fold in males from 5 to 17.5 years of age (Malina 1969). On a proportional basis, muscle mass represents about 40% and 42% of body mass in females and males respectively during mid-childhood and 42% and 54% of body mass in females and males during late adolescence (see figure 9.6). These developmental changes in absolute and proportional muscle mass probably account for a large portion of the age- and gender-associated differences in strength during childhood.

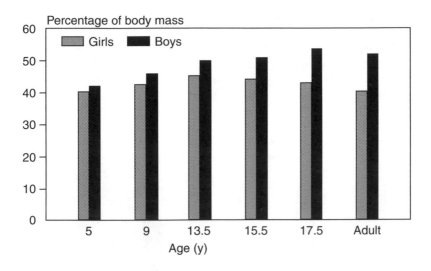

Figure 9.6 Age- and gender-associated changes in development of proportional (percentage of body mass) muscle mass.

Data from Malina and Bouchard 1991.

Muscle Size

Correlations between muscle breadths or widths (determined by radiography) and strength range from low to moderate and vary considerably across different muscle groups (Blimkie 1989; Malina 1975). Correlations between muscle cross-sectional area—determined by anthropometry, ultrasound, or computerized tomography—and maximal voluntary strength in children have been summarized recently (Blimkie 1989) and are generally moderate to strong in both sexes across a variety of muscle groups. Studies by Davies (1985) and Ikai and Fukunaga (1968) demonstrated a fairly linear increase in maximal voluntary strength with increasing muscle cross-sectional area between mid-childhood and late adolescence. The gender difference in muscle size is small until mid-puberty, increases progressively with age during late puberty and adolescence, and reaches its peak difference during early adulthood (Johnston and Malina 1966). The gender difference in muscle size becomes more marked in upper limbs than lower limbs with advancing age so that compared to males females have only about 50% of the upper limb, but about 70% of the lower limb muscle size by late adolescence (Sale and Spriet 1996).

Age- and gender-associated differences in strength were wholly eliminated when absolute strength measures were normalized for muscle cross-sectional area (Davies 1985; Ikai and Fukunaga 1968). These findings provide compelling evidence that muscle cross-sectional area, rather than age and gender per se, is the most important factor influencing strength development during childhood.

Muscle Fiber Characteristics

Besides the influence of gross muscle size, changes in muscle fiber number and differentiation (e.g., changes in fiber type distribution and size) might also influence strength development during childhood. Muscle fiber number is generally believed to be largely genetically determined and fixed in humans at birth (Gollnick et al.

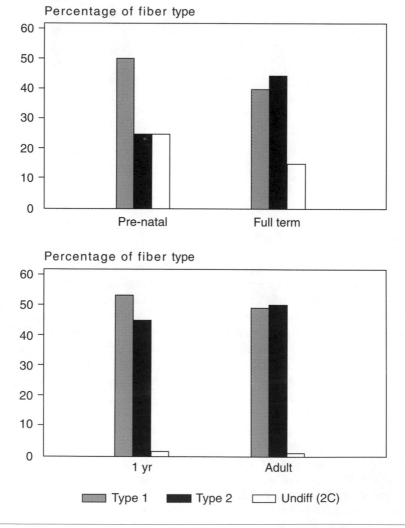

Figure 9.7 Development of muscle fiber type distribution in the vastus lateralis muscle of humans.

Data from Oertel 1988.

1981), although fiber number may increase for a short time after birth, depending on the child's maturity status (Malina and Bouchard 1991). In young adults, males generally have a greater number of muscle fibers (not always a significant difference) than females in the upper limbs, which exhibit the greatest gender difference in muscle cross-sectional area and mass (Alway et al. 1989; Miller et al. 1993; Sale et al. 1987; Schantz et al. 1983). Whether and when this gender difference in fiber number is established remains to be determined.

As shown in figure 9.7, there is considerable differentiation of muscle fiber types in utero from pre- to full-term and from birth to one year of age. From about one year of age, however, the fiber type distribution of the child has attained near adult proportions, and there does not appear to be any clear gender difference in fiber type distribution during childhood (Colling-Saltin 1980; Elder and Kakulas 1993; Hedberg and Jansson 1986; Malina 1986; Oertel 1988). The percent distribution of type 2 fibers is lower for both sexes in early and mid-childhood compared to adulthood and attains adult proportions during late adolescence, mostly from conversion of the undifferentiated type 2C fibers (Colling-Saltin 1980; Fournier et al. 1982; Hedberg and Jansson 1986). Adolescent males tend to exhibit greater individual variability in muscle fiber type distribution than females and may also have a slightly higher proportion of type I fibers than females during this stage of development (Glenmark et al. 1992; Komi and Karlsson 1978; Saltin et al. 1977).

Muscle fibers undergo a tremendous increase in size during childhood (see figure 9.8). Fiber diameter increases by about 75% from birth to one year of age and then continues to increase by a magnitude of about 3.5 fold in girls and 4-5 fold in boys from early childhood to adolescence (Colling-Saltin 1980; Oertel 1988). The magnitude of increase may vary between upper and lower limb muscles. Lower limb muscle fiber area has been reported to increase in the order of 20 fold, compared with the 7-12 fold increase in upper limb fibers (Aherne et al. 1971). There is apparently no gender difference in fiber diameter until adolescence (Brooke and Engel 1969; Oertel 1988). In girls, fiber diameter reaches its peak during adolescence, and adolescent girls have the same fiber size as adult females. In boys, however, fiber diameter continues to increase during adolescence and achieves its peak size only during late adolescence or early adulthood (Oertel 1988). Moreover, males apparently exhibit a relatively greater size increase in type 2 fibers, and more specifically the type 2B fibers, compared with females during adolescence. This preferential growth effect results in greater 2B/1 and 2A/1 fiber type ratios in males compared to females during adolescence and early adulthood (Glenmark et al. 1992).

Type 2B and 2A fibers of the adult human quadriceps have recently been shown to have 10 times (in males) and 3 times (in females) the maximum shortening velocity of type 1 fibers (Larsson and Moss 1993). Differences of this magnitude in shortening speed might be expected to influence velocity-dependent strength and power performance of muscle composed of varying distributions of type 1 and 2 fibers. If these contractile characteristics of the various fiber types are present at all stages of development, then the increase in type 2 fiber type distribution in both sexes with increasing age might confer an advantage to older children compared

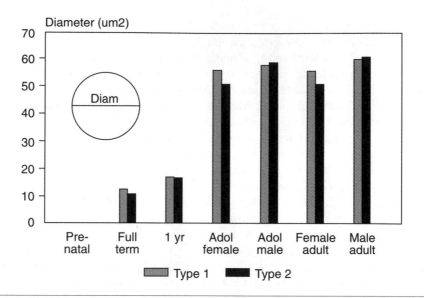

Figure 9.8 Age- and gender-associated changes in muscle fiber diameter in the vastus lateralis (VL) of humans from childhood to adulthood.

Data from Oertel 1988.

with younger children in high speed strength and power activities. Likewise, during adolescence females might be afforded a slight advantage in these types of activities compared with boys because of their higher proportion of type 2 fibers. In the latter instance, however, the potential advantage due to an increased proportion of type 2 fibers may be offset by relatively greater increases in the size of the type 2 fibers in males compared with females during the adolescent period. The degree to which these fiber type adaptations account for age- and gender-related changes in strength during childhood and adolescence remains to be determined.

Chemical and Ultrastructural Characteristics

Changes in the chemical composition of muscle also occur during childhood that might contribute to the age- and gender-related changes in muscle strength. Sodium and chloride ion concentrations decrease and potassium ion and phosphorus content increases dramatically during the first year of life. They change slowly from this time onward towards a chemically mature state, which is achieved in early adolescence (Boileau et al. 1985; Malina and Bouchard 1991). At the ultrastructural level, there is apparently little difference between children and adults. The relative proportion of the muscle fiber occupied by myofibrils (83%), cytoplasm (11.5%), mitochondria (5%), and lipid droplets (0.5%) are similar in children and young adults (Bell et al. 1980). Whether, and to what degree, these changes influence strength development and contribute to the gender difference in strength during childhood remains to be determined.

Puberty and Maturation

Maturity differences have little effect on strength development in the prepubescent years but become more strongly manifest with the encroachment of and during puberty (Beunen et al. 1980). Early maturing boys are generally stronger than average or late maturing boys at each age during puberty. The maturity effect diminishes after mid-puberty, and there is virtually no difference in strength among maturity groups at the end of puberty. These observations clearly demonstrate the average group effect of varying rates of maturation on strength development during puberty, but they provide little detail about the dynamics of strength development of individuals in relation to maturity status.

Velocity curves that represent yearly increments in strength expressed in relation to established markers of sexual or somatic maturity provide important information about the dynamic features of individual strength development during puberty that are not discernable from age-based distance curves. It is clear from the velocity curves in figure 9.9 that there are definite developmental strength spurts in both sexes and that these spurts occur after the peak growth spurt in height in both boys and girls. Although not the case in this figure, if comparable strength data sets were available, there is little doubt that males would have a larger magnitude of strength gain during their spurt than females.

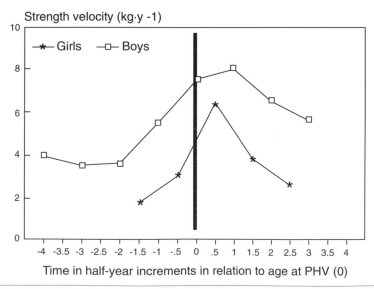

Figure 9.9 Composite isometric strength development in relation to pubertal status.

Data from Blimkie 1989.

How does the timing of the strength spurt relate to the development of muscle mass or size? For many muscle groups in males, the peak rate of gain in muscle cross-sectional area coincides with the peak rate of gain in height (at age of PHV) and precedes the peak strength gain by a few months (Blimkie 1989; Malina and Bouchard 1991). In females, however, there is more variability in the timing of the spurt in muscle cross-sectional area, and the peak gains in strength appear to be more closely temporally related than in boys (Blimkie 1989; Malina and Bouchard 1991). The temporal dissociation in boys, between the timing of the spurts in muscle cross-sectional area and strength development, suggests that some other factor besides muscle size itself (perhaps a lag in neuromotor maturation) exerts an important regulatory influence on the force-generating capacity of muscle during this brief period of rapid growth.

Lastly, how consistent are the timing characteristics of peak strength gains among individuals and between sexes? Peak strength gains occur for the majority (72%) of boys after the age at PHV (see figure 9.10). Many boys (23%), however, experience peak strength gain before or at the same time as the peak spurt in height (Faust 1977; Stolz and Stolz 1951). For girls, the situation is more variable. In one study (Faust 1977), fewer than half (49%) of the girls had their peak strength spurt following the age at PHV, but for the remaining girls peak strength gain occurred before or at the same time as age at PHV.

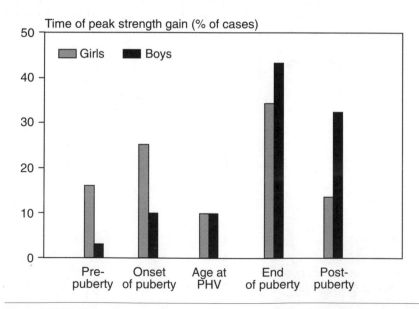

Figure 9.10 Variation (percentage distribution of cases) in the timing of individual spurts in strength in relation to age at peak height velocity (age at PHV) and developmental status.

Data from Blimkie 1989.

Hormonal Effects on Strength

Age- and gender-associated changes in muscle size and strength during puberty have been attributed largely to hormonal influences and more specifically to changes in testosterone secretion that occur during this period. Testosterone, which is a potent anabolic agent, increases modestly (4 fold) during the early stages of puberty and then increases rapidly by another 20 fold between mid- and late puberty in males. In girls, testosterone secretion increases linearly between early and late puberty, but the magnitude of the entire increase is only 4 fold, and peak levels are 15 fold lower than in boys by the end of puberty (Blimkie 1989).

Testosterone is believed to be the most active stimulator of muscle growth, and by its direct influence on the development of muscle mass is probably the most important factor influencing the development of strength and sexual differentiation in strength during puberty. Besides its effect on muscle mass, testosterone may also influence the developmental pattern for strength through more subtle influences by regulating neurotransmitter release (Souccar et al. 1982) and muscle fiber type conversion (Kelly et al. 1985).

Testosterone is not the only hormone, however, capable of influencing anabolic processes and muscle growth. Growth hormone, the somatomedins, insulin, and the thyroid hormones are all known to be important regulators of normal somatic and muscle growth (Florini 1987). Furthermore, muscle growth and strength performance may be ultimately determined by the balance between hormone-regulated anabolic and catabolic processes. Cortisol in particular, and the glucocorticoids in general, are considered catabolic in nature and may have actions that oppose the anabolic hormone effects on muscle growth and strength. While these hormones play a supportive role in muscle development and may have subtle influences on strength development during puberty, they do not exhibit the dramatic sex difference evident for testosterone secretion during this period. In normal healthy children, these hormones are probably relatively less important than testosterone in influencing strength development during puberty.

Physical Activity

Sociocultural and behavioral influences such as age- and gender-associated differences in level of physical activity might also influence the development of strength during childhood. There is some indication based on energy expenditure data (Saris 1986) and physical activity participation rates (Canada Fitness Survey 1983) that boys may be slightly more active than girls in early and mid-childhood and that boys are more likely than girls to participate in activities that require a high degree of muscular strength. There is also some evidence that participation rates in general (Canada Fitness Survey 1983) and total energy expenditure (Verschuur and Kemper 1985) decrease for girls during adolescence, and either do not change (Canada Fitness Survey 1983) or increase in males (Beunen et al. 1988) during the same period.

The significance of these differences in explaining strength development has been largely unexplored and remains to be determined. In a recent study (Beunen et al. 1992), however, differences in the level of general physical (sport) activity did not appear to influence either the shape or magnitude of strength development in boys from puberty to late adolescence. Although differences in the amount of physical activity may be evident across ages, between sexes, and among individuals, perhaps other factors, including the type and intensity of participation in physical activity, play a more important role in influencing the development of strength during childhood.

Heritability

Human performance is determined by environmental and genetic influences and their interaction. Based on rather limited data, there appears to be a low to moderate degree of heritability for isometric strength of selected muscle groups (Kovar 1983), little or no genetic effect for others (Kimura 1956; Komi and Karlsson 1978; Komi et al. 1973), and a moderate heritability for composite isometric strength (Engstrom and Fischbein 1977; Mizuno 1956; Sklad 1973). There are no available studies of the heritability of isokinetic strength in children, but a strong genetic effect has been reported for dynamic strength and power (Jones and Klissouras 1986; Komi and Karlsson 1979; Kovar 1975).

Whatever its magnitude, the heritability of strength could be mediated by genetic determination of muscle fiber number, composition, distribution, and fiber size within a muscle. There appears, however, to be little concensus regarding the genetic influence on muscle fiber differentiation and development. An early study (Komi and Karlsson 1979) indicated a high heritability for slow twitch (type 1) fibers of the vastus lateralis, whereas a more recent study (Bouchard et al. 1986) indicated that there was no significant genetic effect for either fiber type distribution or fiber area in the vastus lateralis in either sex. Animal studies have demonstrated a strong gender-linked genetic influence over the determination of muscle fiber number with males having a larger number of fibers than females, at least in rodents (Rowe and Goldspink 1969). Adult females may also have fewer muscle fibers than adult males (Alway et al. 1989; Miller et al. 1993; Sale et al. 1987; Schantz et al. 1983; Wells and Plowman 1983). There are no studies to our knowledge, however, of gender differences in fiber number during childhood or of the heritability of muscle fiber number in humans.

Neurological and Biomechanical Influences on Strength

There is some, albeit limited, indirect (Asmussen and Heeboll-Nielsen 1955) as well as direct evidence (Blimkie 1989, Davies 1985) for reduced muscle activation ability in younger children compared with older children for some muscle groups. The importance of this influence in terms of strength differentiation across ages and between gender needs further investigation.

The biomechanical effects of musculoskeletal changes with growth on strength development have not been extensively addressed in children. Changes in muscle pennation with increased muscle size during growth may influence force output and contribute to age and gender differences in strength, especially during puberty and adolescence. As shown in figure 9.11, muscle pennation angle, as reflected by ultrasonic measurements of muscle fascicles, increases substantially from childhood to early adulthood in both sexes (T. Fukunaga and Y. Kawakami, personal communication) for the vastus lateralis and gastrocnemius medialis. Fascicle angles appear to plateau in females during late adolescence but continue to increase in

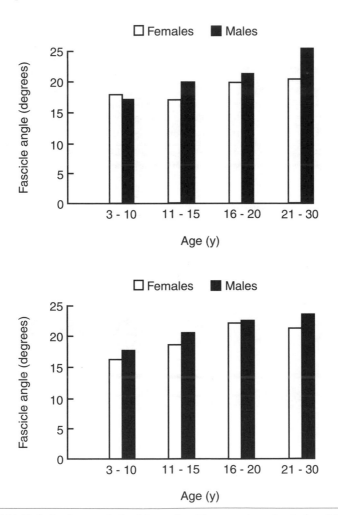

Figure 9.11 Variation in muscle fascicle angle with age and gender during childhood as determined by ultrasonography for the vastus lateralis and gastrocnemius medialis.

Data from T. Fukunaga and Y. Kawakami.

males until early to mid-adulthood. The effects of these pennation changes, and their relative importance to age- and gender-related strength development curves during childhood need to be investigated.

Stability of Strength

Inferences about stability are derived from correlational studies of the relationship between strength measures at different times during childhood. As shown in figure 9.12, stability in strength is highest when the measurement interval is short and does not overlap adjacent developmental stages, e.g., one year intervals between either 7-8 or 17-18 years of age, during the discrete developmental stages of early childhood and late adolescence. Stability becomes progressively poorer as the age range and number of developmental stages included in the comparison increases, e.g., stability is higher between late puberty and late adolescence, spanning an interval of 3 years and 2 developmental stages, than between late childhood and late adolescence, which spans 3 developmental stages and 6 years. The poor stability in strength, particularly across the circumpubertal years, is most likely due to the interindividual variability in rates of maturation in the previously established determinants of strength. With such variability, it is impossible to

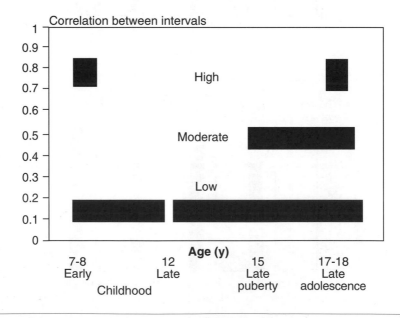

Figure 9.12 Stability of strength measures in relation to measurement interval during childhood.

Data from Malina and Bouchard 1991.

confidently predict individual strength performance during adolescence based on measures made during early or late childhood. Predictions will generally be more accurate and less problematic, however, if made over a narrow age interval and if confined to discrete developmental stages.

Strength Trainability During Childhood

The effectiveness, benefits, and risks of strength training for children have not been as extensively studied and documented as for adults. However, considerable new information on this topic has arisen during the past decade. A brief review of the key findings relating to the effectiveness of strength training, the trainability of children compared with adults, the persistence of training induced strength gains during detraining, and the mechanisms underlying strength changes during training and detraining will be provided in this chapter.

Effectiveness of Resistance Training

Initial studies that failed to demonstrate any increase in strength with resistance or strength training during childhood either utilized fairly modest training loads by today's standards, and/or were of very short duration (Ainsworth 1970; Docherty et al. 1987; Kirsten 1963; Vrijens 1978). Studies that have controlled for the confounding effects of growth and motor skill acquisition on strength gain and that have incorporated moderate to high training loads, however, provide rather convincing evidence that strength training can result in substantial and significant increases in strength during pre-adolescence (Blimkie et al. 1989b; Faigenbaum et al. 1993; Hassan 1991; Mersch and Stoboy 1989; Nielsen et al. 1980; Ozmun et al. 1994; Pfeiffer and Francis 1986; Ramsay et al. 1990; Sailors and Berg 1987; Sewall and Micheli 1986; Weltman et al. 1986). The results from one of the longest studies (20 weeks) involving children, which incorporated high intensity training loads, are summarized in figure 9.13.

Results from the majority of recent training studies provide compelling evidence that strength training can be effective in increasing strength during the pre-adolescent period. The effectiveness of training appears, as it also does in adults, to be dependent primarily on the provision of a sufficient training intensity and volume, and to a lesser degree on training duration. Strength improvements have been reported using isometric, isotonic, and isokinetic training methods involving high intensity loading. The optimal combination of training method, intensity, volume, and duration of training for maximal strength gain during pre-adolescence, however, has yet to be established. There are no adequately controlled studies, to our knowledge, that have investigated gender differences in the trainability of strength in pre-adolescents.

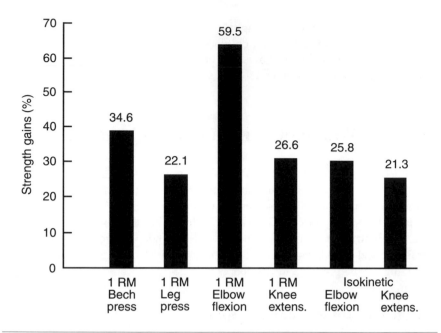

Figure 9.13 Effects of 20 weeks of heavy resistance training on a variety of maximum strength measures in prepubescent boys.

Data from Ramsay et al. 1990.

Comparative Trainability

Comparative trainability can be considered either in terms of percentage (relative) or absolute strength gain, compared with pre-training levels. Earlier studies in this area suggested that pre-adolescent children had either the same or lower relative trainability and lower absolute trainability for some muscle groups compared with adolescents and adults (Hettinger 1958; Kirsten 1963; Vrijens 1978). More recent studies, however, that have incorporated moderate to high training intensities and volumes and that have separated groups more clearly on the basis of maturity level have consistently reported comparable, and sometimes greater, relative strength trainability in pre-adolescents compared with adolescents and adults (Nielsen et al. 1980; Pfeiffer and Francis 1986; Sailors and Berg 1987; Sale 1989; Westcott 1979). A summary of the results from one of these studies is provided in figure 9.14. There is less information about the trainability of absolute strength in children, but it appears that children are probably less trainable in terms of absolute strength gains than adolescents and adults (Sailors and Berg 1987; Sale 1989). Additional studies that include distinct maturity groups, comparable training intensity, and control for age- and gender-associated differences in background level of physical activity are required, however, before the question of comparative strength trainability is unequivocally resolved.

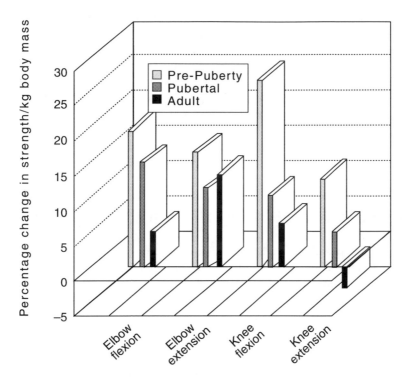

Figure 9.14 Comparative trainability of relative strength changes (percentage improvement) during prepuberty, puberty, and adulthood.

Data from Pfeiffer and Francis 1986.

Persistence of Strength Gains

Since training appears to be effective in increasing strength, the question arises as to whether prior training induced strength gains will be maintained or lost during periods of reduced training or complete detraining in children. This is a difficult question to answer, since growth-related increases in strength during the detraining period may be wholly or partially masked by the effect of reduced training on strength levels achieved by the prior training. Only two studies, to our knowledge, have investigated this question with the inclusion of a control group to account for the effects of growth on strength changes during the detraining period (Blimkie et al. 1989a; Faigenbaum et al. 1996). In the earlier study (Blimkie et al. 1989a), the majority of strength measures in the previously trained group converged toward the control values, suggesting that strength gains during pre-adolescence were probably impermanent. Similar results were observed in a more recent study by Faigenbaum et al. (1996) for leg extension and chest press strength. In this study, however, even after evident strength loss, chest press strength remained significantly increased in the previously trained group compared with the control group at the end of the post-detraining phase.

Likewise, only one study (Blimkie et al. 1989a) has investigated the question of maintenance strength training during pre-adolescence. A once weekly high intensity strength training session was not sufficient in this study to conserve prior training induced strength gains in this group of pre-adolescent boys. Clearly, no firm conclusion can be made about the persistence of strength gains induced from strength training or the requirements for maintenance training during pre-adolescence based on the available literature. These issues are also unresolved for the pubertal and adolescent child.

Mechanisms Underlying Strength Changes

What are the physiological adaptations and the mechanisms underlying strength changes during training and detraining during pre-adolescence? Are the adaptations and mechanisms similar in children and adults?

Morphological Adaptations

Training induced changes in gross limb morphology, and by inference changes in muscle size, have been assessed using indirect anthropometric measurement techniques. In short, there is no evidence from any of the studies that reported significant increases in strength of resistance training-induced muscle hypertrophy during pre-adolescence (Blimkie et al. 1989b; Hassan 1991; McGovern 1984; Ozmun et al. 1994; Ramsay et al. 1990; Sailors and Berg 1987; Siegel et al.1989; Weltman et al. 1986).

The effect of strength training on muscle size in children has also been studied using fairly precise imaging techniques such as soft-tissue roentgenography, computerized axial tomography, and magnetic resonance imaging (Mersch and Stoboy 1989; Ramsay et al. 1990; Vrijens 1978). Despite demonstrating significant improvements in muscle strength, Ramsay et al. (1990) found no evidence of upper arm or thigh muscle hypertrophy measured by computerized tomography in pre-adolescent boys following 20 weeks of high intensity strength training. Using roentgenography, Vrijens (1978) likewise found no evidence of strength training induced muscle hypertrophy in the upper arm or thigh in pre-adolescent boys. This is perhaps not all that surprising, since this study failed to demonstrate a significant training induced strength improvement.

In contrast to these studies, however, recent studies by Fukunaga et al. (1992), and Mersch and Stoboy (1989) reported significant strength training induced increases in both strength and muscle cross-sectional area of the thigh and upper arm, respectively, in pre-adolescent children. Muscle area was measured by the highly precise technique of magnetic resonance imaging in the study by Mersch and Stoboy (1989), but measurements were made on only two pre-adolescent subjects. In the other study (Fukunaga et al. 1992), muscle and bone area was measured in larger numbers of pre-adolescent subjects of both sexes using the less precise technique of ultra-sonography. The results from the latter study are curious, however, since the training program that was based on isometric elbow flexion exercises had a greater effect on elbow extension than flexion strength. In fact, elbow flexion strength increases were more common in the control groups than in the trained groups, and only one of the six sub-populations in this study (1st grade girls) demonstrated a training-associated increase in elbow flexion strength.

It is difficult, given the small sample in the study of Mersch and Stoby (1989) and the non-specificity of the training adaptation in the study by Fukunaga et al. (1992) to totally discount the largely negative results from all the other studies in this area. Nevertheless, these results leave open the possibility of strength training induced muscle hypertrophy even during pre-adolescence.

Whether muscle hypertrophy is possible or not, however, it is evident from the results of all of these studies, including Fukunaga et al. (1992) and Mersch and Stoboy (1989), that the magnitude of this morphological adaptation is small in comparison to the reported strength gains and in comparison to adults. Therefore, other factors besides changes in muscle size must account predominantly for the strength gains observed in these studies.

Neurological Adaptations

By inference, and based solely on the lack of evidence for muscle hypertrophy, both Hassan (1991) and Weltman et al. (1986) attributed the strength increases in their studies of pre-adolescent boys to undefined neurological and neuromotor adaptations. A more direct means of neurological assessment, the twitch interpolation technique (Belanger and McComas 1981), has been used by Blimkie et al. (1989b) and Ramsay et al. (1990) to assess the contribution of changes in motor unit activation (MUA) to training-induced strength increases in pre-adolescent boys. MUA of the elbow flexors and knee extensors increased by 9% and 12%, respectively, after 10 weeks of training, and an additional 10 weeks of training resulted in much smaller increases of only 3% and 2%, respectively. The percentage increases in MUA were less than the increases in strength for both muscle groups. Most recently, Ozmun et al. (1994) used electromyography to measure strength-training induced changes in neuromuscular activation of the elbow flexors in pre-adolescent boys and girls. Eight weeks of training resulted in significant increases in both integrated EMG amplitude (16.8%), and maximal isokinetic strength (27.8%). Results from these studies provide direct evidence that training-induced strength gains in pre-adolescents, especially during the early stages of strength training, are attributable at least in part to increases in neuromuscular activation.

Since the magnitude of the changes in neuromuscular activation are generally smaller than the observed increases in strength, it appears that other factors besides increased neuromuscular drive may also play a role in the determination of training-induced strength gains. It is likely that part of the strength gain may also be attributed to improved motor coordination. Improved movement coordination is probably a more important contributor to strength gains in more complex multi-joint exercises, e.g., the one repetition maximum (1RM) arm curl or leg press exercises, than in less complex and more isolated actions such as those involved in isometric strength assessment of the elbow flexors or knee extensors. Results from the studies by Blimkie et al. (1989b) and Ramsay et al. (1990) indirectly support this contention, since training resulted in larger percent improvements in 1RM arm curl and leg press strength (specific exercises performed during training) than in non-specific isometric elbow flexion and knee extension strength.

Adaptations In Evoked Contractile Properties

Training-induced changes in evoked contractile properties of muscle could also account for part of the observed increase in strength in pre-adolescents following strength training. In the only study that investigated this issue in pre-adolescents (Ramsay et al. 1990), twitch torque, a measure of muscle strength uninfluenced by voluntary effort, increased significantly for both the elbow flexors and knee extensors after 20 weeks of strength training. Since there were no corresponding increases in muscle size, these results indicate an improvement in twitch-specific tension (strength per cross-sectional area). If the increase in twitch-specific tension was also accompanied by an increase in tetanic-specific tension (which was not assessed in this study due to the discomfort associated with the technique), then changes in contractile properties may account for some of the unexplained increase in training-induced maximal voluntary strength gains evident in pre-adolescents. This finding suggests that undefined qualitative adaptations in the muscle may account in part for the training-induced strength gains evident in children following strength training.

Adaptations During Detraining

In adults, strength training-induced increases in muscle size and neural drive decay during detraining at about the same rate as they increase during training (Narici et al. 1989). Detraining in adults is apparently characterized by a relatively rapid reduction in neuromuscular activation, and a more gradual reduction in muscle size (Narici et al. 1989). Since strength training appears to have little, if any, effect on muscle size during pre-adolescence, it is probable that the decrement in training-induced strength gains in this group during detraining are attributable predominantly to changes in the level of neuromuscular activation and motor coordination.

Only one study has investigated the physiological adaptations during maintenance (reduced) training and detraining during pre-adolescence (Blimkie et al. 1989a). Eight weeks of detraining had no significant effect on the magnitude of change in estimated (by anthropometry) lean upper arm or thigh cross-sectional areas among groups of maintenance trained, detrained, and control pre-adolescent boys. The maintenance trained and detrained groups had completed 20 weeks of heavy strength training prior to detraining. The lack of change in muscle size with detraining in this study was not surprising, however, since, in contrast with adults, there was no evidence of muscle hypertrophy at the end of the training program. Results from this single study suggest that any loss in strength during reduced training or total detraining in pre-adolescents is probably not attributable to a reduction in muscle size.

In the same study (Blimkie et al. 1989a), there was a trend towards reduced neuromuscular drive (reduced MUA) in both the maintenance-trained and totally detrained groups. The reductions were considerably larger in the totally detrained group than in the maintenance-trained group. These results suggest that the loss of strength gains during detraining in pre-adolescents is attributable in part to a reduction in neuromuscular activation, as it is also in adults. Although it has never been assessed directly, it is likely that part of the decrement in strength during detraining, especially for more complex, multi-joint strength maneuvers may also be attributed to a loss in motor coordination. Clearly, more information is required about detraining and the physiological adaptations that accompany this process during pre-adolescence.

Directions for Future Research

Our understanding of the effects of growth and maturation on strength development and the effectiveness of strength training during childhood has increased tremendously over the past few decades. Numerous questions remain, however, and need to be examined in future studies. Following is a list of some of the more important issues that we feel need to be addressed in future research. Resolution of these issues will permit better preparation of young athletes and will ensure continued safe and high participation rates in youth sport.

- Investigations of the relationship between the functional strength requirements of activities of daily living and strength capabilities of healthy children and children with chronic diseases or disabilities must be undertaken.
- Investigations of the relationship between muscle and strength development during childhood and health status during both childhood and adulthood, e.g., the importance of muscle mass and strength for optimal bone mineral development and the minimization of fractures during the growth spurt period and during the post-menopausal years in females must likewise be explored.
- Investigating the roles of various anabolic hormones—including testosterone, estrogen, and growth hormones—on strength and muscle development between the sexes and at different stages of development would yield worthwhile information.
- The absolute and relative importance of morphological, neuromuscular, biomechanical, and endocrinological determinants of strength at different stages of development and between genders must also be investigated.

- Age-, sex- and maturity-based practical and safe weight training guidelines for strength improvement and maintenance must be established.
- The importance of strength and strength training for improved sports performance and the prevention and rehabilitation of sport related injuries must be determined.

Summary

Strength increases naturally and dramatically from birth to adulthood, and its development is influenced mostly by biological maturation and sexual differentiation. Strength gains during childhood are closely related to changes in somatic growth, muscle size, neurological development, and biomechanical changes associated with growth. Rapid increases in strength occur during the pubertal growth spurt, and gender differences that become evident at this time are probably associated with maturational awakening and sexual differentiation of the neuroendocrine axis. Strength differences between children of similar age and strength development during childhood are also influenced by heredity and lifestyle factors, including physical activity and sports participation.

Strength training has the potential of improving sport performances, enhancing body composition, and reducing the rate of sport injury and rehabilitation time following injury. These potentially beneficial effects of strength training remain, however, largely unproven for the pre-adolescent (Blimkie 1992; Blimkie 1993). Strength training is also a potentially risky activity for the child in that it may induce temporary or permanent musculoskeletal injury, and it may have detrimental effects on cardiorespiratory fitness and cardiovascular function. Yet with appropriate technique instruction and proper exercise prescription and supervision, strength training does not appear to be a particularly risky activity for most children in terms of health and injury outcome, and it seems to have no detrimental effect on either cardiorespiratory fitness or blood pressure (Blimkie 1992; Blimkie 1993) in normal healthy children. Caution is warranted, however, for children with physical, mental, and medical handicaps, and strength training for these groups should be closely supervised by an adult and monitored by a physician. Moreover, because it is such a highly specialized type of exercise, strength training should be recommended as only one of a variety of physical activities and sport pursuits for the child, regardless of health status.

References

Aherne, W., Ayyar, D.R., Clarke, P.A., Walton, J.N. 1971. Muscle fibre size in normal infants, children and adolescents: An autopsy study. *J. Neurolog. Sci.* 14: 171-182.

Ainsworth, J.L. 1970. The effect of isometric-resistive exercises with the Exer-Genie on strength and speed in swimming. Unpublished Doctoral thesis. University of Arkansas.

Alway, S.E., Grumbt, W.H., Gonyea, W.J., Stray-Gunderson, J. 1989. Contrasts in muscle and myofibers of elite male and female bodybuilders. *J. Appl. Physiol.* 67: 24-31.

Asmussen, E. Growth in muscular strength and power. In: Rarick, G.L., ed. 1970. Physical activity human growth and development. New York, Academic Press, 60-79.

Asmussen, E., Heeboll-Nielsen, K. 1955. A dimensional analysis of physical performance and growth in boys. *J. Appl. Physiol.* 7: 593-603.

Belanger, A.Y., McComas, A.J. 1981. Extent of motor unit activation during effort. *J. Appl. Physiol.* 51: 1131-1135.

Bell, R.D., MacDougall, J.D., Billeter, R., Howald, H. 1980. Muscle fiber types and morphometric analysis of skeletal muscle in six-year-old children. *Med. Sci. Sports Exerc.* 12: 28-31.

Beunen, G.P., Lefevre, J., Claessens, A.L., et al. 1992. Age-specific correlation analysis of longitudinal physical fitness levels in men. *Europ. J. Appl. Physiol.* 64: 538-545.

Beunen, G., Malina, R.M. 1988. Growth and physical performance relative to the timing of the adolescent spurt. *Exerc. Sport Sci. Rev.* 16: 503-540.

Beunen, G.P., Malina, R.M., Van't Hof, M.A., Simons, J., Ostyn, M., Renson, R., Van Gerven, D. 1988. Adolescent growth and motor performance: a longitudinal study of Belgian boys. HKP Sport Science Monograph Series. Champaign, IL: Human Kinetics.

Beunen, G., Simons, J., Ostyn, M., Renson, R., Van Gerven, D.. Learning effects in repeated measurements designs. In Berg, K., Eriksson, B.O., eds. 1980. Children and exercise IX. Baltimore: University Park Press: 41-48.

Blimkie, C.J.R. Age- and sex-associated variation in strength during childhood: Anthropometric, morphologic, neurologic, biomechanical, endocrinologic, genetic, and physical activity correlates. In Gisolfi, C.V., Lamb, D.R., eds. 1980. Perspectives in exercise science and sports medicine. vol. 2. Indianapolis: Benchmark Press: 99-163.

Blimkie, C.J.R. 1992. Resistance training during pre- and early puberty: Efficacy, trainability, mechanisms, and persistence. *Can. J. Sport Sci.* 17: 264-279.

Blimkie, C.J.R. Benefits and risks of resistance training in children. In Cahill, B.R., Pearl, A.J., eds. 1992. Intensive participation in children's sports. Champaign, IL: Human Kinetics: 133-165.

Blimkie, C.J.R. 1993. Resistance training during preadolescence: Issues and controversies. *Sports Med.* 15: 389-407.

Blimkie, C.J.R., Martin, J., Ramsay, J., Sale, D., MacDougall, D. 1989a. The effects of detraining and maintenance weight training on strength development in prepubertal boys. *Can. J. Sport Sci.* 14: #102P.

Blimkie, C.J.R., Ramsay, J., Sale, D., MacDougall, D., Smith, K., Garner, S. Effects of 10 weeks of resistance training on strength development in prepubertal boys.

In Oseid, S., Carlsen, K-H., eds. 1989b. Children and exercise XIII. Champaign, IL: Human Kinetics: 183-197.

Boileau, R.A., Lohman, T.G., Slaughter, M.H. 1985. Exercise and body composition of children and youth. *Scand. J. Sports Sci.* 7: 17-27.

Bouchard, C., Simoneau, J.A., Lortie, G., Boulay, M.R., Marcotte, M., Thibault, M.C. 1986. Genetic effects in human skeletal muscle fibre type distribution and enzyme activities. *Can. J. Physiol. Pharmacol.* 64: 1245-1251.

Brooke, M., Engel, W. 1969. The histograph analysis of human muscle biopsies with regard to fibre types. *Neurology* 19: 591-605.

Cahill, B., ed. 1988. Proceedings of the conference on strength training and the prepubescent. Chicago: American Orthopaedic Society For Sports Medicine.

Canada fitness survey. 1983. Canadian youth and physical activity, Ottawa, ON: Fitness and Amateur Sport.

Canada fitness survey. 1985. Physical fitness and Canadian youth, Ottawa, ON: Fitness and Amateur Sport.

Carron, A.V., Aitken, E.J., Bailey, D.A. Untitled. In Lavallee, H., Shephard, R.J., eds. 1977. Frontiers of activity and child health. Ottawa, ON: Editions Du Pelican: 139-143.

Carron, A.V., Bailey, D.A. 1974. Strength development in boys from 10 through 16 years. Monographs of the Society for Research in Child Development, 39: 4, Serial No. 157.

Clarke, H.H. 1971. Physical and motor tests in the Medford boy's growth study. Englewood Cliffs, NJ: Prentice-Hall.

Clarke, H.H., Degutis, E.W. 1962. Comparison of skeletal age and various physical and motor factors with the pubescent development of 10, 13, and 16 year old boys. *Res. Quart.* 33: 356-368.

Colling-Saltin, A-S. Skeletal muscle development in the human fetus and during childhood. In Berg K., Eriksson, B.O., eds. 1980. Children and exercise IX. Baltimore: University Park Press: 193-207.

Davies, C.T.M. 1985. Strength and mechanical properties of muscle in children and young adults. *Scand. J. Sports Sci.* 7: 11-15.

Docherty, D., Wenger, H.A., Collis, M.L., Quinney, H.A. 1987. The effects of variable speed resistance training on strength development in prepubertal boys. *J. Hum. Movement Stud.* 13: 377-382.

Elder, G.C.B., Kakulas, B.A. 1993. Histochemical and contractile property changes during human development. *Muscle Nerve* 16: 1246-1253.

Engstrom, L.M., Fischbein, S. 1977. Physical capacity in twins. *Acta Genet. Med. Gemellol.* 26: 159-165.

Faigenbaum, A.D., Westcott, W.L., Micheli, L. J., Outerbridge, A.R., Long, C.J., LaRosa-Loud, R., Zaichkowsky, L.D. 1996. The effects of strength training and detraining on children. *J. Strength and Cond. Res.* 10: 109-114.

Faigenbaum, A.D., Zaichkowsky, L.D., Westcott, W.L., Micheli, L.J., Fehlandt, A.F. 1993. The effects of a twice-a-week strength training program on children. *Ped. Exerc. Sci.* 5: 339-346.

Faust, M.S. 1977. Somatic development of adolescent girls. Monograph. Society For Research In Child Development, 42(1): 1-90.

Florini, J.R. 1987. Hormonal control of muscle growth. *Muscle and Nerve* 10: 577-598.

Forbes, G.B. 1965. Toward a new dimension in human growth. *Pediatr.* 36: 825-835.

Fournier, M., Ricca, J., Taylor, A.W., Ferguson, R.J., Montpetit, R.R., Chaitman, B.R. 1982. Skeletal muscle adaptation in adolescent boys: sprint and endurance training and detraining. *Med. Sci. Sports Exerc.* 14: 453-456.

Froberg, K., Andersen, B., Lammert, O. Maximal voluntary isometric strength in differently trained boys during puberty. In Coudert, J. and Van Praagh, E., eds. 1992. Paris: Masson: 162.

Froberg, K., Lammert, O. Development of muscle strength during childhood. In The child and adolescent athlete. Bar-Or, O., ed.,1996 .The encyclopedia of sports medicine. vol. IV. London: Blackwell Scientific: 25-41.

Fukunaga, T., Funato, K., Ikegawa, S. 1992. The effects of resistance training on muscle area and strength in prepubescent age. *Ann. Physiol. Anthrop.* 11: 357-364.

Glenmark, B., Hedberg, G., Jannson, E. 1992. Changes in muscle fibre type from adolescence to adulthood in women and men. *Acta Physiol. Scand.* 146: 251-259.

Gollnick, P.D., Timson, B.F., Moore, R.L., Riedy, M. 1981. Muscular enlargement and numbers of fibers in skeletal muscles of rats. *J. Appl. Physiol.* 50: 936-943.

Hassan, S.E.A. 1991. Die Trainierbarkeit der Maximalkraft bei 7- bis 13 jahrigen Kindern: Leistungssport 5: 17-24.

Hedberg, G., Jansson, E. 1986. Skelettmuskelfiber-komposition. Kapacitet och intresse for olika fysiska aktiviteter blandelever: Gymnasieskolan. Rapport 54, Pedagogiska Institute: Umea. Cited in Malina, 1986.

Hettinger, T.H. 1958. Die Trainierbarkeit menschlicher Muskeln in Abhängigkeit vom Alter und Geschlecht. *Internationale Zeitschrift für angewandte Physiologie einschliesslich Arbeitsphysiologie* 17: 371-377.

Ikai, M., Fukunaga, T. 1968. Calculations of muscle strength per unit cross-sectional area of human muscle by means of ultrasonic measurement. *International Zeitschrift für angewandte Physiologie einschliesslich Arbeitsphysiologie* 26: 26-32.

Johnston, F.E., Malina, R.M. 1966. Age changes in composition of the upper arm in Philadelphia children. *Hum. Biol.* 38: 1-21.

Jones, B., Klissouras, V. Genetic variation in the force-velocity relation of human muscle. In Malina, R.M., Bouchard, C., eds. 1986. Sports and human genetics. Champaign, IL: Human Kinetics: 155-163.

Jones, H.E. 1949. Motor performance and growth. Berkley: University of California Press.

Kelly, A., Lyons, G., Gambki, B., Rubinstein, N. 1985. Influences of testosterone on contractile proteins of the guinea pig temporalis muscle. *Adv. Exper. Biol. Med.* 182: 155-168.

Kemper, H.C.G. Health and fitness of Dutch teenagers: a review. In Day, J.A.P., ed. 1986. Perspectives in kinanthropometry. Champaign, IL: Human Kinetics: 61-80.

Kimura, K. 1983. The study on physical ability of children and youths: On twins in Osaka City. *Jinrui Idengaku Zasshi* 64: 172-196. Cited in Bouchard and Malina, 1983.

Kirsten, G. 1963. Der Einflus Isometrischen Muskeltrainings auf die Entwicklung der Muskelkraft Jugendlicher. *Internationale Zeitschrift für angewandte Physiologie einschliesslich Arbeitsphysiologie* 19: 387-402.

Komi, P.V., Karlsson, J. 1978. Skeletal muscle fibre types, enzyme activities and physical performance in young males and females. *Acta Physiol. Scand.* 103: 210-218.

Komi, P.V., Karlsson, J. 1979. Physical performance, skeletal muscle enzyme activities, and fibre types in monozygous and dizygous twins of both sexes. *Acta Physiol. Scand.* 462 (Suppl.): 1-28.

Komi, P.V., Klissouras, V., Karvinen, E. 1973. Genetic variation in neuromuscular performance. *International Zeitschrift für angewandte Physiologie einschliesslich Arbeitsphysiologie* 31: 289-304.

Kovar, R. 1975. Motor performance in twins. *Acta Genet. Med. Geme Illolog.* 24: 174.

Kovar, R. 1983. Human variation in motor abilities and its genetic analysis. Prague: Charles University. Cited in Bouchard and Malina, 1983.

Larsson, L., Moss, R.L. 1993. Maximum velocity of shortening in relation to myosin isoform composition in single fibres from human skeletal muscles. *J. Physiol.* 472: 595-614.

Maglischo, C.W. 1968. Bases of norms for cable-tension strength tests for upper elementary, junior high and senior high school girls. *Res. Quart.* 39: 595-603.

Malina, R.M. 1969. Quantification of fat, muscle and bone in man. *Clin. Orthop. Rel. Res.* 65: 9-38.

Malina, R.M. 1975. Anthropometric correlates of performance. *Exerc. Sport Sci. Rev.* 3: 249-274.

Malina, R.M. Growth of muscle tissue and muscle mass. In Falkner, F, Tanner, J.M., eds. 1978. Human growth. vol. 2. New York: Plenum Press: 273-294.

Malina, R.M. Growth of muscle tissue and muscle mass. In Falkner, F, Tanner, J.M., eds. 1986. Human growth: A comprehensive treatise 2. New York: Plenum Press: 77-99.

Malina, R.M., Bouchard, C. 1991. Growth, maturation and physical activity. Champaign, IL: Human Kinetics.

Malina, R.M., Johnston, F.E. 1967. Relations between bone, muscle and fat widths in the upper arms and calves of boys and girls studied cross-sectionally at ages 6 to 16 years. *Hum. Biol.* 39: 211-223.

McGovern, M.B. 1984. Effects of circuit weight training on the physical fitness of prepubescent children. Dissertation Abstracts International 45(2): 452A-453A.

Mersch, F., Stoboy, H. Strength training and muscle hypertrophy in children. In Oseid, S., Carlsen, K-H., eds. 1989. Children and exercise XIII. Champaign, IL: Human Kinetics: 165-182.

Miller, A.E.J., MacDougall, J.D., Tarnopolsky, M.A., Sale, D.G. 1993. Gender differences in strength and muscle fiber characteristics. *Eur. J. Appl. Physiol.* 66: 254-262.

Mizuno, T. 1956. Similarity of physique, muscular strength and motor ability in identical twins. Bulletin of The Faculty of Education. Tokyo: Tokyo University. 1: 190-191. Cited in Bouchard and Malina, 1983.

Narici, M.V., Roi, G.S., Landoni, L., Minetti, A.E., Cerretteli, P. 1989. Changes in force, cross-sectional area and neural activation during strength training and detraining of the human quadriceps. *Eur. J. Appl. Physiol.* 59: 310-319.

Nielsen, B., Nielsen, K., Behrendt-Hansen, M., Asmussen, E. Training of "functional" muscular strength in girls 7-19 years old. In Berg, K., Eriksson, B.D., eds. 1980. Children and exercise IX. Champaign, IL: Human Kinetics: 69-78.

Oertel, G. 1988. Morphometric analysis of normal skeletal muscles in infancy, childhood and adolescence. An autopsy study. *J. Neurol. Sci.* 88: 303-313.

Ozmun, J.C., Mikesky, A.E., Surburg, P.R. 1994. Neuromuscular adaptations following prepubescent strength training. *Med. Sci. Sports Exerc.* 26: 510-514.

Parker, D.F., Round, J.M., Sacco, P., Jones, D.A. 1990. A cross-sectional survey of upper and lower limb strength in boys and girls during childhood and adolescence. *Ann. Hum. Biol.* 17: 199-211.

Pfeiffer, R.D., Francis, R.S. 1986. Effects of strength training on muscle development in prepubescent, pubescent, and postpubescent males. *Phys. Sportsmed.* 14: 134-143.

Ramsay, J.A., Blimkie, C.J.R., Smith, K., Garner, S., MacDougall, J.D., Sale, D.G. 1990. Strength training effects in prepubescent boys. *Med. Sci. Sports Exerc.* 22: 605-614.

Rowe, R.W.D., Goldspink, G. 1969. The growth of five different muscles in both sexes of mice. *I. Normal mice. J. Anat.* 104: 519-530.

Sailors, M., Berg, K. 1987. Comparison of responses to weight training in pubescent boys and men. *J. Sports Med.* 27: 30-36.

Sale, D.G. Strength training in children. In Gisolfi, C.V., Lamb, D.R., eds. 1989. Perspectives in exercise science and sports medicine. vol. II. Indianapolis: Benchmark Press: 165-222.

Sale, D.G., MacDougall, J.D., Alway, S.E., Sutton, J.R. 1987. Voluntary strength and muscle characteristics in untrained men and women and male bodybuilders. *J. Appl. Physiol.* 62: 1786-1793.

Sale, D.G., Spriet, L.L. Skeletal muscle function and energy metabolism. In Bar-Or, O., Lamb, D.R., Clarkson, P., eds. 1996. Exercise and sports medicine. vol. 9. Carmel, IN: Cooper Publishing Group: 289-363.

Saltin, B., Henriksson, J., Nygaard, E., Andersen, P., Jansson, E. 1977. Fibre types and metabolic potentials of skeletal muscles in sedentary man and endurance runners. *Ann. New York Acad. Sci.* 301: 3-29.

Saris, W.H.M. 1986. Habitual physical activity in children: methodology and findings in health and disease. *Med. Sci. Sports Exerc.* 18: 253-263.

Saris, W.H.M., Elvers, J.W.H., Van't Hof, M.A., Binkhorst, R.A. Changes in physical activity of children aged 6 to 12 years. In Rutenfranz, J., Mocellin, R., Klimt, F., eds. 1986. Children and exercise XII. Champaign, IL: Human Kinetics: 121-130.

Schantz, P., Randall-Fox, E., Hutchisin, W., Tyden, A., Astrand, P.-O. 1983. Muscle fibre type distribution, muscle cross-sectional area and maximal voluntary strength in humans. *Acta Physiol. Scand.* 117: 219-226.

Sewall, L., Micheli, L.J. 1986. Strength training for children. *J. Pediat. Orthop.* 6: 143-146.

Siegel, J.A., Camaione, D.N., Manfredi, T.G. 1989. The effects of upper body resistance training on prepubescent children. *Ped. Exerc. Sci.* 1: 145-154.

Sklad, M. 1973. Rozwoj fizyczny: motorycznosc blizniat. Materialyi Prace Antropologiczne 85: 3-102. Cited in Bouchard and Malina, 1983.

Souccar, C., Lapa, A.J., do Valle, J.R. 1982. The influence of testosterone on neuromuscular transmission in hormone sensitive mammalian skeletal muscles. *Muscle and Nerve* 5: 232-237.

Stolz, H.R., Stolz, L.M. 1951. Somatic development of adolescent boys. New York: Macmillan.

Verschuur, R., Kemper, H.C.G. Habitual physical activity in Dutch teenagers measured by heart rate. In Binkhorst, R.A., Kemper, H.C.G., Saris, W.H.M., eds. 1985. Children and exercise XI. Champaign, IL: Human Kinetics: 194-202.

Vrijens, J. 1978. Muscle strength development in the pre- and post-pubescent age. *Med. Sport* 11: 152-158.

Wells, C.L., Plowman, S.A. 1983. Sexual differences in athletic performance: biological or behavioral? *Phys. Sportsmed.* 11: 52-63.

Weltman, A., Janny, C., Rians, C.B., Strand, K., Berg, B., Tippitt, S., Wise, J., Cahill, B.S., Katch, F.I. 1986. The effects of hydraulic resistance strength training in prepubertal males. *Med. Sci. Sports Exerc.* 18: 629-638.

Westcott, W.L. 1979. Female response to weight training. *J. Phy. Educ.* 77: 31-33.

10

CHAPTER

Isokinetic Strength During Childhood and Adolescence

Vasilios Baltzopoulos
Eleftherios Kellis

This chapter focuses on the following objectives:

- To review the findings on muscle function in children assessed using isokinetic dynamometry
- To explain the difficulties and problems in performance of isokinetic measurements in children and the necessary adjustments and correction methods
- To highlight the differences between isolated isokinetic joint tests and functional activities and the implications for training and performance prediction in young athletes

Strength is a general concept used to describe the ability of the muscles to exert force under various testing conditions or movements. The force exerted by muscles causes the rotation of the segments around joints. Consequently, strength in this text refers to the rotational effect of force (moment).

Isokinetic dynamometers allow the assessment of muscle and joint function under constant joint angular velocity conditions. This is accomplished by adjusting the force exerted on the limb so that the acceleration of the system is zero. This also allows maximum moment exertion by the muscles throughout the range of motion. The resultant joint moment can be evaluated at angular velocities ranging from 0 to $500° \cdot s^{-1}$ for concentric movements and from 0 to $300° \cdot s^{-1}$ for eccentric movements. However, it must be noted that isokinetic angular velocity refers to the velocity of the dynamometer lever arm and the body segment and not to the linear shortening or lengthening velocity of the muscle(s) involved.

One of the most important features of isokinetic dynamometry is the accurate assessment of muscle function. In addition, the range of motion and angular velocity can be adjusted depending on the subject's ability to exert force. The results of an isokinetic test can be stored and compared with those of other tests in order to monitor strength improvements.

Most of the research in this area has focused on the evaluation of isokinetic parameters in adults (Baltzopoulos and Brodie 1989; Kellis and Baltzopoulos 1995). The examination of strength development with age has not been extensively pursued using isokinetic dynamometry. In this chapter the basic principles of isokinetics and their particular application for the assessment of muscle function during childhood are presented. The problems that may arise in examining children and some basic correction methods are presented. In addition, research findings on the use of isokinetic exercise in training programs are discussed.

Isokinetic Parameters

A typical isokinetic dynamometry test involves measurement of the resultant or net moment during isolated joint movement(s) at a preselected joint angular velocity. After the test, appropriate corrections of the dynamometer-recorded moment are performed in order to calculate the joint moment during the isokinetic (constant angular velocity) range of movement. From these data sets (moment-angular position or moment-time at different angular velocities), a number of different parameters are calculated in order to quantify various aspects of muscle function such as maximum strength, endurance, joint balance, etc. These parameters are described in detail in the pages to follow.

Maximum Joint Moment

The most common isokinetic parameter is the maximum moment, and although there is no commonly accepted standard, the number of repetitions for maximum moment measurement ranges from two to six (Gaul 1996). The moment at a predetermined angular position or the average moment from a number of repetitions is also used as an indicator of muscle function.

Studies that have examined isokinetic strength characteristics in preadolescents focused mainly on the maximum moment output at a single point and over a range of angular velocities (Alexander and Molnar 1973; Molnar, Alexander, and Gutfield 1979; Burnie and Brodie 1986; Burnie 1987; Mohtadi et al. 1990). Gaul (1996) presented a comprehensive review of isokinetic measurement protocols for the evaluation of muscular strength in pediatric populations. Tables 10.1 and 10.2 summarize the results of the major, most recent studies that have examined isokinetic function of the knee extensors and flexors in different pre- and postpubertal age groups. The concentric maximum moment of knee extensors is generally greater

Table 10.1 Concentric Knee Extension Moment (Nm) at Different Angular Velocities as Reported in Some of the Main Studies on Isokinetic Strength in Childhood and Adolescence

Study	N	Sex	Mass (kg)	Age	0.52 / 30	1.05 / 60	1.57 / 90	1.74 / 100	2.09 / 120	3.14 / 180	4.01 / 230	5.24 / 300	I.D.	G	ROM (deg)	Rep
												rad/s				
												deg/s				
Calmers et al. 1995	9	F	28.7	11.3		**74.9** *19.5*			**61.1** *11.1*				Cybex 6000 C	+		6
Merlini et al. 1995	12	M	27.2	7.1				**40.1** *12*					Lido	+	0-100	5
Russell et al. 1995	22	M	42	13.4			**91.4** *23.2*				**70.9** *15.6*		KinCom	+	0-90	6
	18	M	55	15.4			**131** *25.8*				**98.5** *22.1*					
	11	M	61.7	17.5			**163** *27.3*				**115.1** *18.6*					
Kanehisha et al. 1994	30	M	24	7.7		**141*** *4.6**				**93.4*** *4.9**		**58.7*** *3.8**	Cybex II	N/A	0-90	5
	30	F	23.8	7.8		**130*** *5.1**				**72.4*** *4.1**		**43.6*** *2.5**				
Docherty & Gaul 1991	23	M	37.6	10.8	**80.8** *20.3*					**44.5** *12.4*			Cybex II	N/A	N/A	4
	29	F	39.7	11.1	**82.8** *14.9*					**41.8** *10.6*						
Mohtadi et al. 1990	12	M	37.8	11.3		**83.2** *11.6*							KinCom	+	20-80	3
Docherty et al. 1987	11	M	43.8	12.6	**78.4** *16.8*								Cybex II	N/A	N/A	N/A
Weltman et al. 1988	10	M	27.9	8.2	**38** *6*		**32** *7*						KinCom	N/A	10-90	N/A

Note. Numbers in italics represent one standard deviation. (N: number of subjects; M: male; F: female; I.D.: isokinetic dynamometer; G: gravity correction; ROM: range of movement; Rep: number of repetitions; N/A: not available. *: These values represent force N and must be multiplied by the length of the moment arm (i.e., distance between the point of attachment of the dynamometer on the leg and the axis of rotation) in meters in order to obtain comparable moment (Nm) values.)

Table 10.2 Concentric Knee Flexion Moment (Nm) at Different Angular Velocities as Reported in Some of the Main Studies on Isokinetic Strength in Childhood and Adolescence

Study	Subject				Concentric knee flexion							Protocol			
	N	Sex	Mass (kg)	Age	0.52 / 30	1.05 / 60	1.57 / 90	1.74 / 100	2.09 / 120	3.14 / 180	4.01 / 230	I.D.	G	ROM (deg)	Rep
Calmers et al. 1995	9	F	28.7	11.3		**38**			**35.8**			Cybex 6000 C	+		6
						3.4			*4.9*						
Merlini et al. 1995	12	M	27.2	7.1				**25.2**				Lido	+	0-100	5
								8.7							
Russell et al. 1995	22	M	42	13.4			**44.4**				**36.5**	KinCom	+	0-90	6
							12.5				*9.6*				
	18	M	55	15.4			**64.2**				**51.1**				
							16.1				*14.4*				
	11	M	61.7	17.5			**79.5**				**61.9**				
							15.5				*10.9*				
Docherty & Gaul	23	M	37.6	10.8	**61**					**38.7**		Cybex II	N/A	N/A	4
					10.7					*9.7*					
1991	29	F	39.7	11.1	**56.9**					**34.1**					
					11.7					*10.6*					
Docherty et al. 1987	11	M	43.8	12.6	**89.9**					**67.5**		Cybex II	N/A	N/A	N/A
					20.2					*18.5*					
Weltman et al. 1986	10	M	27.9	8.2	**16.7**		**11.8**					KinCom	N/A	10-90	N/A
					20		*1.1*								

Note. Numbers in italics represent one standard deviation. (N: number of subjects; M: male; F: female; I.D.: isokinetic dynamometer; G: gravity correction; ROM: range of movement; Rep: number of repetitions; N/A: not available.

than that of knee flexors. This reflects the differences in muscle size and function of these two muscle groups.

The maximum concentric moment in children is significantly lower than the eccentric moment output (Mohtadi et al. 1990; Kawakami et al. 1993). This is in agreement with findings based on adults or isolated muscles (Kellis and Baltzopoulos 1995) and indicates that the muscle is able to generate greater force when it is stretched, irrespective of the age or gender of the subjects examined. The difference between concentric and eccentric strength can be mainly attributed to the different contribution of the active and passive components of the muscle. The force generated by the active component, through cross-bridge formation and breakage, requires less energy and is greater under eccentric as compared to concentric actions. The passive forces produced by the stretch of the connective tissues are also significantly greater under eccentric actions when the length of the musculotendinous unit is increased.

In adults, it is known that the maximum moment decreases as concentric angular velocity decreases, whereas eccentric strength is maintained at a similar level or decreases with increasing angular velocity (Baltzopoulos and Brodie 1989; Kellis and Baltzopoulos 1995). Similar findings have been reported in preadolescents for both concentric and eccentric moments (Kawakami et al. 1993; Calmers et al. 1995).

The selection of the type of strength test (eccentric, concentric, or isometric) should be specific to the function of the muscle during the activity under examination. Eccentric testing in children, however, is difficult because of the movement control required. Special care is required, with appropriate instructions and explanations, to ensure that the child understands the requirements of the eccentric test; it is also important to allow adequate time for familiarization.

Reciprocal Muscle Group Ratio

The antagonist-to-agonist moment ratio is another important isokinetic parameter. Findings on the relationship between isokinetic strength imbalances and injury are conflicting, as some studies have found significant correlation whereas others have found no correlation (for a review see Baltzopoulos and Brodie 1989; Kellis and Baltzopoulos 1995). However, it should be noted that injury or joint abnormality may be a result of a wide range of factors, not just reduced strength of some muscles compared to others.

The reciprocal muscle group ratios around different joints in different populations have been examined in a large number of studies (Baltzopoulos and Brodie 1989; Kellis and Baltzopoulos 1995). In preadolescents, the knee flexor-to-extensor ratio was reported to range from 0.45 (Alexander and Molnar 1973) to 0.90 (Burnie 1987). Extensor-to-flexor moment ratios for the elbow, hip, and shoulder of 0.90, 0.65 (Burnett, Betts, and King 1990), and 0.90 (Brodie et al. 1986), respectively, have been reported. The reciprocal ratios for ankle dorsiflexion to plantarflexion movements can range from 0.27 to 0.31 (Tabin, Gregg, and Bonci 1985). In general, reciprocal ratios in preadolescents increase with increasing angular velocity.

These results should be carefully interpreted, as in most studies (Tabin, Gregg, and Bonci 1985; Brodie et al. 1986; Burnie and Brodie 1986; Burnie 1987) gravitational moment correction was not implemented. In this case, the moments of the antigravity muscles are less than their actual values, whereas the opposite is the case for the moment of the muscles facilitated by gravity. This may significantly affect the reciprocal muscle group ratios, especially when testing subjects with limited strength capacity such as children (Baltzopoulos and Brodie 1989; Kellis and Baltzopoulos 1995).

As many natural movements consist of alternating sequences of antagonist and agonist activities producing eccentric and concentric work, it appears more reasonable to examine ratios that account for the different action of the muscles during the activity or sport in which the child participates than to examine the reciprocal ratio under isolated concentric or eccentric conditions. One of these parameters is the antagonist eccentric-agonist concentric maximum moment ratio (Kellis and Baltzopoulos 1995). Examination of the relationship between this parameter and injury in young athletes may provide essential information on the mechanisms responsible for injury. This will also allow the design of more effective rehabilitation and injury prevention programs.

Bilateral Muscle Group Ratio

The comparison of the moment exerted by the same muscle group between the left and right sides is also used as an indicator of imbalance of one side relative to the other (Burnie and Brodie 1986; Burnie 1987; Baltzopoulos and Brodie 1989). The use of bilateral ratios is limited by the lack of normative data for a given population and the specificity of subject characteristics and methodology used. Therefore, bilateral ratios are more applicable in practice than in research, as they can provide a direct and immediate evaluation of weakness of a muscle group (Henderson et al. 1993).

Bilateral moment differences for the knee extensor and flexor muscle groups in healthy children are relatively small (Burnie and Brodie 1986; Burnie 1987; Mohtadi et al. 1990; Capranica et al. 1992), but values as high as 53% have been reported (Henderson et al. 1993). Specific sport (soccer) training at these ages does not appear to result in greater strength of one limb relative to the other (Capranica et al. 1992; Calmers et al. 1995).

The age and the level of strength of subjects can significantly affect the bilateral moment ratio. Children with a lower level of strength demonstrate higher bilateral ratios compared to children with greater moment output (Henderson et al. 1993; Calmers et al. 1995). The protocol used for the assessment of muscle moment should be the same for both legs; otherwise the validity of the results is significantly reduced.

Interpretation of bilateral ratios should consider the effects of dominance and the specific activities of the children examined. Healthy subjects can demonstrate bilateral differences that can be characterized as abnormal. Similarly, children with neuromuscular disorders or injury can produce similar moment output between the affected and the unaffected limb. Muscle strength, as measured by the dynamometer, is the product of the interaction of several neuromuscular mechanisms and can also be affected by the mechanics of the joint examined. Consequently, what is initially considered as bilateral deficit may just be due to the variability of the force production mechanism.

Muscular Endurance

Muscular endurance in isokinetic dynamometry is the ability of the muscle to exert maximum moment at a specific angular velocity for a predetermined period of time. An endurance test usually quantifies the moment (or other parameter such as work or power) decrease during a predetermined number of repetitions (30 to 50) or over a standard period of time. The indicator of muscle endurance (fatigue index) is then estimated as the percentage decline of the peak moment during the final period of the test as compared with the peak moment during the first repetitions. Alternatively, the time or number of repetitions until the moment decreases to a certain percentage of the maximum (usually 50%) can be used as the fatigue index (Baltzopoulos and Brodie 1989; Kellis and Baltzopoulos 1995).

It appears that young boys demonstrate different muscular endurance characteristics than adults (Kawakami et al. 1993). Studies in adults have indicated that, for a given number of repetitions, eccentric moment decline is significantly lower compared to that of the corresponding concentric moment (Kellis and Baltzopoulos 1995). In contrast, in preadolescents, no differences in the decline of moment during 50 actions between eccentric and concentric tests were found (Kawakami et al. 1993).

The findings described suggest that children are unable to develop maximum eccentric strength for a long period of time. This can be attributed to a reduced ability to fully activate the muscles, especially under eccentric conditions, and reduced reliance on glycolysis (Kawakami et al. 1993; Kanehisa et al. 1995). However, the limited number of studies in this area does not permit general conclusions on muscle fatigue characteristics in children. The effects of age, gender, and level of strength on isokinetic endurance parameters have to be established.

Reliability and Validity of Isokinetic Dynamometry

The reliability of moment measurements is a very important issue in isokinetics. A test is reliable when similar moment measurements are obtained with repeated tests over a certain time interval. Poor reliability of the measurements may lead to erroneous conclusions about the parameter examined.

The validity of the isokinetic parameters indicates whether these quantities are an accurate measure of the relevant muscle and joint function characteristics. As the reliability and validity of measurements are closely linked, it is essential to minimize the factors affecting them and ensure valid and reliable estimates of isokinetic muscle and joint function.

Reliability of Isokinetic Testing

Isokinetic strength tests in adult populations demonstrate high reliability, depending on the joint examined and the testing protocol used (Kellis and Baltzopoulos 1995). Research on reliability of isokinetic measurements in preadolescents is limited (Merlini, Dell'Accio, and Granata 1995) and indicates that, in general, there is good reliability even for children in the 6-8-year-old group. The most reliable isokinetic concentric tests are those involving the knee joint (Molnar, Alexander, and Gutfield 1979; Weltman et al. 1986; Gross et al. 1990). Isokinetic tests of the elbow flexors and extensors and shoulder muscles demonstrate moderate to high reliability (Molnar, Alexander, and Gutfield 1979; Weltman et al. 1988). Finally, findings on the reliability of concentric moments during hip movements are conflicting, as some studies have reported minimal test-retest variation (Molnar, Alexander, and Gutfield 1979) whereas others have found poor to moderate reliability (Burnett, Betts, and King 1990).

In preadolescents, the reliability of the measurements is affected, to a greater extent than in adults, by neuromuscular differences (e.g., muscle coordination) that exist between children and adults. It seems that younger children can produce consistent isokinetic results that are similar to those for older children (Burnett, Betts, and King 1990). But especially at young ages, children may be afraid to exert maximal moment during the test, a difficulty that is also often observed in adults, especially in injured individuals. Problems may also arise when one examines joints in cases in which the positioning and limits of motion are more difficult to set. In addition, special attention is necessary in examination of isokinetic eccentric strength because it is difficult for children to understand the nature of the movement and what is required during the test (Kellis and Baltzopoulos 1995). The problems mentioned can be effectively overcome by providing precise and detailed instructions on what the child has to do. The instructions should also be very simple; the examiner needs to avoid any technical details and try to provide examples of movements that are already known to children to help them understand what they are required to do, such as:

1. This machine measures the strength of your legs, so you must try your best.
2. You must kick with your leg all the way to the end until your knee is straight and then pull your leg back. You must do this as hard and as fast as you can (concentric test).
3. The machine will pull your leg up and then down. You must try to stop the machine from pulling your leg. Try as hard as you can (eccentric test).

4. During the test the machine draws a graph of your strength on the computer. Watch the computer and try to make the line go near the top of the computer by trying harder.
5. If you start feeling any pain in your legs or start feeling sick or dizzy then stop straight away.

Demonstration of the movement at a variety of speeds followed by submaximal repetitions could also familiarize the child with the dynamometer, thus increasing the validity and reliability of the testing. The factors just mentioned are particularly important when examining children with neuromuscular, brain, or joint disorders.

Validity of Isokinetic Testing

The accuracy of isokinetic dynamometers can be influenced by several mechanical and procedural factors, and appropriate correction methods are required. The movement consists of the acceleration of the limb until the predetermined velocity is achieved, the constant-velocity (isokinetic) phase, and the deceleration of the limb (see figure 10.1).

The duration of the constant-velocity (isokinetic) period depends on the preset (target) angular velocity, the range of motion, and the capabilities of the subject. The faster the preset speed, the shorter the isokinetic part of the movement. Similarly, the greater the range of motion the greater the constant-velocity period. Because the dynamometer moment is not equal to the joint moment during acceleration and deceleration of the system, these nonconstant-velocity periods should not be in-

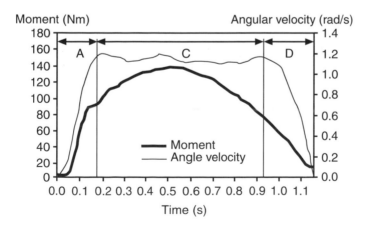

Figure 10.1 Moment and angular velocity graphs from an isokinetic knee extension at a preset velocity of 1.05 rad/s. The graph illustrates the different phases of the movement: A (acceleration), C (constant velocity or isokinetic) and D (deceleration). The movement is performed mainly in constant-velocity conditions (C), and the maximum moment was recorded during this isokinetic phase.

cluded in the analysis. Otherwise, appropriate moment correction equations based on the mechanics of the system, which account for the angular acceleration rates and the inertial characteristics of the limb, should be applied (Baltzopoulos 1995). Failure to correct this error may lead to erroneous estimation of muscle properties and use of inappropriate parameters, such as the moment exerted during the first 0.125 ms of the movement (torque acceleration energy). Furthermore, it is likely that even the corrected maximum moment is exerted under nonconstant-velocity (i.e., nonisokinetic) conditions, especially in high-preset-velocity tests (see figure 10.2).

In these cases, if the angular velocity is not checked, then the maximum moment reported may have been recorded at a different (usually lower) velocity and therefore does not represent muscle strength at the preset velocity. These factors are especially important when one examines joints with a very limited range of motion and weak muscle groups where the movement may consist only of acceleration and deceleration movements. For these reasons it is particularly important to consider the kinematics of the movement when testing children.

The forces due to the weight of the limb(s) and the lever arm of the dynamometer also affect the resultant joint moment produced during movements that are performed on the sagittal plane. For example, during concentric knee extension-flexion movements, the knee flexors are facilitated by the gravitational forces whereas the knee extensors are antigravity muscles. This results in overestimation of the knee flexion moment and underestimation of the knee extension moment. The effects of gravity are greater for subjects with limited strength capacity, such as children and patients with neuromuscular disorders. Current gravity correction methods require

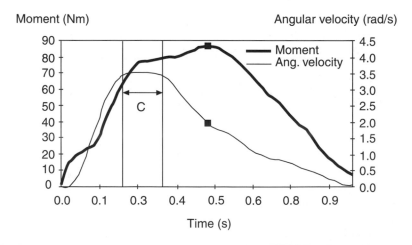

Figure 10.2 Moment and angular velocity data during a knee extension test at a preset angular velocity of 3.15 rad/s. Notice the shorter constant-velocity phase and the longer acceleration and deceleration periods. The maximum moment indicated by the square marker is clearly outside the isokinetic phase, and was recorded when the angular velocity of the joint was decreasing and it was approximately 2 rad/s.

measurement of the gravitational moment of the limb-lever arm system at an angular position. This can be performed either with the limb at a static position or during its passive fall against the resistance provided by the dynamometer at a very slow angular velocity. However, the accuracy of these methods can be affected by the tension of the muscle-tendon units and the ability of subjects to relax their limbs. Correction of the moments using anthropometric data is more accurate and simpler, as it is not affected by elastic tension effects and muscle relaxation (Kellis and Baltzopoulos 1996 a and b). This is especially important in the testing of children, because it may be more difficult for the examiner to explain the gravity correction procedure and for children to relax their limb during the correction procedure. After its estimation, the gravitational moment is added to the recorded moment of the muscles opposed by gravity and subtracted from the recorded moment of the muscles facilitated by gravity.

The ability of children to perform maximally during a test can also be affected by motivational factors. When children have feedback on the muscular output, they attempt to perform better during the test. Most common dynamometers offer real-time visual feedback on the moment exerted throughout the range of motion. The implementation of visual feedback leads to significant improvements on maximum strength output under both concentric (Baltzopoulos, Williams, and Brodie 1991) and eccentric (Kellis and Baltzopoulos 1995) conditions. Given the general suggestion that children cannot fully activate the motoneuron pool and perform maximally (Kawakami et al. 1993), the use of visual feedback in isokinetic testing protocols is necessary. The effects of verbal encouragement on maximum moment output are not known; if used, it is recommended that encouragement be standardized. All motivational techniques should be explained to the child in detail in the form of standardized pretesting instructions.

Isokinetic Training and Performance Considerations

The unique advantages of isokinetic dynamometry have led to widespread applications in both training and assessment of muscle and joint function. However, it is important to recognize that muscle function, muscle length, and velocity of contraction during isolated isokinetic joint movements is different from those in most functional activities and sports. Isokinetic dynamometry is a safe and effective training and assessment method for muscle and joint function, but the differences in neuromuscular mechanics between isokinetic and other functional joint movements must be considered carefully. This is particularly important when one attempts to use isokinetics for specific training or indeed prediction of performance in sport activities that have little or no neuromuscular or biomechanical similarity.

The following sections address some of the important issues in isokinetic training and assessment and their relationship to anthropometric and functional activities.

Effects of Gender and Age on Isokinetic Strength Measurements

Isokinetic dynamometry has been used to examine strength changes as the child grows up. In general, isokinetic moment output is greater with increasing age. However, there are some differences in strength development among various muscles examined.

Children 13 years old produce concentric elbow or knee flexion moment that is 2.5 times greater than that of 8-year-old subjects (Sunnegardh et al. 1988). Similarly, elbow extension and flexion strength increases from 15 to 17 years of age (Gilliam et al. 1979). Alexander and Molnar (1973) reported that isokinetic strength increases from 7 to 10 years of age, decreases or remains similar from 11 to 13 years, and increases linearly after 14 years of age.

Balageu et al. (1993) examined the isokinetic strength of trunk extensors and flexors of 117 children. The maximum trunk flexor strength decreased from the ages of 10 to 13. In contrast, the extensor moment increased or remained similar from the ages of 10 to 13 years. Isokinetic moment of all muscles increased in children older than 13 years. These findings can be attributed to changes in mass, height, and other anthropometric factors as the child grows up. In addition, neuromuscular maturation and hormonal changes also contribute to strength increases.

Gender differences in isokinetic muscle strength are also age dependent. Eight-year-old males and females produce similar concentric strength scores, whereas 13-year-old males perform better than females (Sunnegardh et al. 1988). The development of strength with age is different in girls as compared to boys. Girls develop strength until the age of 12; strength is then maintained constant until the age of 14 and decreases at 15 years (Balageu et al. 1993). One of the main factors affecting these differences is the strength per cross-sectional area unit (CSA) of the muscles involved (Sunnegardh et al. 1988).

The limited amount of research and available data do not permit definite conclusions on the effects of age and gender on isokinetic strength development. Very few research studies so far have included eccentric isokinetic tests in their protocols. The effects of factors such as neuromuscular loading, muscle coordination, and physiological changes on isokinetic moment output at different ages can provide essential information on the mechanisms underlying strength development in children.

Anthropometric and Functional Activity Parameters

Evaluation of muscular performance under isokinetic conditions provides information on strength development at a particular age. When evaluated along with other measurements, it is also possible to establish the contribution of anthropometric and physiological factors on strength performance.

It appears that CSA in preadolescents is significantly correlated to isokinetic strength (Kawakami et al. 1993; Kanehisa et al. 1994). However, after a muscle endurance test, this relationship becomes nonsignificant (Kawakami et al. 1993). This indicates that the muscle characteristics of children are significantly altered by muscle fatigue conditions. Findings on the strength-to-CSA ratio are conflicting, as some studies have found higher ratios in adults compared to children (Kanehisa et al. 1994) whereas others (Davies 1985) have reported the opposite. A factor that may affect the strength-to-CSA ratio is the inability of children to fully activate their muscles during a maximal isokinetic test. Some studies in children have reported that anthropometric parameters such as age, height, mass (or weight), body composition, and flexibility are not significantly correlated to isokinetic strength (Berg, Miller, and Stephens 1986; Weltman et al. 1988). On the other hand, others (Tabin, Gregg, and Bonci 1985; Balageu et al. 1993) found significant correlation between maximum concentric strength of ankle, knee, or trunk muscles and body weight (Tabin, Gregg, and Bonci 1985) or age and gender (Balageu et al. 1993). A nonsignificant correlation between daily physiological activity (Sunnegardh et al. 1988) and a 30 m sprint performance (Berg, Miller, and Stephens 1986) with isokinetic concentric strength was also reported.

Training Adaptations

Isokinetic dynamometers can also be used for improving muscle strength in healthy children. Isokinetic exercise at a specific angular velocity improves strength at the training velocity. Concentric training at intermediate velocities results in improvements at slow and fast angular velocities (for a review see Kellis and Baltzopoulos 1995). In adults, the training improvements following isokinetic training are related to possible metabolic alterations and recruitment of more motor units. Muscle hypertrophy and changes to muscle CSA and neural mechanisms may also contribute to strength improvements.

Isokinetic testing has been used only to evaluate strength-training programs in preadolescents (Ramsay et al. 1990; Ozmun, Mikesky, and Surburg 1994). Training with open kinetic chain exercises of elbow or knee muscles demonstrated significant increases in isokinetic or isotonic maximum moment measurements (Ramsay et al. 1990; Ozmun, Mikesky, and Surburg 1994). These increases were associated with increases in motor unit activation in some studies (Ozmun, Mikesky, and Surburg 1994), whereas others (Ramsay et al. 1990) reported no significant increases in CSA and motor unit activity at the end of the training program.

Isokinetic programs in children should be applied at a number of velocities and combined with electromyographic and anthropometric measurements. This will provide information on the changes in neuromuscular responses induced by isokinetic training programs.

Directions for Future Research

Research on isokinetic parameters in children is very limited. The moment-velocity characteristics have to be examined under eccentric and concentric conditions. Since children's limited strength capacity is related to neural factors, the application of electromyographic techniques would provide essential information on differences in force production mechanisms between adults and children or between younger and older children. This could also provide information on muscle coordination in preadolescents. More information on the effects of gender and age on isokinetic eccentric and concentric strength is also necessary. The reliability of testing around a wider range of joints should be reported. In addition, future isokinetic studies should consider the effects of inertia, gravity, and other methodological factors when establishing maximum moment and reciprocal or bilateral ratio characteristics in children. More studies that account for the effects of these factors on isokinetic parameters are necessary in order to establish a large database that can be used for performance or clinical applications. Finally, the training adaptations following an isokinetic exercise program in childhood need to be established.

Summary

Isokinetic dynamometry allows accurate and objective quantification of muscle strength. Preadolescents demonstrate isokinetic moment-velocity characteristics that are similar to those observed in adults. Eccentric moment is greater as compared to concentric. The isokinetic moment decreases with increasing concentric angular velocity and decreases or remains similar with increasing eccentric angular velocity. Concentric strength increases as the child grows up. This increase is different between males and females. In general, gender differences are minimal between 7 and 11 years of age, whereas after 13 years of age boys tend to produce greater isokinetic moment output than girls. Reciprocal ratios differ with the joint tested and can range from 0.62 to 0.90 for knee and elbow extension-flexion, respectively. Bilateral moment differences are not evident in children, even for athletes involved in specific sports. The muscle endurance characteristics are different in adults and preadolescents, especially under eccentric conditions where a high moment decline has been observed. The reliability of isokinetic measurements in preadolescents is greater than adults for the knee joint and lowest for the hip joint. The reliability and validity of an isokinetic strength test can be affected by several factors, and appropriate correction methods are necessary especially when testing children. From several parameters, body weight and CSA appear to correlate significantly with isokinetic strength. Finally, there is no detailed information on the effects of isokinetic training programs on muscular performance in preadolescents.

References

Alexander, J., and Molnar, G. 1973. Muscular strength in children: preliminary report on objective standards. *Arch. Phys. Med. Rehabil.* 54: 424-427.

Balageu, F., Damidot, R., Nordin, M., Parnianpour, M., and Waldburger, M. 1993. Cross-sectional study of the isokinetic muscle trunk strength among school children. *Spine* 18: 1199-1205.

Baltzopoulos, V. 1995. Muscular and tibiofemoral joint forces during isokinetic knee extension. *Clin. Biomech.* 10: 208-214.

Baltzopoulos, V., and Brodie, D.A. 1989. Isokinetic dynamometry: applications and limitations. *Sports Med.* 8: 111-116.

Baltzopoulos, V., Williams, J.G., and Brodie, D.A. 1991. Sources of error in isokinetic dynamometry: effects of visual feedback on maximum torque measurements. *J. Orthop. Sports Phys. Ther.* 13: 138-142.

Berg, K., Miller, M., and Stephens, L. 1986. Determinants of 30 meter sprint time in pubescent males. *J. Sports Med. Phys. Fitness* 26: 225-231.

Brodie, D., Burnie, J., Eston, R., and Royce, J. 1986. Isokinetic strength and flexibility characteristics in preadolescent boys. In *Children and exercise XII,* ed. J. Rutenfranz. Champaign IL: Human Kinetics: 309-319.

Burnett, C.N., Betts, E.F., and King, W. 1990. Reliability of isokinetic of hip muscle torque in young boys. *Phys. Ther.* 70: 244-249.

Burnie, J. 1987. Factors affecting selected reciprocal muscle group ratios in preadolescents. *Int. J. Sports Med.* 8: 40-45.

Burnie, J., and Brodie, D.A. 1986. Isokinetics in the assessment of rehabilitation: a case report. *Clin. Biomechanics* 1: 140-146.

Calmers, P., Borne, I.V.D., Nellen, M., Domenach, M., Minaire, P., and Drost, M. 1995. A pilot study of knee isokinetic strength in young, highly trained, females gymnasts. *Isokinetics Exerc. Sci.* 5: 69-74.

Capranica, L., Cama, G., Fanton, F., Tessitore, A., and Figura, F. 1992. Force and power of preferred and non-preferred leg in young soccer players. *J. Sports Med. Phys. Fitness* 32: 358-363.

Davies, C.T.M. 1985. Strength and mechanical properties of muscle in children and young adults. *Scand. J. Sports Sci.* 7: 11-15.

Docherty, D., and Gaul, C.A. 1991. Relationship of body size, physique and composition to physical performance in young boys and girls. *Int. J. Sports Med.* 12: 525-532.

Docherty, D., Wenger, H.A., Collis, M.L., and Quinney, H.A. 1987. The effects of variable speed resistance training on strength development in prepubertal boys. *J. Hum. Mov. Stud.* 13: 377-382.

Gaul, C. 1996. Muscular strength and endurance. In *Measurement in pediatric exercise science*, ed. D. Docherty. Champaign, IL: Human Kinetics: 225-258.

Gilliam, T., Sady, S., Freedson, P., and Villanacci, J. 1979. Isokinetic torque levels for high school football players. *Arch. Phys. Med. Rehabil.* 60: 110-114.

Henderson, R., Howes, C., Erikson, K., Heere, L., and DeMasi, R. 1993. Knee flexor-extensor strength in children. *J. Orthop. Sports Phys. Ther.* 18: 559-563.

Kanehisa, H., Ikegawa, S., Tsunoda, N., and Fukunaga, T. 1994. Strength and cross-sectional area of knee extensor muscles in children. *Eur. J. Appl. Physiol.* 68: 402-405.

Kanehisa, H., Ikegawa, S., Tsunoda, N., and Fukunaga, T. 1995. Strength and cross-sectional areas of reciprocal muscle groups in the upper arm and thigh during adolescence. *Int. J. Sports Med.* 16: 54-60.

Kawakami, Y., Kanehisa, H., Ikefawa, S., and Fukunaga, T. 1993. Concentric and eccentric muscle strength before, during and after fatigue in 13 year-old boys. *Eur. J. Appl. Physiol.* 67: 121-124.

Kellis, E., and Baltzopoulos, V. 1995. Isokinetic eccentric exercise: a review. *Sports Med.* 19: 202-222.

Kellis, E., and Baltzopoulos, V. 1996a. Gravitational moment correction in isokinetic dynamometry using anthropometric data. *Med. Sci. Sports Exerc.* 28: 900-907.

Kellis, E., and Baltzopoulos, V. 1996b. Resistive eccentric exercise: effects of visual feedback on maximum moment of knee extensors and flexors. *J. Orthop. Sports Phys. Ther.* 23: 120-124.

Merlini, L., Dell'Accio, D., and Granata, C. 1995. Reliability in dynamic strength knee muscle testing in children. *J. Orthop. Sports Phys. Ther.* 22: 73-76.

Mohtadi, N.G.H., Kiefer, G.N., Tedford, K., and Watters, S. 1990. Concentric and eccentric quadriceps torque in pre-adolescent males. *Can. J. Sport Sci.* 15: 240-243.

Molnar, G., Alexander, J., and Gutfeld, N. 1979. Reliability of quantitative strength measurements in children. *Arch. Phys. Med. Rehabil.* 60: 218-221.

Ozmun, J.C., Mikesky, A.E., and Surburg, P.R. 1994. Neuromuscular adaptations following prepubescent strength training. *Med. Sci. Sports Exerc.* 26: 510-514.

Ramsay, J.A., Blimkie, C.J., Smith, K., Garner, S., McDougall, J.D., and Sale, D. 1990. Strength training effects in prepubescent boys. *Med. Sci. Sports Exerc.* 22: 605-614.

Russell, K.W., Quinney, H.A., Hazlett, C.B., and Hillis, D. 1995. Knee muscle strength in elite male gymnasts. *J. Orthop. Sports Phys. Ther.* 22: 10-17.

Sunnegardh, J., Bratteby, L.E., Nordesjo, L.O., and Nordgren, B. 1988. Isometric and isokinetic muscle strength, anthropometry and physical activity in 8 and 13 year old Swedish children. *Eur. J. Appl. Physiol.* 58: 291-297.

Tabin, G., Gregg, J., and Bonci, T. 1985. Predictive leg strength values in immediately prepubescent and postpubescent athletes. *Am. J. Sports Med.* 13: 387-389.

Weltman, A., Janney, C., Rians, C.B., Strand, K., Berg, B., Tippitt, S., Wise, J., Cahill, B., and Katch, F. 1986. The effects of hydraulic resistance strength training in pre-pubertal males. *Med. Sci. Sports Exerc.* 18: 629-638.

Weltman, A., Tippet, S., Janney, C., Strand, K., Rians, C., Cahill, B., and Katch, F. 1988. Measurement of isokinetic strength in prepubertal males. *J. Orthop. Sports Phys. Ther.* 9: 345-351.

11

CHAPTER

Power and Speed Training During Childhood

Antti Mero

This chapter focuses on the following objectives:

- Understanding the factors that influence power and speed in children and adolescents
- Assessing speed-strength and power development and trainability
- Assessing speed development and trainability

Healthy children normally play games, and the games involve a great deal of short-term speed-strength output (e.g., hopping, stepping, jumping). This means that they are doing high-power muscular work. Short sprints are also involved in games demanding sprint characteristics (stride rate, stride length, and other sprint skills) that will develop and provide a substantial basis for training in adolescence and adulthood.

Very few controlled studies are available on the trainability of muscular speed-strength, speed, or power at different young ages. Because prepubescent, pubescent, and postpubescent girls (Nielsen et al. 1980) and boys (Pfeiffer and Francis 1986; Weltman et al. 1986; Mero, Vuorimaa, and Häkkinen 1990) can all respond to appropriate resistance training with an increase in muscular strength, such training may also induce increases in speed-strength, speed, and power (Mero, Vuorimaa, and Häkkinen 1990). In practice, physical educators and coaches know from experience that training can improve children's performance in activities that require high muscular power or speed.

Of special interest to physical educators and coaches, for example, are factors influencing speed-strength, speed, and power in children and adolescents. An outline of such relationships, as well as a discussion of speed-strength, speed, and power training based on research data and practical experience, will be given in this chapter.

Factors Influencing Power and Speed in Children and Adolescents

During growth and development, many factors affect performance capacity. In this chapter some of them (nervous system, motor units, connective tissue and bone, elastic potentiation, motor coordination, flexibility, hormonal factors, nutrition, energy production, training) will be discussed with regard to speed-strength, speed, and power in children and adolescents.

The Nervous System

The application of strength to various sport activities demands skill, and skill is dependent on the nervous system. In order to understand the development of skill and its subsequent performance parameter, speed, we need to be familiar with some characteristics of the nervous system during growth and development.

It is believed that after the sixth month of fetal life no new nerve cells are formed and that subsequent growth of the nervous system depends on an increase in the size of existing cell bodies (Sinclair 1989). There are enlargement, ramification, and myelination of the processes, as well as auxetic and multiplicate growth of the specialized connective tissue cells that support the nerve cells; and progressively more complex connections and assemblies are formed between nerve cells. Once formed, a nerve cell can increase in mass up to 200,000 times. The diameter of the myelinated nerve fibers in peripheral nerve trunks increases considerably during growth. By the age of 5 or 6 years the nervous system has reached about 90% its adult size. From the age of 12-13 years, it develops very slowly and is very near final maturation. This early maturation of the nervous system makes it possible to train coordination and skill from birth. During the first decade, skill training can be emphasized and subsequently speed is improved rapidly.

Motor Units

The motor unit consists of the motoneuron, its motor axon, and the muscle fibers supplied by the motoneuron. Today the classification of Burke (1981) is widely accepted among physiologists (Kernell 1986). According to this classification, developed from animal models and based on contractile speed and sensitivity to fatigue during a fused tetanus, three types of motor units can be distinguished: (1) fast-twitch, fatigue sensitive; (2) fast-twitch, fatigue resistant; and (3) slow-twitch, the most resistant to fatigue (see Burke, Levine, and Zajac 1971).

Types of Human Muscle Fiber

In human muscles, a characterization of motor units based on their physical properties is difficult to achieve, and in most studies a classification based on histochemical criteria has been used. Human muscle fibers can be classified as follows:

Type I: slow-twitch fibers, fatigue resistant—suitable for long-lasting, low-level force production

Type IIA: fast-twitch fibers, fatigue resistant—suitable for prolonged and relatively high force output

Type IIB: fast-twitch fibers, fatigue sensitive—suitable for high force production, for example during fast sprinting

Type IIC: intermediary fibers, between types I and II—histochemically reactive with both fast-twitch and slow-twitch antimyosins

Skeletal Muscle Differentiation and Training

Skeletal muscle differentiates during the postnatal period into slow, fast, or mixed muscles. This differentiation is based on a complex trophic and neurophysiological interaction between motoneurons and muscle fibers. Buller, Eccles, and Eccles (1960) demonstrated the importance of the motoneurons for the expression of the contractile properties of a muscle. In the cat's hind limb, cross reinnervation of the nerve supply to the slow soleus muscle and the fast flexor digitorum longus muscle altered the contractile properties of the reinnervated muscles: the fast muscle acquired properties of the former slow muscle and vice versa. It is well established today that not only the biomechanical properties change, but also that many of the histochemical, mitochondrial, and structural differences between fast and slow muscles are under neuronal control. Dum et al. (1985) have demonstrated that transformation from a fast to a slow muscle is much easier to achieve following cross reinnervation than the reverse.

According to Kernell (1986) regarding chronic nerve stimulation experiments, and as discussed by Noth (1992), the role of training can be suggested as follows. The transformation of a slow muscle into a fast muscle by training programs involving short periods of maximal muscle actions is probably impeded by the normal daily use of these muscles in postural activity. On the other hand, the transformation of a fast muscle into a muscle with slow contractile properties must involve maximal actions, because motor units with fast contracting properties have the highest threshold for recruitment.

For the training of children and adolescents, the discussion just referred to produces many questions. For example, what happens in the neuromuscular system of children after birth if they perform many very fast movements and then during the first decade of their lives their activity is very strongly characterized by fast movements and locomotion? Will they as a result maintain a greater proportion of fast-twitch fibers in their active muscles? Will they even increase the fast-twitch proportion in their muscles?

Training and Motor Unit Recruitment

Force output is positively related to the discharge rate of a motor unit in the frequency range of the unfused tetanus. Additionally, the force output may be graded by the recruitment of higher-threshold motor units. The "size principle" discovered by Henneman, Somjen, and Carpenter (1965) states that during reflex and voluntary activation of motoneurons, those with the smallest cell bodies have the lowest threshold and the largest cells have the highest threshold. Motoneurons with small spikes innervate motor units with little force output, whereas motoneurons with large spikes generate high amounts of tension. Thus, the Henneman principle also predicts a positive correlation between recruitment threshold and twitch tension. In practice, this means that endurance-type training achieves recruitment of slow-twitch fibers with low-level force production, and that sprint and jump training achieves recruitment of fast-twitch fibers with high force output. It has been shown in animal studies that during very rapid movements, such as paw shaking, high-threshold units can be activated without the firing of small low-threshold units (Smith et al. 1980). This would support the idea of developing the fast part of the neuromuscular system by performing only rapid movements and locomotion. Another question will also arise: Are training effects more efficient in children than in adults?

Muscle Fiber Characteristics During Training

Skeletal muscle is known to be an extremely heterogenous tissue in humans, and muscle fiber distribution between muscles varies greatly (see, e.g., Johnson et al. 1973). Thus, fiber distribution in one muscle is a poor representative of that in all muscles. However, the studies that have involved muscle fiber characteristics have mainly used one muscle (often the vastus lateralis muscle). A number of cross-sectional studies comparing sedentary subjects to well-trained adult athletes have shown that the best endurance athletes have a high percentage of slow-twitch fibers in their vastus lateralis, gastrocnemius, or deltoideus muscles (Gollnick et al. 1972; Costill et al. 1976; Burke et al. 1977; Saltin et al. 1977). In contrast, excellent sprinters, jumpers, and weight lifters have been found to have a high percentage of fast-twitch fibers in their thigh muscles (Gollnick et al. 1972; Thorstensson et al. 1977; Mero et al. 1981). Table 11.1 presents the muscle fiber distribution of the vastus lateralis muscle in Finnish trained athletic boys and girls representing various sport events. The trend was similar to that of adults (for endurance runners, 45% fast-twitch fibers; for sprinters, 59% among 11-12-year-old boys). The greatest amount of fast-twitch fibers (83%) was measured in a sprinter, and the greatest amount of slow-twitch fibers (75%) in a tennis player. In the study by Mero, Jaakola, and Komi (1991), young athletic boys were divided into two groups according to muscle fiber distribution. The "fast" group comprised 10 subjects (sprinters, weight lifters, tennis players) with more than 50% fast-twitch fibers, and the "slow" group comprised 8 subjects (endurance runners,

Table 11.1   Muscle Fiber Distribution in the Vastus Lateralis Muscle of Young Boys and Girls in Various Sport Events (Means; Data From Mero, Vuorimaa, and Häkkinen 1990)

Sport event	n	Gender (B = boys G = girls)	Age (years)	Fast-twitch fiber distribution (%)
Sprint running	4	B	11	59
Tennis	7	B	12	48
Weight lifting	4	B	13	51
Endurance running	4	B	12	45
Sprint running	8	B	15	52
Jumping	13	B	15	48
Sprint running	14	G	15	51
Jumping	12	G	15	47

tennis players, one weight lifter) with more than 50% slow-twitch fibers in their vastus lateralis muscle. The fast group had $59.2 \pm 6.3\%$ and the slow group had $39.4 \pm 9.8\%$ fast-twitch fibers. Other clear differences between the groups were observed regarding reaction time, rate of force development, and rise of the body's center of gravity in the squatting jump. For these variables, the fast group was superior to the slow group. Muscle fiber distribution (% fast-twitch fibers) correlated negatively with reaction time. Muscle fiber area (% fast-twitch fibers) correlated negatively with reaction time and positively with chronological age, height, mass, serum testosterone, force production, and blood lactate in the 60 s maximal anaerobic test. There were no significant correlations between muscle fiber characteristics and maximal oxygen uptake. The study assumed that heredity partly affects the selection of sporting events. Growth, development, and training are associated with muscle fiber area, which affects the physical performance capacity of the neuromuscular system in trained boys.

In order to investigate skeletal muscle fiber characteristics and anaerobic work during a 2-year regular many-sided training period, 18 junior (at the age of 12.6-14.6 years) athletes (runners, weight lifters, and tennis players) were studied (Mero 1992). The training consisted of strength, speed, endurance, and event-specific exercises. Six boys participating in sport activities only at school served as the control group (CG) for the athletic group (AG). At the beginning of the study the AG had greater anaerobic work capacity than the CG in both the 15 s and 60 s maximal bicycle ergometer tests. During the 2 years the AG increased their anaerobic work in the 15 s test and in the 60 s test, but the CG did not. The two groups did not differ from each other in muscle (vastus lateralis) fiber distribution or area, either before or after the training period.

However, the AG increased in relative muscle fiber area of the fast-twitch (FT) fibers from 48.1 ± 4.7% to 52.0 ± 5.3% (p < 0.05) during the 2 years. Serum testosterone level increased markedly in both groups (in AG from 5.8 ± 5.6 nmol/L to 20.4 ± 8.9 nmol/L and in CG from 1.8 ± 1.5 nmol/L to 21.2 ± 3.4 nmol/L) and correlated positively and significantly (r = 0.56, p < 0.05) with muscle fiber area (%FT) in the AG after the 2 years. In the AG a significant correlation (r = 0.52, p < 0.05) was found between muscle fiber distribution (%FT) and peak blood lactate in the 15 s test after 2 years. In addition, the muscle fiber area (%FT) correlated significantly with anaerobic work (r = 0.59, p < 0.05) and peak lactate (r = 0.70, p < 0.01) in the 15 s test of the AG after the training period. These data indicated that regular, many-sided training increases the relative skeletal muscle area of the fast-twitch fibers in pubertal boys, reflected in an enhanced anaerobic work capacity.

In another study by Mero (1993), neuromuscular performance and skeletal muscle fiber characteristics were investigated during a 2-year training period in male (n = 29) and female (n = 29) pubertal (at the age of 13.9-15.9 years) power athletes (sprinters and jumpers). The training consisted of strength, speed, and event-specific exercises. The total amount of training was 4.6 ± 1.3 times per week for males and 4.7 ± 1.1 times per week for females during the 2 years. During the 2-year training period, serum testosterone level increased both in males (from 23.1 ± 8.1 nmol/L to 30.3 ± 5.1 nmol/L) and in females (from 2.3 ± 1.6 nmol/L to 3.7 ± 1.9 nmol/L). At the same time in males, maximal isometric force of the leg extensor muscles increased 7.8%, counter-movement jump 10.5%, and reactive power in jumping 12.0%. In females the respective increases (6.6%, 1.4%, and 4.6%) were nonsignificant. Maximal sprinting speed increased in males 3.4% (from 8.70 ± 0.36 m/s to 9.00 ± 0.26 m/s) but was unchanged in females (8.19 ± 0.24 m/s vs. 8.21 ± 0.41 m/s) during the training period. Biopsies from the vastus lateralis muscle were taken at the beginning of the study. The fast-twitch (FT) fiber distribution was 49.5 ± 9.9% for males and 49.7 ± 7.7% for females. The relative muscle fiber area of the FT fibers was greater (p < 0.01) in males than in females (50.3 ± 3.7% vs. 44.7 ± 4.5%). The muscle fiber distribution (%FT) correlated positively with countermovement jump in females (r = 0.48, p < 0.01). In addition, the muscle fiber area (%FT) correlated positively with maximal velocity in the sprinters (r = 0.64, p < 0.01). These data indicated that neuromuscular performance in power athletes increases more in males than in females in late puberty when the amount of training is similar. One important reason for this is the 8-10-fold serum testosterone level in males compared to females. Fast-twitch fiber distribution and the area of cross-sectional active muscles also have positive effects on jumping and sprinting performances.

Musculoskeletal System

Connective Tissue

The literature contains little about the growth of connective tissue. The thickness of a tendon, and thus the number of collagen fibers developed in it, appears to depend on the severity and duration of the stresses to which it is subjected (Sinclair 1989). In practice this means, for example, that all games and training during childhood and adolescence have effects on connective tissue; however, what we know is mostly from practical experience. One general experience is that during puberty the knee and Achilles tendons of athletic boys and girls are often sore and painful. Key solutions in those cases are proper periodization of training and rest.

Bone

A great deal more is known about the growth of human bone than about the growth of any other human tissue (Sinclair 1989). Bones have both biomechanical and metabolic functions, which are to bear loads and mechanical stress and to provide a dynamic store for functionally and metabolically essential substances such as calcium and phosphate (Bailey and McCulloch 1990; Wasnich et al. 1989). Bone is an adaptive tissue that develops in structure and function in response to mechanical forces and metabolic demands during growth and development. The importance of physical stress and weight-bearing exercises in bone modeling and remodeling, and consequently in maintaining bone mineralization, is generally accepted. The evidence on the type, intensity, and duration of exercise necessary to influence bone mineral density in humans is, however, inconclusive. Slemenda et al. (1991) have suggested that increments in skeletal mass may result from physical activity during childhood in the radius and femur/hip but not in the spine. Nilsson and Westlin (1971) suggested that within an athlete group, sport activities involving a heavy load on the lower limbs were associated with higher bone density at the distal end of the femur. Swimmers did not differ significantly from nonathletes when both exercising and nonexercising controls were included in the comparison. It could be concluded that in childhood and adolescence, strength and power training (especially bounding exercises) is very effective with regard to increasing bone density.

Elastic Potentiation

The most important part of muscular elastic elements for the functioning of active muscle is the series elastic component (SEC). The parallel elastic component (PEC) consists of muscle fascia, connective tissue, and the sarcolemma of the muscle. The SEC component is located in the tendinous structures and the cross bridges of the muscle fibers (Morgan 1977; Proske and Morgan 1984, 1987), and it contributes to performance as elastic potentiation (see, e.g., Huijing 1992). Because locomotion and muscular exercises seldom involve pure forms of isolated isometric, concentric, or eccentric actions, physical activities are mostly a combination of eccentric and concentric actions. This is a natural type of muscle function called a stretch-shortening cycle or SSC (Norman and Komi 1979; Komi 1984). With the SSC it is possible to make the final action (concentric phase) more powerful than that resulting from concentric action alone. In jumping it has been shown that a countermovement jump rises higher than a static jump (Asmussen and

Bonde-Petersen 1974; Komi and Bosco 1978). The difference in the height of the jumps has been suggested to be elasticity. It plays an important role in enhancing both effectiveness (speed and power) and the efficiency of human performance (Komi 1984). A short and rapid stretch with a short coupling time and a high force at the end of pre-stretch creates a good precondition for utilizing tendomuscular elasticity (Cavagna, Dusman, and Margaria 1968; Bosco et al., "Neuromuscular Function," "Store and Recoil," 1982). The force attained at the end of the stretching period depends on the amplitude and the velocity of the stretch. During stretching, three types of mechanisms may exist that explain simultaneous force enhancement: (1) an increase in the number of attached cross bridges (Colomo, Lombardi, and Piazzesi 1986), (2) an increase in the force developed by each cross bridge (Sugi and Tsuchiya 1981), and (3) a recruitment of additional force-bearing elements (Edman, Elzinga, and Noble 1978). Also muscle fiber distribution has been shown to be related to elasticity. Subjects with more fast-twitch fibers benefit more from the rapid stretch with a small amplitude than their slow-type counterparts. On the other hand, slow-twitch fibers have a longer cross-bridge cycle time (Goldspink 1978) that allows them to better utilize long and slow stretches (Bosco et al. 1982).

The elasticity-age curve (Bosco and Komi 1980) is similar to the strength-age curve (Hettinger 1968), showing that both elasticity and strength potential reach the highest level at the age of 20-30 years in both genders. In the two jumping tests (countermovement jump and static jump), a difference of about 5-15% (elasticity) has been measured in the rise of the jumps in adults (Bosco 1982) and in young athletic and nonathletic boys (Mero, Vuorimaa, and Häkkinen 1990). Can training therefore increase elasticity? Are training effects similar in childhood and adolescence to those in adulthood? According to the scientific data mentioned earlier and practical knowledge, it is obvious that sprint-type running, jumping, and playing games, for example, are good exercises to improve elasticity in leg extensor muscles. Because we do not have conclusive training studies, these questions are still open. However, it has been shown in animal experiments that special training can modify the tendomuscular elasticity, especially the elastic properties of connective tissue (Suominen, Kiiskinen, and Heikkinen 1980; Woo et al. 1981). In the skeletal muscle these adaptations are manifested by increased tensile strength and stiffness (Kovanen, Suominen, and Heikkinen 1984). However, many-sided physical activity and training in childhood and adolescence are probably effective in improving elasticity, although scientific data are lacking.

Motor Coordination

In physical activity and sport performance, along with speed-strength, speed, and power, motor coordination plays an important role in the cooperative interaction between the nervous system and the skeletal muscles. The early development of motor coordination provides a large basis on which to improve skills, and especially speed ability, in many sport events.

Five fundamental coordinative capabilities can be distinguished (Hirtz 1981):

1. The ability to orientate spatially
2. The ability to differentiate kinesthetically
3. The ability to react
4. The ability to keep rhythms
5. The ability to maintain balance

According to Tittel (1992), a nonlinear relationship could be seen between biological age and coordinative capabilities in 13-year-old handball players. Individuals who were biologically younger (about 11 years) showed better coordination test results than children biologically aged 13 or 14 years. This result shows that coordinative maturity occurs before sexual maturity. Furthermore, according to Tittel (1992), at the age of 8 or 9 years the spatial component develops as well as maximal motor frequency and speed coordination. During the 11th and 12th years, reactive capability using acoustic and optical signals and rhythmic capacity are fully developed. Gender differences occur during the 12th and 13th year of age, when girls are better than boys, and then once again after the 18th year of age; women are 10% better than men in coordinative capabilities (Rutenfranz and Hettinger 1959). Changing of external conditions (e.g., reducing the weight of shots or adjusting ball sizes) should be considered when training coordinative capabilities during childhood and adolescence (Israel 1976; Willimczik 1979; Winter 1981), but the alteration in weight or size should not be so large as to basically change the characteristics of rhythm or speed and consequently the coordinatory structure.

Flexibility

In most habitual daily activities as well as in sport, flexibility is an important factor for physical performance. Flexibility or range of movement has also been thought to be an important factor for the prevention of injuries in training and competition. There is a high injury risk especially in speed-strength and speed and power training. Furthermore, flexibility is very specific if we consider, for example, a hurdler, a football player, a pole-vaulter, or a swimmer. Each of them requires flexibility, but the quality and intensity of the range of movement in each of the types of sport will be different.

Flexibility is restricted by the bone structure of the joint, cartilage tissue, length of the ligaments, muscles, tendons, and other connective tissues that cross the joints. Other factors that also limit the range of movement are the contact of muscle and fat as well as having the compressed tissue between the articulating segments of the bones removed. Furthermore, age, body type, training, gender, temperature, humidity, warming up, circadian variation, relaxation, and active or passive execution of the movement may affect flexibility (Reilly 1981). The age of 9-12 years (before puberty) is a sensitive phase for flexibility training, and a phase in which it is possible to reach a maximum level in flexibility (Sermejev 1964; Zaciorskij 1973). This is important if we think about elite sports.

Flexibility exercises have to be incorporated in the preparatory part of each speed-strength, speed, and power training session and have to be preceded by a general warm-up (e.g., jogging 10-15 min). Throughout the flexibility training the amplitude of an exercise must be increased progressively. Flexibility exercises to relax muscles to the resting situation after a training session are also suggested. These exercises can be done either immediately after the session or some hours later when muscles have taken up energy and other nutrients and are not so fatigued.

Hormonal Factors

Prepubertal growth and maturation are principally dependent on the stimulation of growth hormone, while pubertal growth and maturation are mainly under the influence of steroid hormones. In the prepubertal phase, muscle mass increases in parallel to body mass. Moderate strength, speed-strength, and power training is recommended, but very high training loads should be avoided because of the sensitivity of the joint structures, especially of the growth zones (epiphysis) of the bones. During prepuberty there are no differences between girls and boys with respect to trainability for strength characteristics. Table 11.2 presents sexual hormone levels before and during puberty. In the development of strength characteristics, the male sexual hormones are very important because of their anabolic (protein incorporating) effects. These facilitate the synthesis of muscle protein. In puberty, all-around training should take place. Adequate strength and speed-strength training is important because of the rapidity with which growth occurs; an optimal musculature stabilizes the rapidly growing skeletal system. On the other hand, puberty is a good time to continue training for elite sports for both genders, but especially for boys. Certain precautions in carrying out speed-strength exercises are warranted. Ossification zones are sensitive and liable to injuries

Table 11.2   Estradiol and Testosterone Concentrations Before and During Puberty

Age (years)	Estradiol[a]		Testosterone[a]		Testosterone[b]	
	Girls	Boys	Girls	Boys	Girls	Boys
8-9	0.4	-	0.8	0.9-1.0	-	-
10-11	0.4-8	0.4	0.4-2.0	1.0-2.0	-	2.9
12-13	0.8-10	0.1-1.2	0.8-3.0	5.0-9.0	-	9.5
14-15	0.6-16	0.2-1.6	0.8-3.0	12.0-24.0	2.4	21.3

Note: Values are nmol/L.

[a]Reiter and Root 1975 (range values).

[b]Mero et al. 1990 (mean values).

and damage; therefore, very heavy loads or faulty techniques should be avoided in order to take care of the cartilage of the epiphysis.

Nutrition

For effective training, nutritional factors are also very important and must be balanced with the training. In speed-strength, speed, and power training in children and adolescents, some nutritional aspects differ from those for endurance training, for example. However, achieving an optimal combination of energy, proteins, vitamins, minerals, and water is the most important task in a day, although we know it is not very easy to carry out this task in practice.

In puberty, during the period of rapid growth, nutritional requirements are substantially increased (Forbes 1981). With respect to the muscle development that occurs in speed-strength, speed, and power training, energy, protein, and some minerals (calcium, magnesium, iron, zinc, and chromium) are very important. Strength training is considered to require less total energy than endurance training. Studies on both adolescents and young adults indicate that heavy strength training also requires very high energy expenditure (Alexandrov and Shishina 1978; Celejowa and Homa 1970; Dragan, Vasiliu, and Georgescu 1985; Laritcheva et al. 1978). There are only a limited number of studies on speed-strength athletes and their nutrition. However, it seems that their total energy intake is not very high (Mero 1994) and that it is clearly lower than in endurance athletes. Strength training increases protein need; during puberty this need must be recognized because of the substantially increased protein need of the age phase. Therefore, the need is probably twofold; it may be over 2.0 g protein/kg body mass per day in children and adolescents. More study is necessary before it is possible to make definitive recommendations regarding protein intake in young athletic boys and girls during speed-strength and speed (power) training. During puberty, in addition to increased energy and protein requirements, calcium, magnesium, and zinc are especially critical because of their role in the development of muscle and skeletal mass (Mahan and Rees 1984). Due to a greater maximal growth rate and larger absolute body size, adolescent males have higher mineral needs than females. Iron is important for blood volume, and chromium for carbohydrate and fat metabolism.

Energy

In performances of short duration and high intensity, energy is provided almost exclusively from the high-energy phosphates adenosine triphosphate (ATP) and creatine phosphate (CP) stored within the specific muscles activated during exercise. Little information on this topic is available regarding children and adolescents in exercise. However, it has been shown that a combined aerobic-anaerobic training program in 11-15-year-old boys induced an increase in muscle substrates such as ATP, CP, and glycogen, as well as in the activity of the glycolytic enzyme

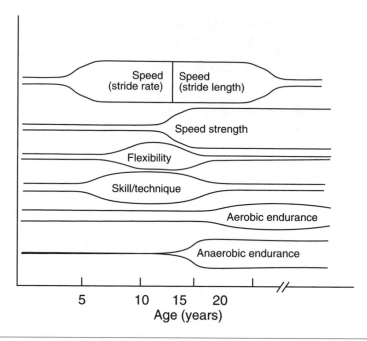

Figure 11.1 The important training areas ("sensitive phases") at different ages.

Adapted from Mero, Vuorimaa, and Häkkinen 1990.

phosphofructokinase (Eriksson 1972). These changes support the notion that anaerobic energy characteristics in children are trainable, perhaps to a similar degree as in adults.

Training

Training and recovery (including sleep) are everyday tasks in athletic boys and girls. Training influences speed-strength, speed, and power more than the other factors mentioned. The next section will present details on training. Figure 11.1 summarizes physical performance capacity and its training at different ages ("sensitive phases").

Speed-Strength and Power Development and Trainability

This section begins with a discussion of how speed-strength and power develop in normal boys and girls and then focuses on speed-strength and power training.

Speed-Strength and Power Development

The literature contains many results for motor fitness tests, including tests in speed-strength and power (e.g., Pate and Shephard 1989). In this specific review, some examples of the test results have been selected to describe speed-strength and power development in children and adolescents. Because it is very difficult to sharply separate trained people from "absolutely" nontrained people, the reader should take this into account when considering the literature. Generally the subjects described are active schoolchildren with more or less variation in physical activity.

Boys begin to jump higher than girls in puberty, at the age of 14 years (Crasselt et al. 1990). Table 11.3 presents results for a countermovement jump in Finnish boys and girls (7-16 years). According to these data boys are also better than girls after the age of 14. During a 5-year follow-up study (Mero, Vuorimaa, and Häkkinen 1990), Finnish athletic boys were better than normal schoolboys in a countermovement jump (see figure 11.2, p. 255), and in both groups strong increases occurred around the age of 14. The standing long jump is very often used as a speed-strength (power)-type motor test. Table 11.4 (p. 256) presents jumping results in a Slovak population aged 7-14 years (Semetka 1982). Power during a reactive jump can be measured (Bosco, Luhtanen, and Komi 1983) if one knows the flight time and the contact time of the jump. Table 11.5 (p. 256) shows results for boys and girls involved in track and field (aged 14-16 years).

The speed-strength and power of muscles other than leg extensor muscles have also been measured with the use of many motor tests. The results of push-ups, pull-ups, sit-ups, and a back muscle test in 30 s showed that both an athletic group and a control group improved their test results during a 5-year follow-up (Mero, Vuorimaa, and Häkkinen 1990). At the age of 11 there was no difference between the groups, but after that age the athletic group was, more or less, better than the controls. However, both groups improved all test results during the 5-year period (from 11 to 16 years).

Speed-Strength and Power Training

In order to plan speed-strength and power training, several factors must be taken into consideration: exercise selection, use of exercise units, periodization, and exercise units and training effects.

Exercise Selection

Children play many kinds of games in which they are running (acceleration, deceleration, constant speed), stepping, hopping, jumping, climbing, wrestling, throwing, pushing, and pulling, and consequently they train their muscles. Often the games are so vigorous that "training" increases speed-strength and power of the activated muscles.

In athletic children and adolescents, the sport events they train in will produce event-specific training effects. If we compare, for example, long jump, football, swimming, and gymnastics, we recognize that the training effects in speed-strength, power, and other physical characteristics differ very clearly. Teachers, coaches, and parents are

Table 11.3 Countermovement Jump (cm) in 7- to 16-Year-Old Boys and Girls

Boys

Age (years)	Very high	High	Middle	Low
7	21	19	16	Below 16
8	22	20	17	Below 17
9	25	23	19	Below 19
10	28	25	21	Below 21
11	30	27	22	Below 22
12	32	29	24	Below 24
13	36	33	27	Below 27
14	43	38	28	Below 28
15	46	40	30	Below 30
16	49	42	33	Below 33

Girls

Age (years)	Very high	High	Middle	Low
7	21	19	16	Below 16
8	22	20	17	Below 17
9	25	23	19	Below 19
10	28	25	21	Below 21
11	30	27	22	Below 22
12	32	29	23	Below 24
13	36	33	24	Below 24
14	38	35	25	Below 25
15	39	36	26	Below 26
16	40	37	27	Below 27

Adapted from Mero, Vuorimaa, and Häkkinen 1990.

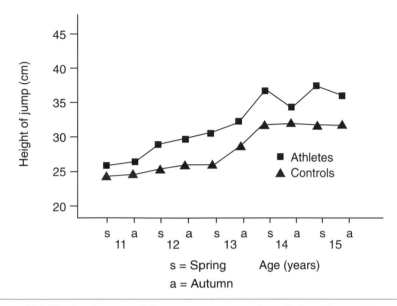

Figure 11.2 The development of the countermovement jump during a 5-year follow-up study in athletic boys (■-■) and in controls (▲-▲).

Adapted from Mero, Vuorimaa, and Häkkinen 1990.

key people who can guide children in many sport events in order to produce multiple training effects.

Puberty provides strong possibilities for increasing speed-strength and power because of hormonal maturation. All-around strength training should take place in athletic boys and girls. Adequate strength training is essential first because of the rapid growth that is occurring, as mentioned earlier. An optimal musculature stabilizes the quickly growing skeleton. Secondly, if we consider an elite athlete career for a boy or a girl, puberty offers possibilities to increase multiple strength and power characteristics that would take a great deal of time to compensate for after puberty. Therefore, in puberty it would be useful to select a number of exercises including "free" weight lifting, use of strength-training machines, jumping (bounding) exercises, sprinting, gymnastics, and use of specific resistance equipment (e.g., medicine balls and shots for throwing). Considering exercises relating to cyclic locomotion, maximal sprint running gives very high power values during contact, whereas force impulses and speed-strength are very high in stepping and hopping (Mero and Komi 1994). In exercise selection the important criteria are effectiveness, safety, and convenience.

The Use of Exercise Units

In goal-oriented athletic training, speed-strength and power exercise units are generally carried out either alone or in combination with the main sport event. The

Table 11.4   Standing Long Jump Results (cm) in 7- to 14-Year-Old Boys and Girls

Age (years)		7	8	9	10	11	12	13	14
Boys	High	169	185	195	204	208	214	223	233
	Middle	147	163	173	182	186	192	201	211
	Low	126	141	151	160	164	170	179	189
Girls	High	163	171	187	193	199	205	216	238
	Middle	141	149	165	171	177	183	194	216
	Low	119	126	143	149	154	161	172	177

Data from Semetka 1982.

Table 11.5   Reactive Power in Jumping During 2 Years of Training in Athletic Boys and Girls (Mean ± SD; Adapted from Mero et al. 1992)

Age (years)	14		15		16	
	Boys	Girls	Boys	Girls	Boys	Girls
Power (W/kg)	49.0 ±7.6	47.6 ±5.4	52.8 ±6.6	48.4 ±4.7	54.9 ±6.4	49.8 ±8.1

Adapted from Mero et al. 1992.

following paragraphs present important principles for conducting speed-strength and power exercise units (Mero, Vuorimaa, and Häkkinen 1990).

Maximal Effort.   In speed-strength and power exercise units, maximal effort is very important to achieve, as striving for maximal effort causes increases in both the recruitment of fast-twitch fibers and their firing rates. This is also "overloading" as in pure strength training, where the load is always very elevated.

Specificity.   It is important that specificity of movement pattern, contraction type, contraction velocity, force, and time to produce force in a selected training exercise are very similar to what they are in the actual sport events in which speed-strength and power will be used.

Load Selection.   In load selection, the recommendation is to use loads of approximately 0-85% of one repetition maximum (1RM). Maximal mechanical power can be gained generally with the use of loads from 20% to 60% of 1RM. Special training backgrounds can influence the percentage value. It is also beneficial to use mixed loads in the same exercise unit to increase training stimuli.

Performance Duration.   In order to use ATP and PC as energy fuels, the duration of one performance (often one series) must be less than 10 s. A longer duration would achieve too much lactate production and lead to pH decreases that have negative effects on force production.

Recovery.   It is recommended that recovery between series be from 2 to 5 min in order to recover ATP and PC stores and also one needs to recover "mentally."

Stimulus Change.   Multiple changes in the exercise unit (load, exercise selection, type of contraction, and so on) are relevant for optimal training of the neuromuscular system, and alterations after 4-6 weeks are recommended.

Progression.   Progression has to occur mainly in the amount of training, because the intensity is always very high (maximal effort).

Periodization of Speed-Strength and Power Development

During prepuberty (age range of 7-11 years), the teaching of mainly strength exercise skills is recommended. Scientific studies show that in this age phase, strength training increases strength and improves motor skill coordination, increases motor unit activation, and produces other undetermined neurological adaptations including better coordination of the involved muscle groups. These adaptations are most likely the major determinants of the strength gains observed (Ramsay et al. 1990). Experience has shown that on average, two speed-strength and power exercise units (one unit is 60 min) a week are suitable for athletic children. When the skills of the exercises have been learned, intensity of the work (power) can be increased.

During puberty (at age 12-16) it is very important to train speed-strength and power in whatever sport event a boy or a girl is practicing. In practice this means two to four exercise units (one unit is 60 min) a week during the training season (Mero, Vuorimaa, and Häkkinen 1990). After puberty the recommendation is that young people train like adults in each sport event.

In nonathletic schoolchildren and adolescents, it is beneficial to train as many sport events as the young people desire; hopefully the children will also activate fast-twitch fibers in their muscles. If they learn to do this, one can hope that later in adulthood they will continue this multiple and "diverse" training and keep the slow and fast-twitch fibers of their large muscles in good shape.

Exercise Units and Training Effects

Training effects can be divided into acute and chronic effects. Both are discussed in the following paragraphs.

Acute Effects. Speed-strength and power exercise units achieve acute effects in the neuromuscular system. These effects occur in the nervous system (recruitment, firing), in skeletal muscle fibers (ATP, PC, enzymes), in elastic elements (SSC), and in the regulatory systems (neural and hormonal system). Following a speed-strength and power unit, both speed-strength and maximal strength decrease in pubertal boys, but they recover quickly because very few hydrogen ions exist in the muscles (Mero et al. 1994).

Chronic Effects. During long-term speed-strength and power training, chronic effects occur in the human neuromuscular system (nervous system, skeletal muscle fibers, elastic elements, and regulatory system), and consequently speed-strength and power increase. In a 5-year follow-up study (Mero, Vuorimaa, and Häkkinen 1990), athletic boys improved speed-strength in the leg extensor muscles (counter-movement jump) by 50% (on average 10% a year) from the ages of 11 to 15. In the control group the respective values were 35% and 7%. In both groups the greatest annual development occurred between the 13th and 14th year (12-14%). Elasticity during the whole period was evaluated by 8-10% (determined by the difference between a static jump and a countermovement jump). Reactive power in jumping increased in boys by 5.9% and in girls by 2.4% per year from the age of 14 to the age of 16 in track and field adolescents (Mero et al. 1992).

Speed Development and Trainability

Here speed development during childhood and adolescence is described first, and then the main focus is on speed training.

Speed Development

Speed development can be described using sprint-type test results. Figure 11.3 presents the development of running speed (during 60 m) in boys and girls aged from 3 to 10 years (Mero, Vuorimaa, and Häkkinen 1990) and shows that the results are very similar for the two genders. It seems that the gender difference occurs at the age of 13-14, as shown in table 11.6, which presents running times during 20 m with a flying start in Finnish boys and girls (7-16 years) (Mero, Vuorimaa, and Häkkinen 1990). The same gender trend can be seen in a Slovak population (see table 11.7, Semetka 1982). During a 5-year follow-up study (from 11 to 15 years), the athletic boys increased their maximum speed (over 20 m) by increasing stride length. Stride rate remained, however, at the same level for 5 years (Mero, Vuorimaa, and Häkkinen 1990). This is mainly related to strength increases in puberty.

Reaction speed develops together with the development of the nervous system. Because the nervous system develops very early, reaction speed (reaction time) is also very near adult values at the age of 10-12. In one study, from the ages of 11 to

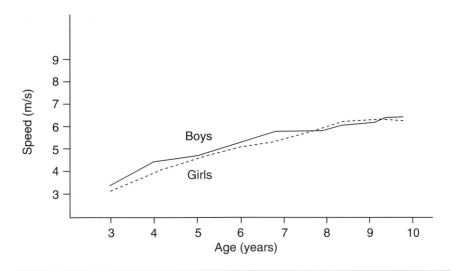

Figure 11.3 The development of running speed (average speed in 60 m) in 3-10-year-old boys (———) and girls (- - - -)

Adapted from Mero, Vuorimaa, and Häkkinen 1990.

15 the reaction speed improved by 4.2% in athletic boys and by 4.7% in controls, with no differences observed between the groups (Mero, Vuorimaa, and Häkkinen 1990).

Speed Training

In speed training, important issues are how to select exercises, how to plan exercise units, how to periodize, and what the possible training effects are.

Exercise Selection

Pure speed training is very event specific. For example, speed training for sprinting is sprint running. In the javelin throw, speed work normally consists of throwing weight implements or throwing lighter javelins than in the competition, as well as sprint running to develop approach run speed. Therefore, exercise selection is event specific, although in children, general speed work, like sprint running, has positive effects on many other sport events.

Speed Exercise Unit

The speed exercise unit is carried out according to a number of principles (Mero, Vuorimaa, and Häkkinen 1990).

Table 11.6   Running Results for 20 m (s) With a Flying Start in 7- to 16-Year-Old Boys and Girls

Boys

Age (years)	Very high	High	Middle	Low
7	3.40	3.60	4.10	Over 4.10
8	3.20	3.35	3.90	Over 3.90
9	3.10	3.30	3.70	Over 3.70
10	2.90	3.15	3.60	Over 3.60
11	2.80	3.00	3.45	Over 3.45
12	2.65	2.85	3.30	Over 3.30
13	2.40	2.65	3.10	Over 3.10
14	2.30	2.45	2.90	Over 2.90
15	2.20	2.35	2.80	Over 2.80
16	2.15	2.30	2.75	Over 2.75

Girls

Age (years)	Very high	High	Middle	Low
7	3.40	3.60	4.10	Over 4.10
8	3.20	3.45	3.90	Over 3.90
9	3.10	3.30	3.70	Over 3.70
10	2.95	3.15	3.60	Over 3.60
11	2.80	3.00	3.45	Over 3.45
12	2.65	2.85	3.30	Over 3.30
13	2.45	2.65	3.10	Over 3.10
14	2.40	2.50	3.10	Over 3.10
15	2.35	2.45	3.05	Over 3.05
16	2.30	2.40	3.00	Over 3.00

Adapted from Mero, Vuorimaa, and Häkkinen 1990.

Table 11.7   Test Results for 50m Run in 7- to 14-Year-Old Boys and Girls

Age (years)		7	8	9	10	11	12	13	14
Boys	High	9.3	8.2	7.9	7.7	7.1	6.8	6.5	6.3
	Middle	10.5	9.2	8.8	8.6	8.0	7.7	7.4	7.2
	Low	11.3	10.2	9.8	9.6	9.0	8.7	8.4	8.2
Girls	High	9.4	8.5	8.2	7.9	7.2	6.9	6.7	6.6
	Middle	10.5	9.6	9.3	9.0	8.3	8.0	7.8	7.7
	Low	11.6	10.6	10.3	10.1	9.4	9.0	8.9	8.8

Data from Semetka 1982.

Performance Speed.   Speed can be submaximal (96-99%), maximal (100%), or supramaximal (over 100%), calculated from the best performance.

Performance Duration.   Duration ranges between 1 and 6 s, when ATP and PC are utilized as energy.

Recovery.   Recovery ranges from 3 to 9 min between repetitions and from 10 to 12 min between sets, allowing ATP and PC stores to recover.

Training Amounts.   In one speed exercise unit there are 5-10 repetitions if performance is maximal or supramaximal. In the case of submaximal repetitions there may be 10-20 repetitions. In sprint running the amounts are lesser than in swimming.

Rest.   The speed exercise unit must be done in a rested state (e.g., after rest day) and not after a lactic speed endurance training day.

Willpower.   Speed performance demands strong willpower, but on the other hand, performance must be relaxed.

Stimulus Change.   Within one speed exercise unit it is beneficial to have stimulus changes that can be achieved, for example, by changing stride length and stride rate and speed, or in throwing events, by changing the mass of the implements thrown.

Periodization of Speed Training

The age phase from 7 to 12 is a sensitive phase for speed development. During this phase the use of exercises to increase stride rate is recommended. Both the devel-

Pediatric Anaerobic Performance

opment of the nervous system and the increasing skills offer possibilities to improve stride rate and consequently speed. Reaction speed should also be almost fully developed in this age phase. There should be two to four training units (one unit is 60 min) per week.

In puberty, strength increases improve stride length and speed. It is also very important to develop stride rate in puberty. This is not an easy task, but regarding elite sport, for example sprint running and swimming, it is necessary. Speed work units including reaction speed should take place about two to five times a week depending on the sport event. After puberty, speed training in adolescents is comparable to adult training.

Speed Exercise Unit and Training Effects

The speed exercise unit achieves acute and chronic effects. Both are discussed here.

Acute Effects.   The speed exercise unit achieves acute effects that are very similar to those for the speed-strength unit in adults (Mero et al. 1995). There are effects on the nervous system, skeletal muscle fibers, elastic elements, and the regulatory systems. Both maximal and fast force production decrease when measured immediately after the unit but recover over some hours. There are no research results available on this topic for children and adolescents.

Chronic Effects.   Chronic effects are also very similar for speed training and speed-strength training with respect to the effects on the human body (Mero, Vuorimaa, and Häkkinen 1990). As a result of these effects, and consequently the changes in the body, the speed level increases.

Unfortunately, the research data on children and adolescents in this regard are very limited. In a 5-year follow-up study (Mero, Vuorimaa, and Häkkinen 1990), running speed increased by 3-5% a year in athletic boys as well as control boys. It is important to note that the athletic boys trained using a multiple program and not exclusively to improve speed. In track and field, running speed of athletes (sprinters, jumpers) improved by 4.0% in boys and by 0.4% in girls after 2 years of training between the ages of 14 and 16 (Mero et al. 1992). This suggests that with athletic children and adolescents, there should be more concentration on the development of speed. However, it is necessary to conduct research, with exact speed programs, regarding the training effects of speed work.

Directions for Future Research

There is a need to describe speed-strength, power, and speed of the main large muscle groups among schoolchildren and also those involved very actively in sport training. The role of coordination in speed development is also very poorly investigated in this age phase.

In adolescence (13-19 years) there are good possibilities for carrying out training studies in field conditions; however, these conditions should be very carefully controlled. Such studies would increase our knowledge of training effects on the nervous system, skeletal muscle fibers, elastic elements, and the regulatory systems and consequently on speed-strength, power, and speed.

Summary

The nervous system, skeletal muscle fibers, connective tissue and bone, elastic potentiation, coordination, hormonal levels, nutrition, energy production, and training influence speed-strength, power, and speed. Coordination, motor skills, and speed develop very well in physically active boys and girls during childhood, together with the rapid development of the nervous system. Boys and girls are similar in speed-strength and maximal running speed during the first decade. At the age of 13-14, boys begin to exceed the level of performance of girls in speed-strength, power, and speed, depending on hormonal maturation. In spite of limited research, it seems clear that training accelerates speed-strength, power, and speed improvements in puberty. Athletic training should be many-sided during puberty, including two to five speed-strength, power, and speed exercise units a week depending on the sport event. In postpuberty, athletic adolescents should train like adult athletes in their respective sport event.

References

Alexandrov, I.I., and Shishina, N.N. 1978. Study in energy metabolism and nutritional status of young athletes. In *Nutrition, physical fitness and health,* ed. J. Parizkova and R.A. Rogozkin, 124-130. Baltimore: University Park Press.

Asmussen, E., and Bonde-Petersen, F. 1974. Apparent efficiency and storage of elastic energy in human muscles during exercise. *Acta Physiol. Scand.* 92: 537-545.

Bailey, D.A., and McCulloch, R.G. 1990. Bone tissue and physical activity. *Can. J. Sports Sci.* 15: 229-239.

Bosco, C. 1982. Stretch-shortening cycle in skeletal muscle function with special reference to elastic energy and potentiation of myoelectric activity. *Stud. Sport Phys. Ed. Health* 15. Jyväskylä, Finland: University of Jyväskyläa.

Bosco, C., Ito, A., Komi, P.V., Luhtanen, P., Rahkila, P., Rusko, H., and Viitasalo, J.T. 1982. Neuromuscular function and mechanical efficiency of human leg extensor muscles during jumping exercises. *Acta Physiol. Scand.* 114: 543-550.

Bosco, C., and Komi, P.V. 1980. Influence of aging on the mechanical behaviour of leg extensor muscles. *Eur. J. Appl. Physiol.* 45: 209-219.

Bosco, C., Luhtanen, P., and Komi, P.V. 1983. A simple method for measurement of mechanical power in jumping. *Eur. J. Appl. Physiol.* 50: 273-282.

Bosco, C., Tihanyi, J., Komi, P.V., Fekete, G., and Apor, P. 1982. Store and recoil of elastic energy in slow and fast types of human skeletal muscles. *Acta Physiol. Scand.* 116: 343-349.

Buller, A.J., Eccles, J.C., and Eccles, R.M. 1960. Interactions between motoneurones and muscles in respect of the characteristic speeds of their responses. *J. Physiol.* 150: 417-439.

Burke, R.E. 1981. Motor units: anatomy, physiology and functional organization. In *Handbook of physiology,* ed. V.B. Brooks. Sec. 1, *The nervous system II,* 345-422. Washington, DC: American Physiological Society.

Burke, R.E., Cerny, F., Costill, D., and William, F. 1977. Characteristics of skeletal muscle in competitive cyclists. *Med. Sci. Sports* 9: 109-112.

Burke, R.E., Levine, D.N., and Zajac, F.E. 1971. Mammalian motor units: physi-ological-histochemical correlation in three types in cat gastrocnemius. *Science* 174: 709-712.

Cavagna, G.A., Dusman, B., and Margaria, R. 1968. Positive work done by a pre-viously stretched muscle. *J. Appl. Physiol.* 24: 21-32.

Celejowa, I., and Homa, M. 1970. Food intake, nitrogen and energy balance in Polish weightlifters, during a training camp. *Nutr. Metabol.* 12: 259-274.

Colomo, F., Lombardi, V., and Piazzesi, G. 1986. The relationship between force, stiffness and velocity of lengthening in tendon-free segments of frog single muscle fibres. *J. Physiol.* 377: 90P.

Costill, D.L., Daniels, J.R., Evans, W., Fink, W., Krahenbuhl, G., and Saltin, B. 1976. Skeletal muscle enzymes and fiber composition in male and female track athletes. *J. Appl. Physiol.* 40: 149-154.

Crasselt, W., Forchel, I., Kroll, M., and Schulz, A. 1990. *Sport of children and adolescents—reality, expectations and tendencies.* Leipzig: Deutsche Hochschule für Körperkultur.

Dragan, G.I., Vasiliu, A., and Georgescu, E. 1985. Effect of increased supply of protein on elite weight-lifters. In *Milk proteins,* ed. T.E. Galesloot and B.J. Tinbergen, 99-103. Wageningen, The Netherlands: Pudoc.

Dum, R.P., O'Donovan, M.J., Toop, J., Tsairis, P., Pinter, M.J., and Burke, R.E. 1985. Cross-innervated motor units in cat muscle. II. Soleus muscle reinnervated by flexor digitorum longus motoneurons. *J. Neurophys.* 54: 837-851.

Edman, K.A.P., Elzinga, G., and Noble, M.I.N. 1978. Enhancement of mechanical performance by stretch during tetanic contractions of vertebrae skeletal muscle fibers. *J. Physiol.* 281: 139-155.

Eriksson, B.O. 1972. Physical training, oxygen supply and muscle metabolism in 11- to 15-year old boys. *Acta Physiol. Scand.* S384: 1.

Forbes, G.B. 1981. Nutritional requirements in adolescence. In *Textbook of pediat-ric nutrition,* ed. R.M. Suskind, 381-391. New York: Raven Press.

Goldspink, G. 1978. Energy turnover during contraction of different types of muscle. In *Biomechanics VI-A,* ed. E. Asmussen and K. Jörgenson, 27-39. Baltimore: University Park Press.

Gollnick, P.D., Armstrong, R.B., Saubert, C.W., Piehl, K., and Saltin, B. 1972. Enzyme activity and fiber composition in skeletal muscle of untrained and trained men. *J. Appl. Physiol.* 33: 312-319.

Henneman, E., Somjen, G., and Carpenter, D.O. 1965. Functional significance of cell size in spinal motoneurones. *J. Neurophys.* 28: 560-580.

Hettinger, T. 1968. *Isometric muscle training.* Stuttgart: Georg Thieme Verlag.

Hirtz, P. 1981. Motor skills: characteristics, the effect of growth and influence possibilities. *Med. Sport* 21: 348.

Huijing, P.A. 1992. Elastic potential of muscle. In *Strength and power in sport,* ed. P.V. Komi, 151-68. Oxford: Blackwell Scientific.

Israel, S. 1976. The early development of coordination. *Körpererziehung* 11: 501-505.

Johnson, M.A., Polgar, J., Weightman, D., and Appleton, D. 1973. Data on the distribution of fibre types in thirty-six human muscles: an autopsy study. *J. Neurolog. Sci.* 18: 111-129.

Kernell, D. 1986. Organization and properties of spinal motoneurones and motor units. In *Progress in brain research,* vol. 64, ed. H-J. Freund, U. Büttner, B. Cohen, and J. Noth, 21-30. Amsterdam: Elsevier Science.

Komi, P.V. 1984. Physiological and biomechanical correlates of muscle function: effects of muscle structure and stretch-shortening cycle on force and speed. *Exerc. Sports Sci. Rev.* 12: 81-121.

Komi, P.V., and Bosco, C. 1978. Utilization of stored elastic energy in leg extensor muscles by men and women. *Med. Sci. Sports Exerc.* 10: 261-265.

Kovanen, V., Suominen, H., and Heikkinen, E. 1984. Mechanical properties of fast and slow skeletal muscle with special reference to collagen and endurance training. *J. Biomech.* 17: 725-735.

Laritcheva, K.A., Yalovaya, N.I., Shubin, V.I., and Smirnov, P.V. 1978. Study of energy expenditure and protein needs of top weight lifters. In *Nutrition, physical fitness and health,* ed. J. Parizkova and V.A. Rogozkin, 155-563. Baltimore: University Park Press.

Mahan, L.K., and Rees, J.M. 1984. *Nutrition in adolescence.* St. Louis: Times Mirror/Mosby.

Mero, A. 1992. Skeletal muscle fiber characteristics and anaerobic work in pubertal boys during training. *Med. Sci. Sports Exerc.* 24: S82.

Mero, A. 1993. Neuromuscular performance and skeletal muscle fiber characteristics in pubertal power athletes during training. *Med. Sci. Sports Exerc.* 25: S47.

Mero, A. 1994. Plasma amino acids in male power athletes during training. XXVth FIMS World Congress of Sports Medicine, Athens, abstract book, 8.

Mero, A., Jaakkola, L., and Komi, P.V. 1991. Relationships between muscle fiber characteristics and physical performance capacity in trained athletic boys. *J. Sports Sci.* 9: 161-171.

Mero, A., and Komi, P.V. 1994. EMG, force and power analysis of sprint-specific strength exercises. *J. Appl. Biomech.* 10: 1-13.

Mero, A., Lehtimäki, M., Mäkelä, J., Levola, M., Helander, E., Rajala, T., Aura, O., Peltola, E., Jouste, P., and Pullinen, T. 1992. Performance capacity of young speed and speed-strength athletes during two years of training. *Sprint Hurdle J.* 3-4: 20-33.

Mero, A., Luhtanen, P., Viitasalo, J.T., and Komi, P.V. 1981. Relationships between the maximal running velocity, muscle fiber characteristics, force production and force relaxation of sprinters. *Scand. J. Sports Sci.* 3: 15-22.

Mero, A., Pullinen, T., Komi, P.V., Pakarinen, A., and MacDonald, E. 1995. EMG, force and hormonal responses to high intensity strength and running exercise units in male power athletes. Paper presented at the XVth Congress of the International Society of Biomechanics, July 2-6, Jyväskylä, Finland.

Mero, A., Pullinen, T., MacDonald, E., and Pakarinen, A. 1994. Acute force and hormonal responses to four strength exercise units in pubertal male athletes. *Proceedings of the International Congress on Applied Research in Sports,* August 9-11, Helsinki, Finland.

Mero, A., Vuorimaa, T., and Häkkinen, K., eds. 1990. *Training in children and adolescents.* Jyväskylä, Finland: Gummerus Kirjapaino Oy.

Morgan, D.L. 1977. Separation of active and passive components of short-range stiffness of muscle. *Am. J. Physiol.* 232: C45-C49.

Nielsen, B., Nielsen, K., Behrendt-Hansen, M., and Asmussen, E. 1980. Training of "functional" muscular strength in girls 7-19 years old. In *Children and exercise IX,* ed. K. Berg and B. Eriksson. Baltimore: University Park Press.

Nilsson, B.E., and Westlin, N.E. 1971. Bone density in athletes. *Clin. Orthop. Rel. Res.* 77: 179-182.

Norman, R., and Komi, P.V. 1979. Electromechanical delay in skeletal muscle under normal movement conditions. *Acta Physiol. Scand.* 106: 241-248.

Noth, J. 1992. Cortical and peripheral control. In *Strength and power in sport,* ed. P. Komi, 9-20. Oxford: Blackwell Scientific.

Noth, J. 1992. Motor units. In *Strength and power in sport,* ed. P. Komi, 21-28. Oxford: Blackwell Scientific.

Pate, R.R., and Shephard, R.J. 1989. Characteristics of physical fitness in youth. In *Perspectives in exercise science and sports medicine,* ed. C.V. Gisolfi and D.R. Lamb. Vol. 2, *Youth, exercise and sport,* 1-43. Indianapolis: Benchmark Press.

Pfeiffer, R., and Francis, R.S. 1986. Effects of strength training on muscle development in prepubescent, pubescent and postpubescent males. *Physician Sports Med.* 14: 134.

Proske, U., and Morgan, D.L. 1984. Stiffness of cat soleus muscle and tendon during activation of part of the muscle. *J. Neurophys.* 52: 459-468.

Proske, U., and Morgan, D.L. 1987. Tendon stiffness: methods of measurement and significance for the control of movement. A review. *J. Biomech.* 20: 75-82.

Ramsay, J.A., Blimkie, C.J.R., Smith, K., Garner, S., MacDougall, J.D., and Sale, D.G. 1990. Strength training effects in prepubescent boys. *Med. Sci. Sports Exerc.* 22: 605-614.

Reilly, T. 1981. The concept, measurement and development of flexibility. In *Sports fitness and sports injuries,* ed. T. Reilly, 61-69. London: Faber & Faber.

Reiter, E.O., and Root, A. 1975. Hormonal changes of adolescence. *Med. Clin. North Am.* 59: 1289.

Rutenfranz, J., and Hettinger, T. 1959. Researches about the correlation of performance with age, sex and maturity. *Z. Kinderheilkunde* 83: 65.

Saltin, B., Henrikson, J.R., Nygaard, E., Andersen, P., and Jansson, E. 1977. Fiber types and metabolic potentials of skeletal muscles in sedentary man and endurance runners. *Ann. New York Acad. Sci.* 301: 3-29.

Semetka, M. 1982. Physical development and motor efficiency of 7 to 14 year old Slovak population. *Tréner* 26: 1.

Sermejev, B. 1964. The influence of specific exercises to flexibility in school-age children. *Theorie und Praxis der Körperkultur* 5: 434-436.

Sinclair, D. 1989. *Human growth after birth.* 5th ed. Oxford: Oxford University Press.

Slemenda, C.W., Miller, J.Z., Hui, S.L., Reister, T.K., and Johnston, C.C., Jr. 1991. Role of physical activity in the development of skeletal mass in children. *J. Bone Min. Res.* 6: 1227-1233.

Smith, J.L., Betts, B., Edgerton, V.R., and Zernicke, R.F. 1980. Rapid ankle extension during paw shakes: selective recruitment of fast ankle extensors. *J. Neurophys.* 43: 612-620.

Sugi, H., and Tsuchiya, T. 1981. Enhancement of mechanical performance in frog muscle fibers after quick increases in load. *J. Physiol.* 319: 239-252.

Suominen, H., Kiiskinen, A., and Heikkinen, E. 1980. Effects of physical training on metabolism of connective tissues in young mice. *Acta Physiol. Scand.* 108: 17-22.

Thorstensson, A., Larsson, L., Tesch, P., and Karlsson, J. 1977. Muscle strength and fiber composition in athletes and sedentary men. *Med. Sci. Sports* 9: 26-30.

Tittel, K. 1992. Coordination and balance. In *The Olympic book of sports medicine,* ed. A. Dirix, H.G. Knuttgen, and K. Tittel, 194-211. Oxford: Blackwell Scientific.

Wasnich, R.D., Ross, P.D., Vogel, J.M., and Davis, J.W. 1989. *Osteoporosis. Critique and practicum.* Honolulu: Banyan Press.

Weltman, A., Janney, C., Rians, C.B., Strand, K., Berg, B., Tippit, S., Wise, J., Cahill, B., and Katch, F.I. 1986. The effect of hydraulic resistance strength training in pre-pubertal males. *Med. Sci. Sports Exerc.* 18: 629-638.

Willimczik, K. 1979. The motor development during childhood and youth. Schorndorf, Germany: Hofmann-Verlag.

Winter, R. 1981. Principles of development in coordination of locomotion. *Med. Sport* 21: 194, 254, 282.

Woo, S.L.-Y., Gomez, M.A., Amiel, D., Ritter, M.A., and Gelberham, R.H. 1981. The effects of exercise on the biomechanical and biochemical properties of swine digital flexor tendons. *J. Biomech. Eng.* 103: 51-56.

Zaciorskij, V. 1973. The physical characteristics of athletes. *Leistungssport* 1: 3-5.

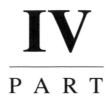

PART

Clinical and Environmental Limitations

12

CHAPTER

Injuries and Anaerobic Performance During Development

Lyle J. Micheli
Sig Berven

This chapter focuses on the following objectives:

- Describing the musculoskeletal system of children and adolescents
- Discussing the characteristics and effects of acute traumatic injuries
- Assessing the risk factors for injury and how they can be reduced

Anaerobic performance demands short and explosive bursts of maximal exertion, translating to tremendous stress on adolescent bone, joints, and soft tissues. In aggressively pursuing the Olympian goals of faster, higher, and stronger, the adolescent athlete exposes himself to mechanical forces that frequently exceed the capacity of an immature musculoskeletal system. There are two general types of injury for which adolescent athletes are at risk: acute traumatic injuries and overuse syndromes. The incidence of acute traumatic injuries appears similar in adolescents at free play and those in organized sport (Jackson, Jarret, and Bailet 1978; Roser and Clawson 1970). In fact, a study of Irish school children found acute traumatic injuries to be twice as common in non-organized sport and playground activity than in organized competition (Zaricznyj, Shatuck, and Mast 1980). It seems clear that in an organized environment, adolescents should be relatively safer than at free play as adequate supervision and control of the playing surface and conditions can be exercised.

However, in the category of overuse injuries, there is clearly a difference in injury rates, with organized sport being the near exclusive domain of overuse syndromes. The rise in overuse injuries in adolescents correlates closely with the organization of children's sports. The National Youth Sports Safety Foundation estimates that 20 to 30 million American children play organized sports out-of-school, and another 25 million participate in interscholastic competitive sports. Many adolescents participating in organized sports are playing under strenuous pressures and expectations from coaches, parents, and peers. Often, these pressures and expectations are put forth without guidance and counselling, leading to a whole new genre of adolescent injuries — overuse syndromes. Once the bane of only the professional athlete or the recreational adult athlete who intermittently overexerts a deconditioned body, overuse injuries are now distinguishing organized adolescent sport from free play among adolescents.

Adolescent athletes are reaching levels of performance that equal and often exceed those of skeletally mature adults. The growing number of overuse injuries in training, and of acute traumatic injuries in training and competition is related to increased participation of adolescents in organized sport, as well as to inadequate supervision and ill-advised training regimens. In order to train and compete safely and effectively without injury, it is important to define the characteristics and the capacity of the immature skeleton, and to identify the patterns of injury that are characteristic of the immature skeleton. This level of understanding of the immature musculoskeletal system is essential for those who intend to design training programs and competitive events that will minimize the risk of injury while allowing for maximum performance.

The Immature Musculoskeletal System

Injury patterns of the immature musculoskeletal system are distinct from those of adults, and relate to special features of the skeleton that permit growth and remodeling. Skeletal growth occurs at three sites about the joint of the child: the epiphyseal plate (growth plate), the apophyses, and the joint surface (see figure 12.1). Injuries and stresses to the developing skeleton involve different structures depending upon the stage of the chondro-osseous maturation. In taking a history and examining a patient it is essential to be aware of his stage of skeletal maturation as this data will clearly determine what structures are at risk from a given mechanism of injury.

There are several factors that make injuries to the immature skeleton distinct from those of the mature skeleton (Ogden, 1982):

1. Fractures are most likely to occur following seemingly minimal trauma.
2. Joint injuries, dislocations, or ligamentous disruptions are much less com mon than in adults.
3. The periosteum of the immature athlete is thicker, stronger, and more biologically active.

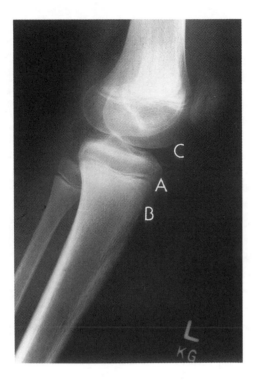

Figure 12.1 Growth cartilage is present at three sites about the joint of a child: (*a*) the epiphyseal plate; (*b*) the apophysis, site of major tendon insertions; and (*c*) the joint surface.

4. Diagnosis presents special difficulty due to variable radiolucency at the epiphyses.
5. Remodeling can correct many residual angular deformities.
6. Injuries to specific growth regions may lead to significant disturbances of growth.
7. Diaphyseal fractures may stimulate longitudinal growth by increasing blood supply to the metaphysis, physis and epiphysis, leading to leg length discrepancy.

The immature musculoskeletal system is characterized by open physes, a separate epiphysis, a thick and active periosteum, thin metaphyseal cortices, and relatively strong tendons, joint capsules, and ligaments compared with developing bone. Longitudinal growth occurs at the cartilage of the epiphyseal plate, which is the weak link of the immature bone (Burstein and Frankle1968). The four layers of the epiphyseal plate are illustrated in figure 12.2. The zone of the hypertrophied cells has relatively less extracellular matrix than the surrounding cartilage and bone, and is therefore more susceptible to separation or fracture (Bright, Burstein, and Elmore

1974). Shear stresses are particularly disruptive to physeal cartilage whereas metaphyseal bone is susceptible to fracture in compression. Temporally, the zone of hypertrophied cells is widest during the periods of rapid growth, and therefore more susceptible to injury during these periods.

The epiphysis of the immature skeleton is the portion of bone defined by a secondary center of ossification. There are two distinct types of epiphysis that are of significance in defining adolescent injuries: the traction epiphysis, or apophysis, and the compression epiphysis or pressure epiphysis (Salter and Harris 1963). The traction epiphysis is the site of insertion or origin of major muscle groups, and is subjected to traction forces. It is non-articular, but subject to large sheer and traction forces during explosive muscle contractions of anaerobic sports, and to repeated stresses during prolonged training and repetitive exertion. Examples of

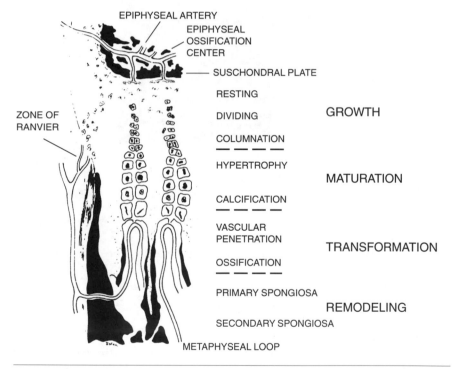

Figure 12.2 The epiphyseal plate is an avascular zone between the epiphyseal ossification center and the metaphyseal ossification center. The four zones of the epiphyseal plate are: (*a*) the resting zone, a region of metabolically inactive chondrocytes in dense concentration; (*b*) the proliferating zone, a region of cellular division with formation of pallisading columns and increased extracellular matrix; (*c*) the hypertrophic zone, a swelling of chondrocytes with minimum extracellular matrix volume, making them susceptible to fracture; and (*d*) the provisional calcification zone, a region of vascular penetration and deposition of mineral phase.

Reprinted from Albright and Brand 1987.

apophyseal injuries include the tibial tubercle in Osgood-Schlatter's Disease, Iliacapophysitis, Sever's Disease (calcaneal apophysitis), and traction apoph ysitis of the elbow. Injuries to the compression epiphysis may be intra-articular or extra-articular (see discussion of epiphyseal plate fractures, p. 283).

The periosteum of the immature skeleton is much thicker and more active than it is in skeletally mature adult. The marked difference is fracture healing capacity in the child compared with the adult and can be attributed largely to the difference in the periosteal bone coverage. Specifically, the child's periosteum is far more likely to elevate in an intact fashion from metaphyseal and diaphyseal bone, maintaining its integrity and osteogenic potential. The thick periosteum of the forearm and tibia also offers protection against open fractures. The interposition of the periosteum between fracture fragments can make fracture reduction more difficult and necessitate open reduction.

The muscle-tendon units and ligamentous structures of adolescents have become an important consideration in injuries of the pediatric population as overuse syndromes and repetitive training regimens have entered the realm of adolescent sport. In general the athlete with open physes is more susceptible to growth plate injuries than to ligament or muscle-tendon injuries, which are characteristic of the adult skeleton (Best 1995). Tensile forces that produce muscle-tendon or ligament injuries in the adult usually result in apophyseal avulsions and growth plate injuries in the growing child. The myotendinous junction is a region of highly folded membranes at the interface between the muscle and tendon, and it is at this transition point that most muscle strains occur. In the growing adolescent, the growth of the skeleton applies a chronic stretch to the musculotendinous junction where muscle fiber growth occurs through addition of sarcomeres. During rapid growth, a mismatch or imbalance may exist between sarcomere length and mechanical requirements, and strain and tears at the musculotendinous junction are more common.

The final anatomic feature of developing bone that is important to consider in understanding injury patterns in the adolescent skeleton is the relative weakness of developing bone in compression compared with mature bone. Developing bone in the metaphysis and diaphysis has a relatively greater porosity than mature bone, composed of woven osteoid matrix rather than lamellar components, and of highly vascular matrix rather than dense mineral. The active growth and remodeling of the metaphysis makes it particularly susceptible to fracture because of its thin cortex and high content of spongy, trabecular bone. While the structural characteristics of developing bone do make it more susceptible to fracture in compression than mature bone, these features also prevent fracture propagation and comminution, and promote rapid healing.

This description of the structural characteristics of the immature skeleton creates a framework for discussion of specific injury patterns seen in children and adolescents. The discussion of patterns of injuries is divided into acute traumatic injuries and overuse injuries.

Acute Traumatic Injuries

Acute traumatic injuries result from a single application of force sufficient to mechanically disrupt the tissues.

Fractures

Tremendous forces are generated by a full impact collision in football, falls from high jump or even pole vaulting heights, and twists in a misplaced step during a 100 m sprint or a landing from the parallel bars. The forces from such occurrences can lead to fracture in both the adult and the adolescent athlete, though the adolescent is far more likely to sustain a bony injury from a stress while the adult is more likely to suffer ligamentous or musculotendinous tear. Bones have a capacity for elastic osseous deformation, with the immature skeleton having more capacity for such change than the mature skeleton. However, overload of the capacity of bone to recoil results in an acute plastic deformation. Kaye Wilkins defines four basic types of fracture patterns to growing bones (Wilkins, 1980).

Plastic Deformation

Plastic deformation is a curvature of diaphyseal bone without cortical disruption. Microfractures may occur within the relatively loose osteoid matrix of developing bone, resulting in bending of bone without a distinct macroscopic cortical interruption. This injury is most commonly seen in the forearm in response to a bending force. Correction can usually be accomplished with a closed reduction and casting, though a large amount of force may be required for reduction as the fracture is relatively stable and the cortex maintains its structural integrity.

Torus Fractures

A torus fracture is a compression injury along the axis of a long bone and can result in a folding of the metaphyseal portion of developing bone. As noted earlier, metaphyseal bone is characterized by porous, vascular, rapidly remodeling woven bone with little lamellar architecture. Reduction is usually not required as the joint surface is not involved and there is no angulation of rotation, but protection with immobilization is essential to prevent further injury and development of deformity.

Green-Stick Fractures

A greenstick fracture is an incomplete cortical disruption. A bending or rotational force applied at each end of a long bone may concentrate a compression or tension force at the mid-diaphyseal region. Failure in compression generally results in less displacement than failure in tension. Angulation of greater than 10 degrees should generally be reduced (Wilkins 1994). The greenstick fracture in tension disrupts the periosteum, and the plastic deformity tends to be recreated during healing if immobilization is inadequate.

Epiphyseal-Plate Fractures

The weakness of the epiphyseal plate in relation to the bone of the surrounding epiphysis and metaphysis has been studied extensively (Bright, Burstein, and Elmore 1974; Burstein and Frankle 1968; Salter and Harris 1963). Ligamentous and fibrous capsular attachments around the joint are two to five times stronger than the weakest area of the epiphyseal plate (Burstein and Frankle 1968). Therefore, a valgus stress to the knee of a skeletally immature adolescent would disrupt the epiphysis rather than the medial collateral ligament, and a valgus stress to the elbow would avulse the medial epicondyle rather than disrupt the medial ligament complex at the elbow. Similarly, the fibrous joint capsule exceeds the strength of the epiphyseal plate so that an injury that may cause a traumatic shoulder dislocation in an adult would lead to a proximal humerus epiphyseal separation in the child.

Approximately 15 percent of all fractures in children involve the physis (Ogden, 1982), with distal radius injuries most common, followed by distal humerus and distal tibia. Physeal injuries are most common during the adolescent growth spurt (Peterson and Peterson 1972) because of thinning of the perichondral ring around the physis (zone of Ranvier) and relative widening of the zone of hypertrophic cells. Salter and Harris define 5 types of injuries to the epiphyseal plate (Salter and Harris 1963):

Type I fractures separate through the epiphyseal plate (see figure 12.3).

Type II fractures involve the epiphyseal plate, and exit through metaphyseal bone.

Type III fractures involve the epiphyseal plate and exit through the epiphysis.

Type IV fractures cross the epiphyseal plate, involving metaphysis and epiphysis.

Type V fractures are crush injuries to the epiphyseal plate, disrupting the normal four zone architecture.

Larson studied 62 epiphyseal plate injuries sustained in athletic activity, recording that 82% were type I or II, and 76% involved the pressure epiphysis while 24% involved the traction epiphysis (Micheli 1987). Growth disturbance is the most worrisome complication of physeal fractures, specifically fractures to the pressure epiphyseal plate. Risk factors for post-traumatic growth disturbance at the physes include the vascular supply to the physis and epiphysis, extent of plate involvement, amount of remaining growth, and the disruption of the physis caused by reduction maneuvers. The femoral head, radial head, distal tibia, distal femur, and the proximal tibia are most susceptible to growth arrest after fracture.

Intra-articular extension of fracture plans are seen in type III and IV physeal injuries. An intra-articular stepoff is particularly important to detect on initial

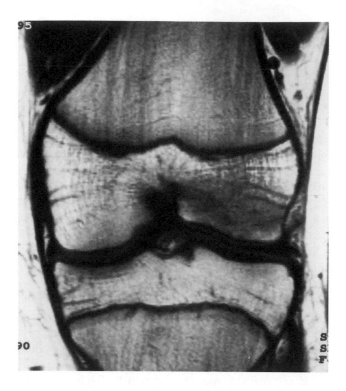

Figure 12.3 Epiphyseal injury of the knee (distal femur) demonstrated by an MRI.

medical evaluation, avoiding the possibility of treating as a sprain an injury that may lead to chronic pain and accelerated osteoarthrosis. The Tillaux fracture (a variant of a Salter-Harris III injury) and the triplane fracture (a variant of a Salter-Harris IV injury) are common examples of physeal injuries with intra-articular extension that are at risk for significant joint disruption. It is essential to study roentgenographs closely for evidence of intra-articular stepoff, and CT evaluation or arthrography may be required to delineate the anatomy. More recently, magnetic resonance imaging (MRI) can demonstrate epiphyseal injury not previously evident by plane radiographs or CT scan (figure 12.3).

Acute Traumatic Dislocations

Traumatic dislocations of joints are far more common in adults than in adolescents because of the strength of the fibrous joint capsule relative to the physeal plate of the immature skeleton. Pathologic conditions including Larson's syndrome, Ehlers-Danlos syndrome (Simonian and Luck 1993), and homocystinuria may lead to multiple and frequent joint dislocations. Dislocations of the elbow are the most common joint dislocation in children, usually occurring after age 10, and accounting for up to 6 percent of elbow injuries in adolescents. Dislocations can also occur of the interphalangeal joints, the metacarpal phalangeal joints, hip, knee, shoulder, radial head, and proximal tibiofibular joint. Patellar dislocation is a relatively rare injury in the skeletally immature athlete, and subluxations or sleeve fractures to the patella are more common mechanisms for patellar injury. McManus reviewed 55 cases of true patellar dislocation and found that most cases involved some underlying dysplasia (McManus, Rang, and Heslin 1979).

Musculotendinous and Ligamentous Injuries: Sprains, Strains, and Contusions

Traumatic injury in the skeletally immature adolescent often spares damage to the developing tendons and ligaments, as the chondro-osseous matrix is the weakest point of bone-tendon or bone-ligament unit. However, despite the differences in skeletal anatomy and physiology discussed that predispose to physeal, apophyseal, and greenstick fractures, soft tissue injuries continue to predominate in athletes between ages 10 and 18 (Watson 1984). Ligamentous disruptions are clearly rare in the skeletally immature athlete, though as the athlete reaches skeletal maturity, the likelihood of ligamentous strain increases with closure of the epiphyseal plate. There is a transition of the weak link of the ligamentous-skeletal unit from bone to ligament with physeal closure (Webber 1988). The knee and the ankle are two joints across which ligamentous injuries are being diagnosed and reported with increased frequency in the adolescent athlete.

With increased participation of adolescents in sports requiring forceful twisting and translation at the knee, ligamentous injuries to the knee appear to be increasing in incidence (DeLee 1994). Historically, avulsion fractures rather than anterior cruciate ligament tears had been the rule in childhood and early adolescence (Ehrlich and Strain 1979; Gronkvist, Hirsch, and Johansson 1984). In 1974, Mercer Rang wrote that ligamentous injuries about the knee do not occur in children (Rang 1974). However, with the advent of arthroscopy for acute evaluation of traumatic hemarthrosis, it has become clear that ligament injury must be considered in the differential diagnosis of the child suffering from knee trauma (Bradley, Shives, and Samuelson 1979; Clanton, DeLee, and Sanders 1979). In diagnostic arthroscopic examination of 70 children ages 7-18 with acute hemarthrosis, 47 percent of preadolescent (age 7-12) and 65% of adolescent (age 12-18) patients had acute anterior cruciate ligament tears (Stanitski, Harvell, and Fu 1993).

At the ankle, ligaments are again relatively spared in skeletally immature athletes, as Salter I and II fractures of the distal fibula are most common (McManama 1988). An inversion injury that would produce a lateral ligamentous injury in the adult would be most likely to disrupt the distal fibula physis in the adolescent athlete. However, in sports demanding significant stresses to the lateral side of the ankle, including gymnastics and basketball, lateral ligament disruption and distal tibiofibular ligament disruption are frequent causes of acute and chronic ankle pain in the adolescent athlete (McManama 1988).

Muscle strain is a soft tissue injury involving a disruption of the membranes at the musculoskeletal junction. Muscle strains are classified into three grades (Webber 1988):

> *First Degree Strain:* Muscle disruption with mild tenderness at the site of the injury with a palpable defect. Pain is elicited by stretch.

> *Second Degree Strain:* Partial tearing at the musculotendinous junction with bleeding and spasm. The patient is unable to fully extend the involved muscle belly.

> *Third Degree Strain:* Complete disruption at the musculotendinous junction with bleeding, spasm, and a palpable defect.

In the skeletally immature athlete a rapid contraction of a musculotendinous unit against resistance will result in an apophyseal avulsion rather than a muscle strain (Best 1995). Specifically, the peripelvic avulsions including the ischial tuberosity as the hamstring origin, the anterior superioriliac spine as the origin of sartorius, and the anterior inferior iliac spine as the origin of rectus femoris are common injuries in the adolescent athlete, caused by forces that would be likely to result in muscle strain in the adult (Paletta and Andrish 1995).

The force of a muscle contracture is transmitted to bony apophysis to produce locomotion through a myotendinous junction. Best has studied the histology of the myotendinous junction and describes a high infolded membrane with a large cross surface area, limiting point forces at the junction (Best 1995). The muscles most susceptible to strain are the muscles that transverse two joints, including hamstrings, quadriceps, biceps, and gastrocnemius, which are subject to eccentric loading patterns. Type II (fast twitch) muscle fibers are also more susceptible to strain than type I. With growth, chronic stretch causes adaptation in the length of both muscle fibers and tendons. The musculotendinous junction is the location of much of longitudinal growth. Imbalances of muscle and tendon length are frequent during rapid growth (Micheli and Smith 1982) leading to relative tightness of muscles and tendons across joints, and an increased incidence of both strains and apophyseal injuries. Weakness and fatigue are clear risk factors for strains to the musculotendinous junction and for apophyseal avulsions. Contracting muscle absorbs more energy than passively stretched muscle (Garrett, Safran, and Seaber 1987). Therefore, stronger muscle can absorb more energy than fatigued muscles, and inadequate strength and aerobic conditioning lead to poor energy absorption by the body of muscle, and strain to the musculotendinous junction. Furthermore, as muscle is composed of 75 percent water and 25 percent protein, its viscoelastic properties lead to an increased compliance with warming (Noonan, Best, and Seaber 1993), suggesting a role for warm-up exercises to prevent strain. Stretching also leads to alteration in mechanical properties of muscle and tendon that may allow for improved energy absorption during contractures (Best, McElhaney, and Garrett 1994).

Whereas muscle strains are injuries to the musculotendinous junction, muscle contusions are injuries resulting from a direct force to the muscle belly. Muscle contusions are probably the most common injury in the adolescent athlete, seen most commonly in the anterior tibialis and quadriceps. A direct force to muscle belly results in hemorrhage, inflammation, and healing both through muscle regeneration and scar formation. In studying muscle contusions in rats, Jarvinen demonstrated that recovery from and healing of muscle contusions was far more rapid in young rats than old (Jarvinen, Aho, and Lehto 1983) and in the rats treated with mobilization after contusions rather than those treated with immobilization (Jarvinen 1975). There is evidence that RICE (Rest, Ice, Compression, Elevation) are appropriate for the treatment of contusions (Jackson and Feagin 1973) though ultrasound, heat, and massage have not been proven to improve recovery (Gross 1994). Of importance, rehabilitation should be carried out slowly with gentle, passive range of motion followed by active range of motion as tolerated by pain. Massage and stretching may increase muscle inflammation and may predispose to development of myositis ossificans. Prevention of contusions can best be accomplished by use of thigh and shin guards in contact sports, especially football and soccer.

Overuse Injuries

Injuries from impact or macrotrauma are common in adolescent play, with little distinction in injury rates between organized sports and free play (Roser and Clawson 1970). However, there is a whole new genre of injuries occurring in children engaged in organized sports that rarely occur in free play. These are the overuse injuries, including tendinitis of the shoulder, elbow, wrist; stress fractures to the tibia or metatarsals; and patellofemoral stress syndrome at the knee (figure 12.4). Overuse injuries are those that occur from the repetitive application of submaximal stresses to otherwise normal tissues. With the volume of training and repetition of exercises required for competitive performance, the normal reparative processes are overwhelmed, and tissue injury and inflammation ensue (Herring and Nilson 1987). Overuse injuries are especially characteristic of anaerobic sports, requiring repetition of short bursts of near maximal power, including gymnastics, figure skating, sprinting, and jumping events. Overuse injuries occur in a variety of tissues including bone (stress fractures) (Yngve 1988), tendons (tendinitis) (Micheli and Fehlandt 1992), musculotendinous junctions (strains) (Gross 1994), bone-ligament junctions (strains) (Micheli and Fehlandt 1992), and bone-tendon junctions (bursitis) (Outerbridge and Micheli 1995). In the skeletally immature athlete, recurrent stress to the epiphysis and the apophysis may lead to epiphyseal changes (Roy, Caine, and Singer 1985) and apophysitises (Micheli 1987). Repetitive microtrauma to the articular cartilage of

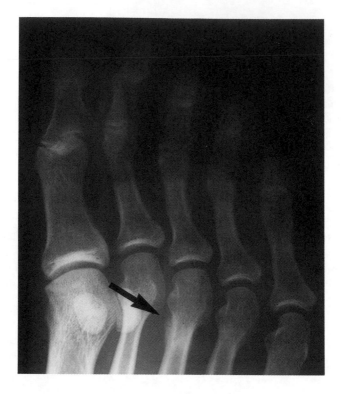

Figure 12.4 Stress fracture of the third metatarsal in a young runner.

the adolescent athlete is another mechanism for overuse and may be causal in the development of chondral and subchondral injury (Federico, Lynch, and Jokl 1990). This profile of injuries represents a mechanism of athletic injury quite distinct from macrotrauma or impact injuries and a profile that is peculiar to organized sports. This observation has important implications for the prevention of overuse injuries.

The epidemic of overuse injuries in adolescent athletes corresponds closely with what has been described as an epidemic of participation of adolescents in organized athletic and competitive sporting programs (Kannus, Nittymaki, and Jarvinen 1988; Micheli and Smith 1982). Pediatric overuse injury rates rise in direct proportion to the level of sports organization (McCarroll, Meaney, and Sieber 1984). Many sports-specific overuse injuries could be prevented if children's participation in sport were gauged by their own desired level of intensity rather than that of coaches or parents (Andrish 1993). While injuries from macrotrauma are difficult to avoid in either free play or organized sport, it is clear that modification of training regimens and an awareness of the risk factors for overuse injuries will stem the rising incidence of the overuse injury pattern.

Risk Factors for Injury and Injury Prevention

Having developed an understanding of the types of injuries characteristic of immature musculoskeletal system, and the anatomical features that predispose the immature skeleton to these injuries, we are better able to define specific risk factors for injury. We have identified two types of injury for which the adolescent athlete is at risk: injuries resulting from a macrotrauma (fractures, avulsions, dislocations), and injuries resulting from repetitive microtrauma (tendinitis, apophysitis, strains, sprains). The risk factors for each type of injury are distinct, as are methods for injury prevention.

Mismatch of athletic participants in terms of size, strength, and skills is an important risk factor for macrotrauma in children. Anaerobic power, muscular strength, and overall sports performance change rapidly during adolescent maturation, with tremendous variation within age groups. Therefore, a method of categorizing adolescents into developmentally appropriate groups rather than age-based groups may serve to "level the playing field" (Andrish 1993) and reduce injuries.

Explosive and forceful interactions are essential to the very nature of the game in many adolescent sports including football, rugby, field and ice hockey, and lacrosse. However, it has been demonstrated that proper protective equipment including helmets and pads significantly reduces injury rates (Saal 1991). Changes in rules are another important mechanism for intervention. In football and rugby, making headfirst tackling, or speartackling, illegal has led to a significant reduction in neck injuries at both a professional and high school level (Saal 1991; Silver and Stewart 1994). Rule changes are also applied to limit overuse injuries in adolescent sports. In baseball, throwing more than 300 skilled pitches per week significantly increases risk of elbow injury (Micheli 1995), and this can be used as a guideline for high school pitching coaches. Similarly, the NCAA restrictions on hours per week of training for swimmers may serve to limit overuse injuries in these athletes.

In assessing overuse injuries, it is useful to identify risk factors for specific injuries in order to determine etiology of a specific injury and to plan prevention of occurrence and recurrence (Micheli 1983). Risk factors for overuse injuries can be divided into intrinsic and extrinsic causes (Standish 1984).

Intrinsic Factors

Following are several factors intrinsic to most injuries.

Anatomic Malalignment

A variety of anatomic factors can predispose to overuse injuries. In the foot, tarsal coalition, excessive foot pronation or supination, or hindfoot malalignment can lead to imbalance of muscle mechanics and injury. Leg length discrepancy and anteversion of the hips or tibial torsion can also create excessive forces to the knee or ankle and predispose to bone, musculotendinous, and ligament injury. Correction of foot and ankle alignment with shoe inserts and orthotics can prevent many injuries due to malalignment.

Growth

In the extremities, longitudinal growth in bones outpaces associated growth of muscle and tendon units. During the adolescent growth spurt, flexibility decreases (Kirschner and Glines 1957) and stress across joint and musculotendinous units is increased (Gross 1994). Preconditioned muscle is capable of absorbing more stress than unconditioned muscle (Safran, Garrett, and Seaber 1988), reducing risk of strain. Conditioning and flexibility have been demonstrated to be effective in preventing morbidity from musculotendinous strains (Heiser, Weber, and Sullivan 1984).

Muscle-Tendon Imbalance

An imbalance of strength, flexibility, or bulk can result from asymmetric use of muscle groups. Swimmers and pitchers may develop an external rotation contracture to the shoulder, reflecting a tight posterior capsule and a loose anterior capsule. This condition may lead to anatomic subluxation of the shoulder, or an impingement syndrome. A well-balanced exercise program will prevent imbalances and resultant asymmetry.

Underlying Disease States and Deconditioning

Occult pathology including slipped capital femoral epiphyses, Legg-Calves-Perthes-Disease, and tarsal coalitions may only be symptomatic during exercise. Athletes recovering from previous injury or fracture are clearly at risk of recurrence. Also, children who arrive at a summer sports camp having spent the summer to date in front of the television are clearly at risk for overuse injuries. Adequate evaluation of participants and modification of training protocols is essential to the prevention of injury in this group.

Extrinsic Factors

These factors are considered extrinsic risk factors, but are no less important to consider than the intrinsic factors discussed above.

Training Errors

Training factors are by far the most common factors predisposing any athlete to an overuse injury (Outerbridge and Micheli 1995). The frequency, volume, and training are all a part of this equation. When the athlete is required to invoke the maximal force of musculotendinous units that are inadequately conditioned or recovered, injury is commonplace. There are two common patterns for overuse injuries due to training errors. First, the athlete who is deconditioned and suddenly begins a strenuous course of exercise, causing inflammation and injury to the musculoskeletal structures. Secondly, the athlete who is pushing towards a peak and is limited by the ultimate breakdown stress that the musculoskeletal system can handle (Gross 1994). Prevention of overuse injury in this population requires a knowledgeable coach or trainer to modify and diversify a training regimen to protect muscle groups from overuse (Stover 1982). Poor technique is another important training error that can lead to injury. In swimming, poor stroke mechanics due to inadequate instruction, or fatigue, places asymmetric stress across joints and musculotendinous units, leading to "swimmer's shoulder" (Richardson, Jobe, and Collins 1980). In skiing, athletes must especially be aware of lapses in technique due to fatigue, as both overuse injury and macrotrauma can result.

Environmental and Equipment Factors

Playing surface, footwear, and equipment are important determinants of stresses transmitted to musculotendinous structures. Inadequate shoe support or less forgiving playing surfaces can lead to stress fractures and apophysitises. Football injuries due to unforgiving qualities of artificial turf have been widely publicized in professional sports. Adolescent athletes are often competing on fields and tracks that are inadequately maintained, and this is an important cause of injury.

Directions for Future Research

Much more must be done to explore risk factors for sports injury occurrence in this age group as a first step in injury prevention. These risk factors include both extrinsic, or environmental, factors and intrinsic, or host, factors. This approach can be productive in the analysis of both acute traumatic injury and overuse injury (Outerbridge and Micheli 1995).

Intrinsic factors include anatomic alignment, muscle-tendon balance, relative fitness level, gender, and stage of physical development. Extrinsic factors include volume and intensity of training; footwear and playing equipment, including mechanical and care factors of playing fields; protective equipment; rules of the game, particularly as applied to altered rules for children; and officiating.

As regards acute traumatic injury in this age group, the major concern, of course, is catastrophic injury. Commotiocordis can serve as an example of a child-specific catastrophic sports injury. A number of reports are found in the medical literature of deaths resulting from projectile blows to the chest of the child participants, including blows from baseballs, softballs, or hockey pucks (Micheli 1987). Whether this chilling injury can be prevented by softer balls or chest protectors is a matter of active debate and clearly an area where laboratory and human study research is needed.

Concerning overuse of training injury, the area of greatest uncertainty is the determination of the minimal and maximal training volume and intensity advisable for this age group. Both ends of this question merit careful attention. What is the minimal threshold required for physical activity, including sports, that is necessary for maximal growth and development? Conversely, what is the maximal value and/ or intensity of training that can safely be done by the growing child without interfering with normal growth and development? This latter question has received wide attention and debate regarding the age, size, and development issues of female gymnasts in the recent 1996 Olympic competition (Abrunzo 1991).

Summary

The adolescent athlete is achieving levels of performance that equal or exceed many adult counterparts. The immature musculoskeletal system is structurally quite different than the mature system, and prone to specific injury patterns, due to both macrotrauma and microtrauma. It is important to recognize the limitations of the immature musculoskeletal system when designing training regimens, modifying rules for sport, and evaluating acute and subacute injury patterns. Macrotrauma occurs with equal frequency in organized sport and free play, and prevention of injuries requires adequate supervision, appropriate matching of competitors, and modification of rules. Overuse injuries due to repetitive microtrauma represent a new spectrum of injury that has arisen with the rise in organized sport for adolescents.

Injury prevention for overuse injuries requires a recognition of the risk factors for injury, and an appropriate modification and diversification of training regimens, an optimization of mechanics with technique and equipment, and adequate conditioning. Adolescents can compete effectively and safely in anaerobic events and competition with supervision and guidance that is responsive to their unique musculoskeletal needs.

References

Abrunzo, T.J.: Commotio cordis. The single, most common cause of traumatic death in young baseball. Am J Dis Child. 145(11): 1279-1282, 1991.

Andrish, J.T.: Pediatric athletic injuries. In MacEwen, G.D., Kasser, J.R., Henrich, S.D. (eds): Pediatric Fractures. A Practical Approach to Assessment and Treatment. Williams & Wilkins, Baltimore, 1993.

Best, T.M.: Muscle-tendon injuries in young athletes. Clin Sports Med. 14(3):669-686, 1995.

Best, T.M., McElhaney, J., Garret, W.E. Jr., et al.: Characterization of the passive response of live skeletal muscle using the quasi-linear theory of viscoelasticity. J. Biomech. 27(4): 413-419, 1994.

Bradley, G.W., Shives, T.C., and Samuelson, K.M.: Ligament injuries in the knees of children. J Bone Joint Surg. 61A(4): 588-591, 1979.

Bright, R.W., Burstein, A.H., and Elmore, S.M.: Epiphyseal plate cartilage. A biomechanical and histological analysis of failure modes. J Bone Joint Surg. 56A(4):688-703, 1974.

Burstein, A.H. and Frankle, V.H.: The viscoelastic properties of biological materials. Ann NY Acad Sci. 146: 158-165, 1968.

Clanton, T.O., DeLee, J.C., Sanders, B., et al.: Knee ligament injuries in children. J Bone Joint Surg. 61A(8): 1195-1201, 1979.

DeLee, J.: Ligamentous injuries of the knee. In Stanitski, C.L., DeLee, J.C., Drez, D. (eds): Pediatric and Adolescent Sports Medicine. W.B. Sanders, Philadelphia, 1994.

Ehrlich, M.G. and Strain, R.E. Jr.: Epiphyseal injuries about the knee. Orthop Clin North Am. 10(1): 91-103, 1979.

Federico, D.J., Lynch, J.K., and Jokl, P.: Osteochondritis dissecans of the knee: A historical review of etiology and treatment. Arthroscopy. 6(3): 190-197, 1990.

Garrett, W.E., Jr., Safran, M.R., Seaber, A.V., et al.: Biomechanical comparison of stimulated and nonstimulated skeletal muscle pulled to failure. Am J Sports Med. 15: 448-454, 1987.

Gronkvist, H., Hirsch, G., and Johannson, L.: Fracture of the anterior tibial spine in children. J Ped Orthop. 4(4): 465-468, 1984.

Gross, R.H.: Acute musculotendinous injuries. In Stanitski, C.L., DeLee, J.C., Drez, D. (eds): Pediatric and Adolescent Sports Medicine., W.B. Saunders, Philadelphia, 1994.

Heiser, T.M., Weber, J., Sullivan, G., et al.: Prophylaxis and management of hamstring muscle injuries in intercollegiate football players. Am J Sports Med. 12(5): 368-370, 1984.

Herring, S.A. and Nilson, K.L.: Introduction to overuse injuries. Clin Sports Med. 6(2): 225-239, 1987.

Jackson, D.W., and Feagin, J.A.: Quadriceps contusions in young athletes. Relation of severity of injury to treatment and prognosis. J Bone Joint Surg. 55A(1): 95-105, 1973.

Jackson, D.W., Jarret, H., Bailet, D., et al.: Injury prediction in the young athlete: A preliminary report. Am J Sports Med. 6:6-16, 1978.

Jarvinen, M.: Healing of a crush injury in rat striated muscle. 2.: A histological study of the effect of early mobilization and immobilization on the repair processes. Acta Pathol Microbiol Scand (Section A, Pathology). 83(3): 269-282, 1975.

Jarvinen, M., Aho, A.J., Lehto, M.., et al.: Age dependent repair of muscle rupture. A histological and microangiographical study in rats. Acta Orthop Scand. 54(1): 64-74, 1983.

Kannus, P., Nittymaki, S., and Jarvinen, M.: Athletic overuse injuries in children. A 30-month follow-up study at an outpatient sports clinic. Clin Pediatr. 27(7):

333-337, 1988.

Kirchner, G. and Glines, D.: Comparative analysis of Eugene, Oregon, elementary school children using the Krauss-Weber Test of Minimum Muscular Fitness. Research Quarterly. 28:16-25, 1957.

McCarroll, J.R., Meaney, C. and Sieber, J.M: Profile of youth soccer injuries. Phys Sportsmed. 12(2): 113-117,1984.

McManama, G.B., Jr.: Ankle injuries in the young athlete.Clin Sports Med. 7(3): 547-562, 1988.

McManus, F., Rang, M., and Heslin, D.J.: Acute dislocation of the patella in children. The natural history. Clin Orthop.139:88-91, 1979.

Micheli, L.J.: Overuse injuries in children's sports: The growth factor. Orthop Clin North Am. 14(2): 337-360, 1983..

Micheli, L.J.: The traction apophysitises. Clin Sports Med. 6(2):389-404, 1987.

Micheli, L.J.: Sports injuries in children and adolescents: Questions and controversies. Clin Sports Med. 14(3) 727-745, 1995

Micheli, L.J. and Fehlandt, A.F.: Overuse injuries to tendons and apophyses in children and adolescents. Clin Sports Med.11(4): 713-726, 1992.

Micheli, L.J., and Smith, A.D.: Sports injuries in children.Curr Problems Ped. 12(9): 1-54, 1982.

Noonan, T.J., Best, T.M., Seaber, A.V., et al.: Thermal effects on skeletal muscle tensile behavior. Am J Sports Med. 21(4): 517-522, 1993.

Ogden, J.: Skeletal injuries in the child. Lea & Febiger, Philadelphi, 1982, pp. 1-25.

Outerbridge, A.R., and Micheli, L.J.: Overuse injuries in the young athlete. Clin Sports Med. 14(3):503-516, 1995.

Paletta, G.A. Jr. and Andrish, J.T.: Injuries about the hip and pelvis in young athletes. Clin Sports Med. 14(3): 591-628, 1995.

Peterson, C.A., and Peterson, H.A.: Analysis of the incidence of injuries to the epiphyseal growth plate. J. Trauma.12(4): 275-281, 1972.

Rang, M., Children's Fractures. J.B. Lippincott, Philadelphia,1974.

Richardson, A.B., Jobe, F.W., Collins, H.R.: The shoulder in competitive swimming. Am J Sports Med. 7(3):259-163,1980.

Roser, C.A. and Clawson, D.K.: Football injuries in the very young athlete. Clin Orthop. 69:219-223, 1970.

Roy, S., Caine, D. and Singer, K.M.: Stress changes to the distal radial epiphysis in young gymnasts. A report of twenty-one cases and a review of the literature. Am J Sports Med. 13(5):301-308, 1985.

Saal, J.A.: Common American football injuries. Sports Med. 12(2):132-147, 1991.

Safran, M.R., Garrett, W.E., Seaber, A.V., et al.: The role of warmup in muscular injury prevention. Am J Sports Med.16(2): 123-129, 1988.

Salter, R.B. and Harris, W.R.: Injuries involving the epiphyseal plate. J Bone Joint Surg. 45A(3): 587-622,1963.

Silver, J.R., and Stewart, D.: The prevention of spinal injuries in rugby football. Paraplegia.32(7):442-453,1994.

Simonian, P.T. and Luck, J.V.Jr.: Synthetic posterior cruciate ligament reconstruction and below-knee prosthesis use in Ehlers-Danlos syndrome. Clin Orthop. 294:314-317, 1993.

Standish, W.D.: Overuse injuries in athletes: A perspective. Med Sci Sports Exerc. 16(1): 1-7,1984.

Stanitski, C.L., Harvell, J.C., and Fu, F.: Observations on acute knee hemarthrosis in children and adolescents. J Ped Orthop. 13(4): 506-510, 1993.

Stover, C.N.: Physical conditioning of the immature athlete. Orthop Clin North Am. 13(3): 528-540, 1982.

Watson, A.W.: Sports injuries during one academic year in 6799 Irish school children. Am J Sports Med. 12(1):65-71, 1984.

Webber, A.: Acute soft-tissue injuries in the young athlete. Clin Sports Med. 7(3): 611-624, 1988.

Wilkins, K.E.: The uniqueness of the young athlete: Musculoskeletal injuries. Am J Sports Med. 8(5): 377-382, 1980.

Wilkins, K.E.: Operative management of the upper extremity fractures in children. AAOS Monograph Series, 1994.

Yngve, D.A.: Stress fracture in the paediatric athlete. In Sullivan, J.A., Grana, W.A. (eds): The Pediatric Athlete. American Academy of Orthopaedic Surgeons, Park Ridge, IL, 1988, pp. 235-240.

Zaricznyj, B., Shattuck, L.M., and Mast. T.J.: Sports-related injuries in school-aged children. Am J Sports Med. 8(5):318-324, 1980.

13

CHAPTER

Neuromuscular Disease and Anaerobic Performance During Childhood

Oded Bar-Or

This chapter focuses on the following objectives:

- To explain the effects of neuromuscular disease on anaerobic performance
- To assess various methodological considerations in measuring anaerobic performance
- To discuss the trainability of children with neuromuscular diseases
- To address several safety considerations that must be followed when testing children and adolescents

There are numerous neuromuscular diseases (NMDs) that affect children and adolescents. For a comprehensive description of these conditions, see Brooke (1986). Each NMD may be accompanied by limitations of a person's muscle performance. However, most research and clinical experience about the anaerobic performance of patients with an NMD has been limited to cerebral palsy (CP) and to progressive muscular dystrophy, mostly of the Duchenne or the Becker type (for a review see Bar-Or 1996). Accordingly, this chapter will focus on these conditions.

The Effects of Neuromuscular Disease on Anaerobic Performance

Physical performance of healthy children and of those with various cardiopulmonary or other diseases is often determined by their maximal aerobic power. In

contrast, motor performance (e.g., ambulation) of children with a NMD may be limited more by fitness components such as muscle strength (Johnson and Braddom
1971; Koch and Simenson 1992; O'Connell, Bernhardt, and Parks 1992; Resnick et
al. 1981), peak muscle power (Bar-Or 1983, 1993; Emons et al. 1992; Parker et al.
1993; Tirosh, Rosenbaum, and Bar-Or 1990), local muscle endurance (Bar-Or 1983,
1986, 1993; Emons et al. 1992; O'Connell, Bernhardt, and Parks 1992; Parker et al.
1993; Tirosh, Rosenbaum, and Bar-Or 1990), and economy of locomotion (Campbell
and Ball 1978; Rose et al. 1989; Unnithan et al., *Med. Sci. Sports Exerc.*, n.d.).

The first to show a reduction in local muscle endurance of patients with NMD
were Hosking et al. (1976), who used a neck flexion test at the supine position (see
also Edwards 1980). Subsequent studies, using the Wingate Anaerobic Test (WAnT),
have shown a considerably lower peak power and mean power in children and
adolescents with spastic CP than in able-bodied children and adolescents (Bar-Or
1986; Parker et al. 1992; Emons et al. 1992). In the Parker et al. (1992) study, the
patients' performance ranged from 2 to 6 SDs below the mean of healthy controls.
Among the patients, those with quadriplegia and hemiplegia scored lower than those
with diplegia when the WAnT was performed with the arms. In another study (Tirosh,
Rosenbaum, and Bar-Or 1990), patients with athetotic CP scored considerably
lower than those with spastic CP, both in mean power and in peak power. Scores for
patients with Duchenne's muscular dystrophy were similar to, or a little higher than,
those for patients with athetotic CP (see figure 13.1).

There are several possible explanations for the low anaerobic performance of children with NMD. The most obvious is the low functional muscle mass in the limbs of

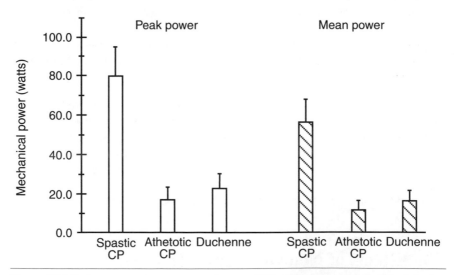

Figure 13.1 Peak power and mean power (mean ± SD) of boys with spastic CP, athetotic
CP, or Duchenne's muscular dystrophy. Subjects performed the arm cranking version of
the Wingate anaerobic test.

Data from Tirosh et al. 1990.

children with atrophic or dystrophic muscles, as well as in those with spastic CP. In CP, this may result from insufficient stretch in the spastic muscles due to an exaggerated tonic reflex (Nash, Nelson, and O'Dwyer 1989). Another possibility is the preferential reduction in type II fibers that may take place in CP (Castle, Reyman, and Schneider 1979; Edstrom 1970) and in other NMDs (McComas et al. 1986). This would reduce performance in high-intensity tasks such as the WAnT (Bar-Or et al. 1980).

Finally, it is possible that mechanical power, as measured with the WAnT (or any other anaerobic test based on performance), underestimates the actual work performed by the muscle. This may result from a deficient synchronization between the agonist and antagonist muscle groups (Berbrayer and Ashby 1990). Using electromyographic analysis, Unnithan et al. (*EMG Clin. Neurophysiol.,* n.d.) found that during treadmill walking, children with spastic CP had a considerably higher coactivation index (a measure of the lack of synchronization between agonist and antagonist muscle groups) than did able-bodied controls. This in turn is a major reason for the considerably higher energy cost of locomotion of such patients (Unnithan et al., *Med. Sci. Sports Exerc.,* n.d.). If one assumes that such lack of synchronization occurs also during anaerobic cycling or arm cranking, the actual work produced by the muscles is higher than that measured with the ergometer. A similar pattern may exist also in athetosis.

In patients with muscular dystrophy, there is no a priori reason to assume lack of synchronization in the activation of agonists and antagonists, but the selective weakness of muscle groups and the contracture of joints may affect the direction of mechanical forces generated by a limb segment, which in turn may cause an underestimation of the actual work performed by the muscles. This possibility is presented as a hypothesis only, one that requires experimental confirmation. Finally, in the child with spastic CP, a mechanical disadvantage may result from the excessive foot pronation, which causes rubbing of the midfoot on the pedal shaft.

Methodological Considerations in Measuring Anaerobic Performance

Conceptually, testing of the anaerobic performance of a person with a NMD is based on principles similar to those used with an able-bodied person. There are, though, special methodological issues to be considered.

Choice of Test

A variety of anaerobic performance tests have been used for able-bodied children (for recent reviews, see Bar-Or 1996; Van Praagh 1996), ranging from vertical jumping and step running, through monoarticular tasks, to all-out cycling. The repertoire of tests for the child with a NMD is much narrower. Fessel, Taylor, and

Johnson (1970) introduced a neck flexion muscle endurance test in which the supine patient was asked to raise his head to 45° from the ground for as long as possible. While feasible in a clinical setting, this test lacks standardization and reliability (Hosking et al. 1976), and it has not received wide recognition.

The only other anaerobic performance test that has been reported for use in children with NMD has been the WAnT (Bar-Or 1986, 1993; Emons et al. 1992; Emons and Van Baak 1993; Janssen et al. 1993; Parker et al. 1992; Tirosh, Rosenbaum, and Bar-Or 1990). For a detailed review of the WAnT's characteristics, see Bar-Or 1987 and Inbar, Bar-Or, and Skinner n.d. The WAnT is feasible for children and adolescents with various NMDs (Parker et al. 1992; Tirosh, Rosenbaum, and Bar-Or 1990), particularly those with CP. As seen in table 13.1, the test is more feasible for use with the arms than with the legs. This reflects the greater difficulty for such patients to perform leg pedaling versus arm cranking, as also seen in aerobic protocols. Because of the anatomic distribution of the degenerative process in Duchenne's muscular dystrophy ("proximal"; thigh muscles start deteriorating at the early phases of the disease), children with this condition find it particularly hard to perform the leg WAnT (Tirosh, Rosenbaum, and Bar-Or 1990).

One of the main features of the WAnT is its very high test-retest reliability and repeatability. This was first shown for able-bodied people of various ages (Bar-Or 1987) and then for children and adolescents with various NMDs (Emons et al. 1992; Tirosh, Rosenbaum, and Bar-Or 1990) and for elderly people with advanced chronic obstructive lung disease (Bar-Or, Berman, and Salsberg 1992). Specifically, Tirosh, Rosenbaum, and Bar-Or (1990) found a test-retest correlation coefficient of 0.98 for fifty-eight 5- to 18-year-old patients with CP, Duchenne's muscular dystrophy, Becker's muscular dystrophy, spinal muscular atrophy, congenital muscular atro-

Table 13.1   Feasibility of the Wingate Anaerobic Test by Diagnostic Group in 5- to 18-Year-Old Boys and Girls (Sexes Combined)

Group	% completing test	
	Arms	Legs
Spastic CP	100	89
Athetotic CP	91	45.5
Duchenne's MD	76.9	15.4
Other neuromuscular diseases	100	60
Total	93.93	60.6

CP indicates cerebral palsy; MD, muscular dystrophy.
Data from Tirosh et al. 1990.

phy, central core myopathy, myotonic dystrophy, and Charcot-Marie-Tooth disease who performed the arm cranking test twice, 1-3 weeks apart. Thirty-eight of them also performed the leg pedaling test twice, with a reliability coefficient of 0.96 (see figure 13.2). It is noteworthy that even patients with athetotic CP (who suffer from an involuntary limb movement) had a test-retest correlation of 0.97 for peak power and of 0.92 for mean power (n = 9) in the arm cranking protocol, but only 0.70 and 0.82, respectively, for leg pedaling. A reliability coefficient of 0.97 was reported by Emons et al. (1992) for twelve 6- to 12-year-old girls and boys with spastic CP who performed the leg pedaling protocol. Eighteen 54- to 84-year-old women and men with an advanced chronic obstructive lung disease had a test-retest reliability of 0.89 when performing an abbreviated version (15 s) of the leg WAnT (Bar-Or, Berman, and Salsberg 1992).

Emons et al. (1992) reported a small, insignificant increase in anaerobic performance between the first and the second test, which might have suggested a learning effect. This, however, was not found in the larger sample studied by Tirosh, Rosenbaum, and Bar-Or (1990).

Another potentially useful anaerobic performance test for children with NMD is the force-velocity test (FVT) (Sargeant et al. 1989; Van Praagh et al. 1989). It requires several very short (5-7 s) all-out cycling or arm cranking sprints. Braking force is changed from one bout to the next in order to construct the person's individual power-force curve, thus identifying the subject's highest peak power. For more details about the FVT, see the chapter by Van Praagh and França in this book.

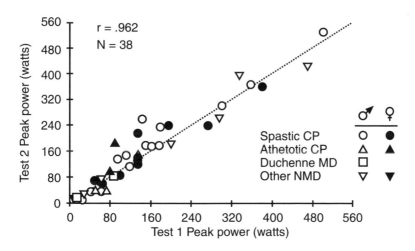

Figure 13.2 Test-retest individual data for peak power in 38 5- to 18-year-old patients with various neuromuscular diseases who performed the leg pedaling version of the Wingate anaerobic test. The broken line denotes identity.

Data from Tirosh et al. 1990.

So far, research using this test has focused on able-bodied people. In a recent study (Van Mil et al. 1996), the upper-limb version of the FVT was performed successfully by children and adolescents with NMD (see discussion later in this chapter). The subjects managed to complete all bouts within one visit to the laboratory. More research is needed, though, to determine the test's feasibility for pedaling, as well as its reliability, when used with this population.

Choice of Ergometer

Because of their low muscle strength and power, some children with a NMD, particularly those at advanced stages of muscular dystrophy or atrophy, may have to pedal or arm crank against an extremely low force. For that purpose an ergometer should be used that has as little as possible power loss between the pedals and the flywheel. In some ergometers, even at "zero" resistance the required power is 15-20 W. This may be too high for some patients. The onus is therefore on the investigator/laboratory technician to calibrate the ergometer and adjust for the lost power. Likewise, an ergometer should be used that allows for very small increments in force. Otherwise it may be impossible to discern small decreases in muscle power due to progression of the disease or to distinguish training-induced improvements. For an example of a simple calibration procedure for mechanically braked ergometers, see Van Praagh et al. (1992).

All studies described by the Wingate group (Bar-Or 1987) and those subsequently performed at the Children's Exercise and Nutrition Centre (Bar-Or 1986, 1993; Parker et al. 1992, 1993; Tirosh, Rosenbaum, and Bar-Or 1990; Van Mil 1996) were done with the Fleisch-Metabo ergometer. This is a mechanical ergometer with a very low (7-10 W) power loss and small increments, which are attained by adding small weights (60 g each) that tighten the belt around the flywheel. Furthermore, the ergometer has a built-in calibration system that continuously adjusts the area of friction between the belt and the flywheel.

In 1981, an isokinetic cycle ergometer was described (Sargeant, Hoinville, and Young 1981) in which force is measured at the pedals by the use of a strain gauge on either side. This allows for a continuous monitoring of the force and the cranking velocity throughout the pedaling cycle. Several anaerobic performance protocols have been used with this "power ergometer," ranging from a single pedal revolution to 60 s all-out cranking. The ergometer, originally constructed for able-bodied people, was subsequently used for adults with NMD (McCartney et al. 1983), but not for children. Isokinetic testing, because of the near-constant angular velocity, can yield basic in situ information on muscle contractile characteristics, particularly force-velocity-power relationships. Such information cannot be achieved by the WAnT, in which velocity drops as the subject fatigues. The disadvantage of this isokinetic ergometer, though, has been its high cost. To the knowledge of this author, the prototype developed by Sargeant, Hoinville, and Young was never manufactured commercially.

Optimal Braking Force

When using the WAnT, FVT, or any other "constant"-force cycling protocol, one ought to select an optimal force that would yield the highest possible power. Optimal forces have been identified for able-bodied children and adults (e.g., Dotan and Bar-Or 1983) based on their body mass. This is a reasonable approach for individuals with a normal lean-to-total body mass ratio, because anaerobic performance is closely related to lean limb mass (Blimkie et al. 1988; Sargeant 1989), but it may not be suitable for an individual with atrophic, dystrophic, hypotonic, or spastic muscles. Two alternative approaches for selecting an optimal braking force for children and adolescents with a NMD have recently been suggested and validated (Van Mil et al. 1996). One is based on an anthropometric estimate of the lean volume of the exercising limb, and the other on the optimal force that yields the highest power in the FVT (Van Praagh et al. 1989). Participants in the latter study were twenty-eight 6- to 16-year-old girls and boys with CP, spinal cord injury, acquired brain damage, muscular dystrophy, or Prader Willi syndrome. The optimal force for the arm cranking WAnT (F_{opt}, Joules per pedal revolution) was $F_{opt} = 0.05$ LAV (ml) + 1.80, in which LAV is lean arm volume determined by anthropometry. Alternatively, $F_{opt} = 0.65\,F_{opt}$FVT (J Arev^{-1}) $- 8.07$, in which F_{opt}FVT is the optimal force for the FVT, taken as 50% of maximal force, when both tests are performed by the upper limbs at the sitting position. In practical terms, the optimal force for the WAnT is two-thirds of that obtained for the FVT. There are no studies that have validated this approach for leg pedaling in this population.

Trainability of the Child With a Neuromuscular Disease

While some studies have documented the aerobic trainability of children, adolescents, and adults with NMD, there is very little information about their anaerobic trainability. Emons (Emons and Van Baak 1993), as part of her doctoral study, trained 6- to 12-year-old girls and boys with spastic CP for 9 months. Training consisted of 45 min aerobic exercise sessions four times per week. Even though peak aerobic power increased during the training program, there was no improvement in anaerobic power. Based on that study alone, it is hard to tell whether anaerobic performance of children with spastic CP is nontrainable or whether the specific aerobic training regimen used did not provide enough anaerobic stimulus.

O'Connell, Bernhardt, and Parks (1992) trained the strength and muscle endurance of three children with CP and three with spina bifida for 8 weeks (circuit training three times per week), using a control group of similar patients. The authors reported an increase in 6RM (repetition maximum) of several muscle groups, an index considered by them to reflect muscle endurance. However, there was no mention of the extent of such an improvement. There was no improvement in 50 m dash.

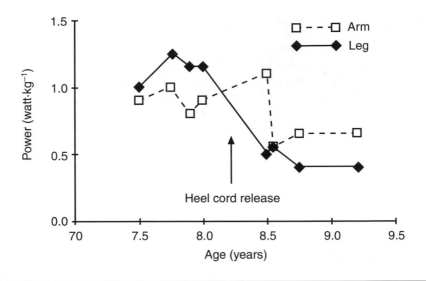

Figure 13.3 Changes over 20 months in peak power of the arms and legs in a boy with Duchenne's muscular dystrophy who periodically performed the Wingate anaerobic test. The arrow denotes time of surgery for a bilateral release of the Achilles tendon. Data from the author's laboratory.

Data from Bar-Or 1993.

Anecdotal data from the author's clinic suggest that performance in the WAnT can be improved in children with Becker's muscular dystrophy, CP, spina bifida, and to a lesser extent, Duchenne's muscular dystrophy. In the latter disease, the peak power and mean power of one child (first seen at age 7.5 years) did not diminish during several months when the patient was physically active, but deteriorated dramatically following several weeks of bed rest subsequent to surgery (see figure 13.3) (Bar-Or 1993).

There are no known explanations why the muscles of a child with a progressive muscle disease can benefit from physical training. The working assumption in the author's clinic has been that motor units that are still functional may respond to training, similarly to those in a healthy muscle. Obviously, more research, using an intervention with randomly assigned controls, is the only means of achieving definitive information about the anaerobic trainability of a child with a NMD.

Safety Considerations for Anaerobic Testing

A person who has completed the WAnT may sometimes complain of nausea and fatigue (and very seldom vomiting) for about 10-20 min. This is particularly evident in tall adolescents who perform the pedaling version. Although no mechanisms have been identified that might underlie this response pattern, it may reflect pooling of blood in the peripheral veins of the legs at the conclusion of pedaling. Indeed, it is extremely rare that such a response occurs with the arm cranking version of the WAnT, which is the test commonly performed with children with NMD. Another safety issue is whether a child whose heart is affected by a NMD (e.g., as in Duchenne's muscular dystrophy or in Friedreich's ataxia) can tolerate a high-intensity exercise task such as the WAnT or the FVT.

One precaution that should be exercised is that subjects/patients warm up prior to performing any anaerobic performance test and taper off (e.g., by cycling backward against a very low braking force) at its conclusion. Another precaution is to let the subject lie down, with the legs elevated, for several minutes after the test, to prevent venous pooling at the lower extremities.

An additional safety issue is whether high-intensity exertion enhances the damage in a diseased muscle. Tradition has it that exertion may enhance the deterioration of muscle fibers in patients with muscular dystrophy. This notion has been based on studies such as that by Bonsett (1963), who reported, using post mortem data on one patient with Duchenne's muscular dystrophy, a greater deterioration in proximal limb and postural muscles than in other muscle groups. The author suggested that those muscles with greater damage had been used more than other muscles during the patient's life. That notion, however, does not explain why respiratory muscles, which work continuously, were not excessively affected. Another indication of possible damage to muscle cells has been that serum creatine kinase increases excessively following exercise in patients with muscular dystrophy. Reports regarding this pattern have been equivocal (Florence et al. 1984; Jackson et al. 1987). Animal (Fowler et al. 1990) and human (Fowler and Taylor 1982) data, as well as clinical experience, suggest that exercise of mild to moderate intensities does not enhance the damage to dystrophic muscles. One study with dystrophic mice (Taylor, Fowler, and Doerr 1976), however, did suggest that training at high intensity was accompanied by a reduction of contractile performance and of longevity, even though there were no histopathological effects.

All in all, there seems to be no definitive conclusion about the safety of high-intensity, anaerobic training in patients with NMD.

Directions for Future Research

One reason for the paucity of information about anaerobic performance and trainability in children with NMD is the *lack of testing methods that are custom-made for each of the various disabilities*. For example, even though the WAnT is highly feasible for children with spastic or athetotic CP, it is considerably less feasible for a patient with an advanced progressive muscular disease (Tirosh, Rosenbaum, and Bar-Or 1990). Testing methods tailored to a specific disability are therefore needed. Studies should be conducted to assess the feasibility, reliability, sensitivity, and specificity of such tests. Ideally, one should also determine their validity. However, the current lack of a "gold standard" for anaerobic performance in this population may render it impossible to conduct validation studies. Magnetic resonance spectroscopy may prove to be a useful gold standard for anaerobic performance, based on recent research with healthy children and adults (Cooper 1995).

Another important research direction is to *determine the anaerobic trainability* of these patients. Randomly assigned intervention studies are required in order to obtain definitive data about trainability. A major challenge is to construct a protocol for the controls that will be ethically justified. Another challenge is to tease out the specific effect of training while the child may be undergoing other therapeutic modalities.

Finally, studies should be conducted to *determine the safety of exercise programs.* The challenge here is that intervention programs in which the endpoint is damage (e.g., enhancement of muscle fiber deterioration in a child with Duchenne's muscular dystrophy) are ethically unjustified. One alternative is to keep a register of the outcomes, positive and negative alike, of clinically based exercise prescription programs. For such a registry the planning, execution, and interpretation should use acceptable statistical and epidemiological methods.

Summary

In children and adolescents with a NMD, muscle performance characteristics such as endurance, strength, peak power, or metabolic cost of locomotion may often limit their daily activities and physical abilities. Indeed, such patients have extremely low anaerobic performance when compared with the general child population. Notwithstanding, most of the research to date on exercise performance and trainability of children and adolescents with a NMD has focused on their O_2 transport system, and much less on their anaerobic fitness. One reason for such lack of information has been the paucity of testing protocols of anaerobic performance custom-made for specific disabilities. Since 1990, the WAnT has been found to be feasible for use in patients with a variety of NMDs and to have a very high test-retest reliability when performed by these patients. While some data suggest that muscle endurance and peak power are trainable in adults with a NMD, no studies have assessed the response of younger patients to anaerobic training. Likewise there is insufficient information about the possible detrimental effects of anaerobic testing or training on these patients.

References

Bar-Or, O. 1983. *Pediatric sports medicine for the practitioner. From physiological principles to clinical applications,* 323-325. New York: Springer-Verlag.

Bar-Or, O. 1986. Pathophysiologic factors which limit the exercise capacity of the sick child. *Med. Sci. Sports Exerc.* 18: 276-282.

Bar-Or, O. 1987. The Wingate Anaerobic Test. An update on methodology, reliability and validity. *Sports Med.* 4: 381-394.

Bar-Or, O. 1993. Noncardiopulmonary pediatric exercise tests. In *Pediatric laboratory exercise testing: clinical guidelines,* ed. T.W. Rowland, 165-185. Champaign, IL: Human Kinetics.

Bar-Or, O. 1996a. Anaerobic performance. In *Measurement in pediatric exercise science,* ed. D. Docherty, 161-182. Champaign, IL: Human Kinetics.

Bar-Or, O. 1996b. Role of exercise in assessment and management of neuromuscular disease in children. *Med. Sci Sports Exerc.* 28: 421-427.

Bar-Or, O., Berman L,, and Salsberg, A. 1992. An abbreviated Wingate anaerobic test for women and men of advanced age. *Med. Sci. Sports Exerc.* 24: S22.

Bar-Or, O., Dotan, R., Inbar, O., Rotshtein, A., Karlsson, J., and Tesch, P. 1980. Anaerobic capacity and muscle fiber type distribution in man. *Int. J. Sports Med.* 1: 89-92.

Bar-Or, O., Inbar, O., and Spira, R. 1976. Physiological effects of a sports rehabilitation program on cerebral palsied and post-poliomyelitic adolescents. *Med. Sci. Sports* 8: 157-161.

Berbrayer, D., and Ashby, P. 1990. Reciprocal inhibition in cerebral palsy. *Neurology* 40: 653-656.

Blimkie, C.J.R., Roche, P., Hay, J.T., and Bar-Or, O. 1988. Anaerobic power of arms in teenage boys and girls: relationship to lean body tissue. *Eur. J. Appl. Physiol.* 57: 677-683.

Bonsett, C.A. 1963. Pseudohypertrophic muscular dystrophy. Distribution of degenerative features as revealed by an anatomical study. *Neurology* 13: 728-738.

Brooke, M.H. 1986. *A clinician's view of neuromuscular diseases.* 2nd ed. Baltimore: Williams & Wilkins.

Campbell, J., and Ball, J. 1978. Energetics of walking in cerebral palsy. *Orthop. Clin. North Am.* 9: 374-377.

Castle, M.E., Reyman, T.A., and Schneider, M.E. 1979. Pathology of spastic muscles in cerebral palsy. *Clin. Orthop.* 142: 223-23.

Cooper, D.M. 1995. New horizons in pediatric exercise research. In *New horizons in pediatric exercise science,* ed. C.J.R. Blimkie and O. Bar-Or, 1-24. Champaign, IL: Human Kinetics.

Dotan, R., and Bar-Or, O. 1983. Load optimization for the Wingate Anaerobic Test. *Eur. J. Appl. Physiol.* 51: 409-417.

Edstrom, L. 1970. Selective changes in the size of red and white muscle fibres in upper motor lesions and parkinsonism. *J. Neurol. Sci.* 11: 537-550.

Edwards, R.H.T. 1980. Studies of muscular performance in normal and dystrophic subjects. *Br. Med. Bull.* 36: 159-164.

Emons, H.J.G., Groenenboom, D.C., Burggraaff, Y.I., Janssen, T.L.E., and Van Baak, M.A. 1992. Wingate Anaerobic Test in children with cerebral palsy. In *Children and exercise XVI,* ed. J. Coudert and E. Van Praagh, 187-189. Paris: Masson.

Emons, H.J.G., and Van Baak, M.A. 1993. Effect of training on aerobic and anaerobic power and mechanical efficiency in spastic cerebral palsied children. *Pediatr. Exerc. Sci.* 5: 412.

Fessel, W.J., Taylor, J.A., and Johnson, E.S. 1970. Evaluating the complaint of muscle weakness: simple quantitative clinical tests. In *First International Congress on Muscle Disease,* ed. J.N. Walton, N. Canal, and G. Scarlato, 544-545. Amsterdam: Excerpta Medica.

Florence, J.M., and Hagberg, J.M. 1984. Effect of training on the exercise responses of neuromuscular disease patients. *Med. Sci. Sports Exerc.* 16: 460-465.

Fowler W.M., Abresch, R.T., Larson, D.B., Sharman, R.B., and Entrikin, R.K. 1990. High-repetitive submaximal treadmill exercise training: effect on normal and dystrophic mice. *Arch. Phys. Med. Rehabil.* 71: 552-557.

Fowler, W.M., and Taylor, M. 1982. Rehabilitation management of muscular dystrophy and related disorders. 1. The role of exercise. *Arch. Phys. Med. Rehabil.* 63: 319-321.

Hosking, G.P., Bhat, U.S., Dubowitz, V., and Edwards, R.H.T. 1976. Measurements of muscle strength and performance in children with normal and diseased muscle. *Arch. Dis. Child.* 51: 957-963.

Inbar, O., Bar-Or, O., and Skinner, J.S. n.d. *The Wingate Anaerobic Test: development, characteristics and applications.* Champaign, IL: Human Kinetics. (1996).

Jackson, M.J., Round, J.M., Newham, D.J., and Edwards, R.H.T. 1987. An examination of some factors influencing creatine kinase in the blood of patients with muscular dystrophy. *Muscle Nerve* 10: 15-21.

Janssen, T.W.J., Van Oers, C.A.J.M., Hollander, A.P., Veeger, H.E.J., and Van Der Woude, L.H.V. 1993. Isometric strength, sprint power, and aerobic power in individuals with a spinal cord injury. *Med. Sci. Sports Exerc.* 25: 863-870.

Johnson, E.W., and Braddom, R. 1971. Over-work weakness in facioscapulohumeral muscular dystrophy. *Arch. Phys. Med. Rehabil.* 52: 333-336.

Koch, B.M., and Simenson, R.L. 1992. Upper extremity strength and function in children with spinal muscular atrophy type II. *Arch. Phys. Med. Rehabil.* 73: 241-245.

McCartney, N., Heigenhauser, G.J.F., Sargeant, A.J., and Jones, N.L. 1983. A constant velocity cycle ergometer for the study of muscle function. *J. Appl. Physiol.* 55: 212-217.

McComas, A.J., Belanger, A.Y., Garner, S.A., and McCartney, N. 1986. Muscle performance in neuromuscular disorders. In *Human muscle power,* ed. N.L. Jones, N. McCartney, and A.J. McComas, 309-24. Champaign, IL: Human Kinetics.

Nash, J., Nelson, P.D., and O'Dwyer, N.J. 1989. Reducing spasticity to control muscle contracture of children with cerebral palsy. *Dev. Med. Child Neurol.* 31: 471-480.

O'Connell, D.G., Bernhardt, R., and Parks, L. 1992. Muscular endurance and wheelchair propulsion in children with cerebral palsy or meningomyelocele. *Arch. Phys. Med. Rehabil.* 73: 709-711.

Parker, D.F., Carriere, L., Hebestreit, H., and Bar-Or, O. 1992. Anaerobic endurance and peak muscle power in children with spastic cerebral palsy. *Am. J. Dis. Child.* 146: 1069-1073.

Parker, D.F., Carriere, L., Hebestreit, H., Salsberg, A., and Bar-Or, O. 1993. Muscle performance and gross motor function in children with spastic cerebral palsy. *Dev. Med. Child Neurol.* 35: 17-23.

Resnick, J.S., Mammel, M., Mundale, M.O., and Kottke, F.J. 1981. Muscular strength as an index of response to therapy in childhood dermatomyositis. *Arch. Phys. Ther. Rehabil.* 62: 12-19.

Rose, J., Gamble, J.G., Medeiros, J., Burgos, A., and Haskell, W.L. 1989. Energy cost of walking in normal children and those with cerebral palsy: a comparison of heart rate and oxygen uptake. *J. Pediatr. Orthop.* 9: 276-279.

Sargeant, A. 1989. Short-term muscle power in children and adolescents. In *Advances in pediatric sports sciences,* ed. O. Bar-Or, 42-65. Champaign, IL: Human Kinetics.

Sargeant, A.J., Hoinville, E., and Young, A. 1981. Maximal leg force and power output during short-term dynamic exercise. *J. Appl. Physiol.: Resp. Environ. Exerc. Physiol.* 51: 1175-1182.

Taylor, R.G., Fowler, D.M., Jr., and Doerr, L. 1976. Exercise effect on contractile properties of skeletal muscle in mouse muscular dystrophy. *Arch. Phys. Med. Rehabil.* 57: 174-180.

Tirosh, E., Rosenbaum, P., and Bar-Or, O. 1990. A new muscle power test in neuromuscular disease: feasibility and reliability. *Am. J. Dis. Child.* 144: 1083-1087.

Unnithan, V.B., Bar-Or, O., Dowling, J.J., and Hoofwijk, M. n.d. Role of cocontraction in the O_2 cost of walking in children with cerebral palsy. *Med. Sci. Sports Exerc.* In press.

Unnithan, V., Dowling, J., Frost, G., Ayub, B., and Bar-Or, O. n.d. Cocontraction and phasic activity during gait in children with cerebral palsy. *EMG Clin. Neurophysiol.* In press.

Van Mil, G.A.H., Schoeber, N., Calvert, R.E., and Bar-Or, O. 1996. Optimization of braking force in the Wingate test for children and adolescents with a neuromuscular disease. *Med. Sci. Sports Exerc.* 28: 1087-1092.

Van Praagh, E. 1996. Testing anaerobic performance. In *The encyclopaedia of sports medicine.* Vol. 6, *The child and adolescent athlete,* ed. O. Bar-Or, 603-16. Oxford: Blackwell Scientific.

Van Praagh, E., Bedu, M., Roddier, P., and Coudert, J. 1992. A simple calibration method for mechanically braked cycle ergometers. *Int. J. Sports Med.* 13: 27-30.

Van Praagh, E., Falgairette, G., Bedu, M., Fellmann, N., and Coudert, J. 1989. Laboratory and field tests in 7-year-old boys. In *Children and Exercise XIII,* ed. S. Oseid and K.H. Carlsen, 11-17. Champaign, IL: Human Kinetics.

14

CHAPTER

Asthma and Anaerobic Performance in Children

François-Pierre J. Counil
Christian G. Préfaut

This chapter focuses on the following objectives:

- Addressing the effects of asthma on physical activity
- Discussing the relationship between aerobic and anaerobic fitness in children with asthma
- Explaining the metabolic adaptations of asthmatic individuals during anaerobic testing
- Assessing the cardiorespiratory adaptations of children and adolescents to anaerobic testing

Questions about exercise ability and athletic performance in childhood asthma are among the everyday concerns of professionals in education and health care. Postexercise bronchospasm, but more often the child's nonspecific complaints of "discomfort" during exercise (dyspnea, fatigue, chest pain, headache, etc.), lead parents, coaches, and physical education teachers to seek medical advice before allowing the asthmatic child to continue or compete in his or her chosen sport. A full evaluation of the patient's condition (severity score, pulmonary function, peak flow monitoring, therapeutic compliance, environmental and psychological assessment; Bar-Or 1983) is necessary in order to give relevant individualized counseling to the patient and family. The importance of regular physical activity should be emphasized at this time, as today we have ample documentation of not only the innocuousness of such activity, but also its substantial beneficial effects (Engström et al. 1991; Orenstein et al. 1995; Ramazanoglu and Kraemer 1985; Varray et al. 1991). Indeed, specific rehabilitation programs have been implemented that are based on such pathophysiological concepts as the ventilatory threshold (Préfaut, Varray, and Vallet

1995). These programs are designed to offer only aerobic training and can be prescribed as part of long-term treatment (Varray and Préfaut 1992).

Parents and the majority of physicians, however, are still reluctant to allow asthmatic children to participate in very intense activities such as anaerobic exercise. Yet in fact the hazardous effect of brief, intense exercise on the stabilized patient has never been demonstrated. Indeed, there are several points in favor of the "anaerobic" approach to exercise in childhood asthma:

1. As a component of athletic performance, anaerobic capacity is a major element in the self-image process during childhood. This is particularly so for asthmatic children (Engström et al. 1991; Fischer and Thompson 1994).
2. Short sprints have been shown to have a preventive effect on postexercise bronchospasm (Bisschop et al. 1992; Schnall and Landau 1980).
3. In our experience, the standard rehabilitation program of exercise, based on individualized aerobic training indexes, is boring to many children. In order to introduce more play activity, the anaerobic component of exercise needs to be increased.

A few years ago, the percentage of asthmatic athletes on the U.S. Olympic teams was reported to be as high as that found in the general population. Even more surprising was the finding that the asthmatic athletes won more medals than the nonasthmatic group (Voy 1986). Although the asthma was probably mild in these athletes, this example indicates that by adapted training, young patients may be able to overcome a limitation to high-intensity exercise.

Asthma and Physical Activity

The overall exercise tolerance of patients with asthma is a function of the disease severity. Dyspnoea and peripheral muscle fatigue are the major components of the limitation. Recently, the scientific basis for recommending exercise rehabilitation for these patients has been established (Préfaut, Varray, and Vallet 1995).

The Asthmatic Child

Characterized as a reversible bronchial obstruction, asthma is the most frequently occurring chronic disease during childhood. Approximately 10% of children experience asthma symptoms. Clinically, bronchial hyperresponsiveness to various stimuli, including exercise, is the most specific sign of asthma. The pathophysiology of asthma has not yet been fully elucidated, but recent work has changed the concept of a primary bronchial spasm toward a broader concept of bronchial inflammation, involving specific cells (eosinophils, mast cells, etc.) and biochemical mediators. The airflow limitation is routinely assessed by pulmonary function tests, the forced expiratory volume in 1 s (FEV_1) being the most reliable parameter of bronchial obstruction.

Exercise and Asthma

The asthmatic child faces several problems when it comes to physical activities. The most commonly cited is the exercise-induced bronchospasm, which is a transient airflow limitation following several minutes of intense exercise. This clinical syndrome is a part of the bronchial hyperresponsiveness and is quite specific to asthma (Clough et al. 1991). Trained asthmatic subjects are less vulnerable to exercise-induced airflow limitation, in spite of much higher exercise intensity, than sedentary persons with similar severity of asthma (Haas et al. 1985). Adapted medication (Virant 1992) and preexercise warm-ups (Virant 1992; Schnall and Landau 1980) are generally prescribed to reduce the incidence of exercise-induced asthma.

Not widely recognized but scientifically documented, the relative unfitness of asthmatic children is now well established, and the underlying mechanisms have been described (Varray and Préfaut 1992). The vicious circle of detraining-hypoactivity encountered in almost every chronic disease (Bar-Or 1983) is not sufficient to explain the unfitness of persons with asthma (Varray and Préfaut 1992). Regarding aerobic fitness, the limitation to exercise is closely linked to the relative hyperventilation of the asthmatic child for a given workload, that is, for a given oxygen consumption. This hyperventilation is deleterious in many respects. Briefly, persons with asthma will reach their maximal ventilation before their maximal potential in terms of muscular power, leading to a ventilatory limitation to aerobic exercise (Préfaut, Varray, and Vallet 1995; Varray and Préfaut 1992). Hyper ventilation will also induce excessive drying and cooling of the airway mucosa, which is thought to be the trigger of exercise-induced asthma (Virant 1992). Last, abnormalities of the ventilatory function, especially overinflation of the asthmatic lung, will impair the cardiac response to exercise (Varray et al. 1993).

Based on this pathophysiological approach, training programs invariably show improvement in the physical fitness of the asthmatic child (Varray and Préfaut 1992). However, all the work done until recently has been applicable only to aerobic exercise.

Anaerobic Fitness in Asthmatic Children

The physiological adaptations to anaerobic exercise in asthmatic children have up to now been a matter of hypothesis based on results obtained by aerobic exercise testing (Varray et al. 1989). In asthmatic children, who are able to develop normal power output during maximal graded exercise testing, the anaerobic fitness was thought to be enhanced as a compensation for the decreased maximal oxygen consumption (Varray et al. 1989). This thinking was based on the premise that asthmatic children have an acquired or genetically determined anaerobic specialization regarding muscle activity. Further research, however, showed that aerobic fitness indexes such as maximal oxygen uptake, maximal power output, and ventilatory threshold are not relevant for predicting anaerobic fitness, and this work was unable to demonstrate anaerobic specialization (Granier et al. 1995). When anaerobic capacity is specifically assessed in asthmatic children, it is lower than in healthy controls.

Testing Guidelines

Anaerobic testing is not yet a part of the routine clinical examination, and guidelines are lacking regarding the indications and counterindications in childhood asthma. Generally, before testing of any asthmatic child for physical fitness level, the following checklist should be completed (Bar-Or 1983; Rossi 1993):

1. Clinical history focusing on the cardiorespiratory system, the normal physical activity, and the symptoms during exercise
2. Basal pulmonary function testing including functional residual capacity measurement in order to assess the severity of the preexercise bronchial obstruction
3. Clinical examination with resting electrocardiogram and blood pressure measurement

A simple mechanically braked bicycle is needed, coupled to a computerized device to record pedal revolution velocity (Mercier, Mercier, and Préfaut 1991). The two tests commonly used are the force-velocity test described by Vandewalle et al. (1987) and the Wingate Anaerobic Test developed by Bar-Or (Bar-Or 1983). As various investigators have noted (Bedu et al. 1991), the sprint activity in these tests is well accepted and easily performed by children, and the overall tolerance is the same as for prolonged, graded exercise tests. Patients in unstable physical condition or with severe bronchial obstruction ($FEV_1 < 60\%$, FEV_1/vital capacity $< 55\%$ of the predicted values) should not be tested (Bar-Or 1983; Rossi 1993).

The question of which asthmatic children would benefit from anaerobic testing has received no clear-cut answers. In our experience, the percentage of asthmatic children enrolled in athletic clubs is similar to that in the general population. For high-level competitors, anaerobic testing is advisable as a complement to the standard aerobic tests. In this case, the anaerobic fitness evaluation should be regarded as both a medical and an athletic performance assessment. Tolerance to high-intensity exercise can then be confirmed with postexercise pulmonary function testing.

Patients in rehabilitation programs with a controlled physical activity of any kind would also benefit from anaerobic evaluation. These children usually have more severe asthma than athletic club members. Thanks to these programs, children experience improved physical fitness and improved everyday exercise tolerance. Indeed, by using objective indexes of anaerobic capacity such as maximal or mean power output, anaerobic testing may help these children to perceive the improvements. Assessment of pulmonary function 15 min after anaerobic testing is also of great value in helping to allay fears of postexercise bronchospasm.

The Results of Testing the Anaerobic Capacity of Asthmatic Children

The average peak power reached by asthmatic children during the force-velocity test is lower than that of controls matched for anthropometric characteristics, sexual maturity, and daily physical activity (see figure 14.1). The peak power reached during the test correlates with the bronchial obstruction parameters (see figure 14.2). Indeed, patients with milder asthma reached higher maximal power than patients with more severe asthma.

During the Wingate test, total energy output, peak power, and mean power output are lower in asthmatic children than in matched controls. The percentage of fatigue is identical in the two groups (see table 14.1). Again, anaerobic fitness as measured by the mean power obtained during this test is negatively correlated with bronchial obstruction (Counil et al. n.d.), whereas daily physical activity is not statistically related to anaerobic fitness (Counil et al. n.d.).

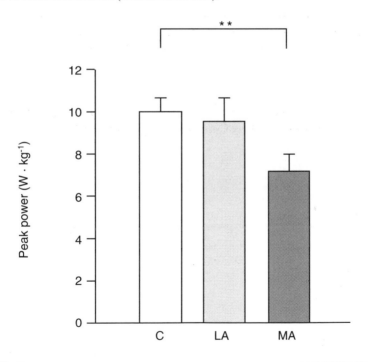

Figure 14.1 Relative peak power reached during the force-velocity test in children with mild asthma (LA, n = 7), moderate asthma (MA, n = 7), and controls (C, n = 14). ** p < 0.01; Wilcoxon-Mann-Whitney test.

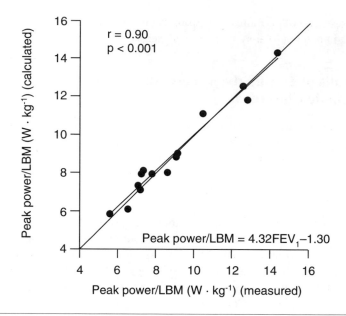

Figure 14.2 Relationship between measured peak power standardized by lean body mass (LBM) and peak power/LBM calculated with the equation of multiple stepwise regression analysis for asthmatic children (n = 14), including only FEV_1.

Table 14.1   Anaerobic Performance Indices During the Wingate Test: Comparison Between Healthy Controls and Asthmatic Children

	Controls (n=7)	Asthmatics (n=8)	
Wtot ($J \cdot kg^{-1}$)	176.9±18.8	140.3±25.5	*
Wtot ($J \cdot kg^{-1}$ LBM)	205.9±23.8	167.5±26.3	*
PP ($W \cdot kg^{-1}$)	7.3±0.5	6±1.1	*
PP ($W \cdot kg^{-1}$ LBM)	8.5±0.8	7.1±1.1	*
MP ($W \cdot kg^{-1}$)	5.9±0.5	4.7±0.8	*
MP ($W \cdot kg^{-1}$ LBM)	6.9±0.8	5.6±0.8	*
Fatigue index	22±11	25±11	NS

Notes: Wtot = Total energy output; PP = maximal power; MP = mean power (means ± SD; *: $p < 0.05$; Wilcoxon-Mann-Whitney test).

Relationship Between Aerobic and Anaerobic Fitness in Asthmatic Children

All the pediatric studies with reference to a control group show that aerobic fitness is markedly decreased in asthmatics (Varray and Préfaut 1992). In our experience, aerobic and anaerobic fitness are correlated. During the Wingate test, the relative contribution of the two metabolic pathways to the total expenditure of mechanical energy is identical for asthmatic and healthy children (see figure 14.3). During the force-velocity test, the linear relationship between force and velocity is not statistically different between the two populations. These results confirm the absence of an anaerobic "specialization" in asthmatic children. Indeed, it would appear that the exercise limitation in these children is due to a simultaneous and parallel decrease in both aerobic and anaerobic fitness. Training status alone cannot explain the overall unfitness of asthmatics. A close link between aerobic fitness and the basal bronchial obstruction has been established (Préfaut, Varray, and Vallet 1995; Varray et al. 1993; Varray and Préfaut 1992), and the same strong correlation was found for anaerobic fitness when daily physical activity was taken into account; that is, the greater the bronchial obstruction, the greater the decrease in anaerobic capacity (refer back to figure 14.2).

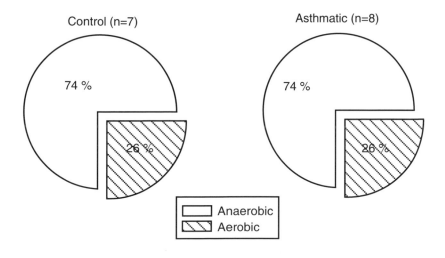

Figure 14.3 Relative contribution of aerobic and anaerobic energy release during the Wingate test in asthmatic and healthy children.

Metabolic Adaptations of Persons With Asthma During Anaerobic Testing

Post-anaerobic exercise plasma acidosis and plasma lactate concentrations are consistently lower in persons with asthma (see figure 14.4). If lactate is taken as an indicator of anaerobic glycolysis (Booth 1988), the lower blood lactate seen in the asthmatic population seems to indicate a lower glycolytic power than in the controls. As shown in figure 14.5, we have also found that epinephrine concentrations tend to be lower in asthmatics during the Wingate test. This finding is interesting because beta-adrenergic stimulation is probably the initiator of anaerobic glycolysis (Booth 1988). A diminished adrenergic response to exercise is a very attractive hypothesis. Although a decrease in sympathoadrenal response to exercise has been reported in asthmatics (Barnes et al. 1981; Belcher et al. 1988; Warren et al. 1982), hyposecretion of catecholamines during exercise is not established in asthmatic children. Up

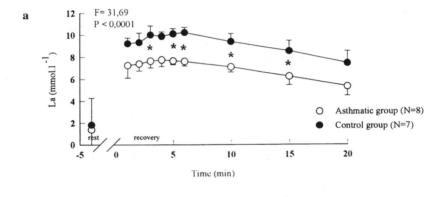

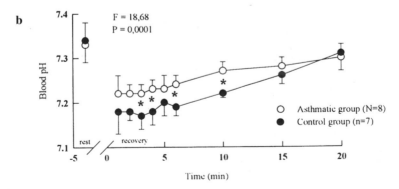

Figure 14.4 Blood lactate concentrations (a) and venous blood pH (b) at rest and after the Wingate test in asthmatic and healthy control children (* $p < 0.05$, contrast method after ANOVA).

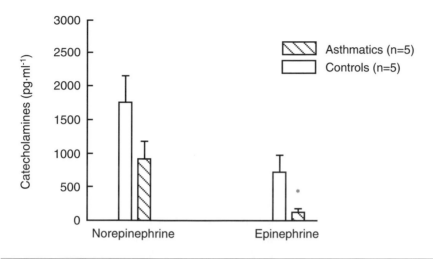

Figure 14.5 Increase in plasma norepinephrine and epinephrine concentrations from resting levels after the Wingate test in asthmatic and healthy control children (* $p < 0.05$; Wilcoxon-Mann-Whitney test).

to now, catecholamine secretion has been studied during submaximal exercise, and data concerning anaerobic exercise are lacking.

Cardiorespiratory Adaptation to Anaerobic Testing

Although the intensities were not precisely described, short, intense warm-ups, such as in sprint running, have been shown to prevent postexercise asthma (Bisschop et al. 1992; Schnall and Landau 1980). Indeed, in our experience, the postexercise bronchospasm is extremely rare after anaerobic testing, and the pulmonary function reveals no significant changes in airflow parameters (see table 14.2).

Table 14.2 Mean Percentage Change in FEV$_1$ Post-Anaerobic Exercise Testing in Asthmatic Children

Test	dFEV$_1$%	SD
Force-velocity (n = 14)	-1.23	5.76
Wingate (n = 8)	3.4	16

Heart rate reached maximal values during the Wingate test, indicating a full involvement of the cardiocirculatory system (Counil et al. n.d.). Heart monitoring, therefore, seems to be a good means for checking the child's level of participation in testing. To our knowledge, no hazardous effects of anaerobic exercise testing have ever been documented.

Directions for Future Research

Physical retraining is an important component of rehabilitation programs for asthmatic children, and its efficiency has been well documented (Clough et al. 1991; Orenstein et al. 1985; Ramazanoglu and Kraemer 1985; Varray et al. 1991). These programs should be based on pathophysiological concepts developed from scientific studies (Préfaut, Varray, and Vallet 1995). The objectives of the current training programs for these children are the following (Bar-Or 1983; Préfaut, Varray, and Vallet 1995; Varray and Préfaut 1992):

1. Improvement of exercise ability (overall physical fitness)
2. Decrease in hyperventilation for a given exercise load
3. Better cardiocirculatory adaptation to exercise
4. Prevention of exercise-induced bronchospasm
5. Increase in peripheral muscle strength
6. Decrease in anxiety and fear of physical activity, improvement of personality disturbances

Aerobic exercise programs have a proven effect on several of these parameters in children with asthma. Anaerobic programs could theoretically achieve objectives 1, 4, 5, and 6 (Fischer and Thompson 1994). The innocuousness of anaerobic activities is further supported by recent studies involving asthmatic children in such activities as judo (Hunnerbein, Achtzehn, and Kriegel 1993) and mountain climbing (Wekesa, Langhof, and Sack 1994). Nevertheless, precise guidelines for anaerobic training in asthmatic children need to be established. Investigators have focused on aerobic training, even though the anaerobic metabolism is elicited in several of the rehabilitation programs under study (Engström et al. 1991; Varray et al. 1991). The results obtained in our laboratory by Varray et al. over a 6-month period of controlled training are highly suggestive (Varray et al. 1991). Indeed, in this study, a group of asthmatic children were trained with an aerobic swimming program for 3 months, followed by a high-intensity training schedule of the same duration. Hereafter, the principal findings of this study related to clinical benefits and effects on physical fitness.

Clinical Benefits

The high-intensity anaerobic training program was well tolerated. No measurable improvements in the frequency of wheezing episodes or the need for regular medication were noted. Lung function also remained unchanged. In contrast, a major subjective improvement was reported by the patients and their parents. The wheezing attacks were less intense, and the children were described as less anxious. These findings are not surprising, as they are the usual effects reported in most studies of exercise rehabilitation programs for asthmatics (Varray and Préfaut 1992).

Effects on Physical Fitness

The anaerobic training that followed the aerobic training period did not further improve aerobic fitness (see figure 14.6), but the gain in aerobic fitness was main-

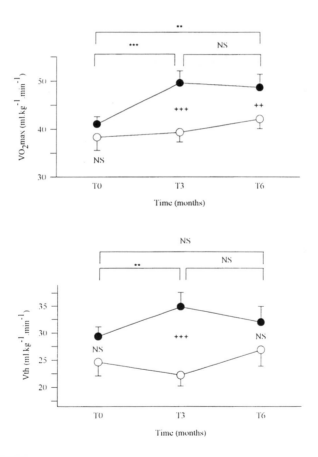

Figure 14.6 Time course of maximal O_2 uptake and ventilatory threshold (Vth) between 0, 3, and 6 months in trained (n = 7, closed circles) and untrained (n = 7, open circles) asthmatic children (** and ++: p < 0.01; *** and +++: p < 0.001; contrast method after ANOVA).

Data from Varray et al. 1989

tained by the anaerobic training. However, the gain in ventilatory threshold obtained with aerobic training was lost following the 3 months of exclusive anaerobic training. This indicates that anaerobic training cannot replace aerobic training in one of its major goals: the increase in the ventilatory threshold, that is, the decrease in relative hyperventilation during exercise (Préfaut, Varray, and Vallet 1995; Varray and Préfaut 1992; Varray et al. 1991). Unfortunately, there are no controlled studies to date on the specific effect of training on anaerobic fitness in childhood asthma.

Summary

In conclusion, anaerobic fitness is altered in asthmatic children. This limitation is correlated with the bronchial obstruction and is of the same magnitude as the aerobic limitation. Although the pathophysiological issues have not been fully elucidated, several observations support the concept of anaerobic training for these children: the anaerobic performance of asthmatic athletes; the strong anaerobic component in children's spontaneous play; the preventive effect of brief, intense warm-up on postexercise bronchospasm; and indeed, the limited anaerobic fitness itself. Anaerobic testing and training are not hazardous. The effect of anaerobic training in childhood asthma needs to be confirmed by controlled studies, but preliminary investigations indicate that there may be substantial benefits to aerobic-anaerobic training. Individualized aerobic training improves the ventilatory limitation in asthmatics during exercise and, indeed, is today the "gold standard" of exercise rehabilitation programs in asthma. Anaerobic training shows promise and seems likely to contribute to the quality of life of asthmatic children in a number of ways: widened spectrum of physical activity, improved muscle power, lower anxiety about high-intensity physical performance, control of postexercise bronchospasm, and improved self-image. The overall result is that these children will be able to fully enjoy athletic involvement.

References

Barnes, P.J., Brown, M.J., Silverman, M., and Dollery, C.T. 1981. Circulating catecholamines in exercise and hyperventilation-induced asthma. *Thorax* 36(6): 435-440.

Bar-Or, O. 1983. *Pediatric sports medicine for the practitioner.* Berlin, Heidelberg: Springer-Verlag.

Bedu, M., Fellmann, N., Spielvogel, H., Falgairette, G., Van Praagh, E., and Coudert, J. 1991. Force-velocity and 30-s Wingate tests in boys at high and low altitudes. *J. Appl. Physiol.* 70: 1031-1037.

Belcher, N.G., Murdoch, R., Dalton, N., Clark, T.J., Rees, P.J., and Lee, T.H. 1988. Circulating concentrations of histamine, neutrophil chemotactic activity and catecholamines during the refractory period in exercise-induced asthma. *J. Allergy Clin. Immunol.* 81(1): 100-110.

Bisschop, C., Desnot, P., Vergeret, J., Calveyrac, P., and Taytard, A. 1992. Short, repetitive and personalized exercise in the prevention of exercise-induced bronchospasm in the asthmatic child. In *Children and exercise XVI, Pediatric work physiology,* ed. J. Coudert J. and E. Van Praagh, 183-186. Paris: Masson.

Booth, F.W. 1988. Perspectives on molecular and cellular exercise physiology. *J. Appl. Physiol.* 65(4): 1461-1471.

Clough, J.B., Hutchinson, S.A., Williams, J.D., and Holgate, S.T. 1991. Airway response to exercise and metacholine in children with respiratory symptoms. *Arch. Dis. Child.* 66: 579-583.

Counil, F.P., Varray, A., Karila, Ch., Hayot, M., Voisin, M., and Préfaut, Ch. n.d. Wingate test performance in asthmatic children: aerobic or anaerobic limitation? *Med. Sci. Sports Exerc.* In press.

Engström, I., Fällström, K., Kalberg, E., Sten, G., and Bjure, J. 1991. Psychological and respiratory physiological effects of a physical exercise programme on boys with severe asthma. *Acta Paediatr. Scand.* 80: 1058-1065.

Fischer, E., and Thompson, J.K. 1994. A comparative evaluation of cognitive-behavioral therapy versus exercise therapy for treatment of body image disturbance. Preliminary findings. *Behav. Modif.* 18(2): 171-182.

Granier, P., Mercier, B., Mercier, J., Anselme, F., and Préfaut, C. 1995. Aerobic and anaerobic contribution to Wingate test performance in sprint and middle-distance runners. *Eur. J. Appl. Physiol.* 70: 58-65.

Haas, F., Pineda, H., Axen, K., Gaudino, D., and Haas, A. 1985. Effect of physical fitness on expiratory airflow in exercising asthmatic people. *Med. Sci. Sports Exerc.* 17(5): 585-592.

Hunnerbein, J., Achtzehn, R., and Kriegel, V. 1993. Judosport in einer trainingsgruppe mit asthmakranken Kindern. *Kinderarztl Prax.* 61(7-8): 264-268.

Mercier, J., Mercier, B., and Préfaut, Ch. 1991. Blood lactate increase during the force-velocity exercise test. *Int. J. Sports Med.* 12: 17-20.

Orenstein, D.M., Reed, M.E., Grogan, F.T., and Crawford, L.V. 1985. Exercise conditioning in children with asthma. *J. Pediatr.* 106: 556-560.

Préfaut, C., Varray, A., and Vallet, G. 1995. Pathophysiological basis of exercise training in patients with chronic obstructive lung disease. *Eur. Resp. Rev.* 5(25): 27-32.

Ramazanoglu, Y.M., and Kraemer, R. 1985. Cardiorespiratory response to physical conditioning in children with bronchial asthma. *Pediatr. Pulmonol.* 1: 272-277.

Rossi, A. 1993. Asthma and sport. *Eur. Resp. Rev.* 3(14): 380-382.

Schnall, R.P., and Landau, L.I. 1980. Protective effects of repeated short sprints on exercise-induced asthma. *Thorax* 35: 828-832.

Vandewalle, H., Pérés, G., Heller, J., Panel, J., and Monod, H. 1987. Force-velocity relationships and maximal power on a cycle ergometer. *Eur. J. Appl. Physiol.* 56: 650-656.

Varray, A., Mercier, J., Ramonatxo, M., and Préfaut, C. 1989. L'exercice physique maximal chez l'enfant asthmatique: limitation aérobie et compensation anaérobie? *Sci. Sports* 4: 199-207.

Varray, A., Mercier, J., Savy-Pacaux, A.M., and Préfaut, C. 1993. Cardiac role in exercise limitation in asthmatic subjects with special reference to disease severity. *Eur. Resp. J.* 6: 1011-1017.

Varray, A., and Préfaut, C. 1992. Importance of physical exercise training in asthmatics. *J. Asthma* 29(4): 229-234.

Varray, A.L., Mercier, J.G., Terral, C.M., and Préfaut, C.G. 1991. Individualized aerobic and high intensity training for asthmatic children in an exercise readaptation program. *Chest* 99: 579-586.

Virant, F.S. 1992. Exercise-induced bronchospasm: epidemiology, pathophysiology, and therapy. *Med. Sci. Sports Exerc.* 24(8): 851-855.

Voy, R.O. 1986. The U.S. Olympic Committee experience with exercise-induced bronchospasm. *Med. Sci. Sports Exerc.* 18: 328-330.

Warren, J.B., Keynes, R.J., Brown, M.J., Jenner, D.A., and McNicol, M.W. 1982. Blunted sympathoadrenal response to exercise in asthmatic subjects. *Br. J. Dis. Chest* 76: 147-150.

Wekesa, M., Langhof, H., and Sack, P. 1994. The asthma six-minute provocation test and mountain climbing in children. *East Afr. Med. J.* 71(1): 51-54.

15
CHAPTER

Malnutrition and Anaerobic Performance in Children

Nicole Fellmann
Jean Coudert

This chapter focuses on the following objectives:

- Discussing the connection between malnutrition and anaerobic performance
- Considering the underlying mechanisms and confounding factors of malnutrition in relation to anaerobic performance
- Explaining how impaired muscle function plays a role in declining anaerobic performance
- Discussing the factors that modulate the effect of malnutrition on performance

Strictly speaking, the term malnutrition applies to overnourished (obese) as well as to undernourished subjects. The present review will be restricted to the effects of chronic undernutrition on anaerobic performances.

Children living in developing countries under poor socioeconomic and hygienic conditions are often exposed to nutritional deprivation. This results in a high incidence of protein-energetic malnutrition of various degrees (mild to severe, depending on the intensity, duration, and timing of the nutritional restriction). Marginal protein-energetic malnutrition is the most widespread form of malnutrition. More than a third of the world's children under 5 years of age are affected, the worst situation being in Asia followed by Africa, Oceania, and Latin America (de Onis et al. 1993). These estimates, which correspond to 192.5 million children, stress the ongoing problem of marginal or mild to moderate malnutrition in developing countries.

During the period of active growth, two adaptive mechanisms are available to children to spare energy and balance a chronic marginal deficiency in energy intake: retardation of physical growth with a concomitant delay in growth spurt and sexual maturation, and a decrease in physical activity (Spurr 1983).

Undernourished children have lower weights and heights than nutritionally normal children of the same chronological age. The reduced body mass is mainly the result of a decrease in body fat mass and muscle mass, which respectively constitute the caloric and protein reserves of the body. In the selection of proteins for energy production, the body first chooses the least critical source, such as muscle, whereas kidneys, heart, and brain are less affected by malnutrition.

In the continuum from mild to severe undernutrition, muscle mass is affected earlier than body fat mass, which changes only in severe stages of undernutrition. Consequently, assessment of anthropometric characteristics probably best reflects the nutritional status. For children, weight and height for age, weight/height ratio, body mass index, and determination of body composition (fat mass and percentage of body weight, lean body mass, muscle cell mass, upper-arm muscle circumference) are useful indications of past malnutrition. Nutritional status can also include biochemical determinations indicative of current malnutrition, such as total plasma proteins, albumin, and prealbumin concentrations (which reflect the body's reserve of protein), to identify the potential for anemia and insulin-like growth factor as a nutritional marker (which has been shown to decrease during protein-energetic malnutrition). Hematological parameters (hemoglobin concentration, hematocrit, and level of iron) to identify the potential for anemia and a dietary history (using the FAO/WHO/UNU [1985] recommendations) of daily energy and protein intakes can also complete the evaluation of the nutritional status.

On the other hand, a dietary deficit can also result in reduced physical activity. A number of investigators have reported that undernourished children are significantly less active than well-fed ones, spending more time in light activities and less in moderate and vigorous activities (Spurr 1990; Spurr and Reina 1995). Moreover, during nutritional recovery from malnutrition, children submitted to a moderate level of physical activity had enhanced development of lean body mass and longitudinal growth as compared to their sedentary peers (Torun et al. 1979). This stresses the interaction between nutrient restriction and physical activity in relation to growth.

Although the primary problem is deficiency of energy and proteins, there are numerous factors that interact in a synergistic manner. Undernourished children always come from a poor socioeconomic background that is often associated with poor hygienic conditions. This results in a high incidence of infectious disease and intestinal parasitosis, which lead to malabsorption of food and worsen the problem of lack of nutrient intake. Additionally, social and cultural factors make it difficult to isolate the effect of actual malnutrition on stunted growth and lower physical performances.

Decreased spontaneous physical activity and reduced body size as an adaptation to marginal malnutrition (low weight for age but normal weight for height), as well as to more severe malnutrition (low weight for height), have a negative effect on the physical fitness and performance of undernourished children. Most studies have focused on measurements of static strength, of motor performances such as sprinting, jumping, and throwing involving motor coordination in addition to dynamic strength, and of and physical working capacity as mainly measured by maximal oxygen consumption (VO_2max). However, little is known of the effect of malnutrition on anaerobic power developed during short-term maximal exercises.

In this chapter, only physical exercises requiring mainly anaerobic metabolism participation will be considered.

Anaerobic Performance and Malnutrition

Because they are inexpensive and simple to administer, field tests are more often used than laboratory tests for assessing anaerobic performance in malnourished children. Very few studies have focused on maximal anaerobic power measurement under laboratory conditions.

Field Tests

Muscle strength is most frequently assessed by high standing jumps or long jumps, ball throwing, handgrip test, or dashes over short distances (30, 50, 60 m) or for short duration (40 s). The results obtained in children suffering from malnutrition are summarized in table 15.1. Only data on mild and moderate undernutrition are available.

All authors agreed in their findings that the absolute strength and motor performance of the malnourished children were significantly below those of their well-fed counterparts. Considering the smaller size of the malnourished subjects, the performances were adjusted for height, weight, and body composition (fat-free mass). The results are conflicting. In some studies the performances remained lower (Bénéfice 1993; Malina and Buschang 1985; Malina 1990; Malina, Little, and Buschang 1991; Sabogal, Malina, and McVean 1979); in some they were similar to those of the well-nourished group (Acevedo 1955; Bénéfice 1993; Ghesquiere and Eeckels 1984; Malina and Buschang 1985; Malina et al. 1987; Malina, Little, and Buschang 1991); and in others they surpassed the performances of the well-fed peers (Ghesquiere and Eeckels 1984; Malina and Buschang 1985; Malina et al. 1987). These discrepancies could result in unsuitable normalization of the data and choice of "control" groups.

It is well established that anthropometric characteristics are mainly responsible for variance in strength and in anaerobic as well as aerobic aptitudes. When the aim of the study is to compare muscular qualities of individuals differing in anthropological characteristics, as is the case in malnourished children, expressing the results per kilogram body mass is not a valid method. Indeed, as discussed earlier, undernourished children have significantly lower muscle mass than normal children. Therefore the power or the strength developed by the muscle should be normalized to the mass, volume, or cross-sectional area of the active muscle during the test. Additionally, correction by using fat-free mass is open to criticism. The

Table 15.1 Strength and Motor Skill Performance (in Absolute Terms and Adjusted for Anthropometric Parameters) of Children Suffering from Mild to Moderate Malnutrition Compared With Well-Nourished Controls

Reference	Country	Age (years)	Sex	Test	Performances in absolute terms	Performances adjusted for body mass
Acevedo 1955	Chile	School children	b-g	grip strength	<	=
Bénéfice 1992	Senegal	9-14	b-g	33-m dash ball throwing standing long jump grip strength	< < < <	
Bénéfice 1993	Senegal	10-11	b-g	33-m dash ball throwing standing long jump	< < <	size < = =
Dekkar et al. 1991	Algeria	5-20	b-g	standing long jump 50-m dash grip strength	< < <	
Ghesquiere and Eeckels 1984	Zaire	6-13	b	grip strength vertical jump ball throwing dash	< < < <	body mass > = = >
Malina and Buschang 1985	Mexico	6-12	b-g	dash jump ball throwing grip strength	< < < <	size = (b); < (g) = (b) > (b)

Reference	Country	Age	Sex	Measure	Comparison	Size / weight
		12-15	b-g	dash	<	size = (b); < (g)
				jump	<	< (b)
				throw	<	> (b)
				grip strength	<	
Malina et al. 1987	Mexico	6-15	b-g	grip strength	<	size =
				dash	<	
				vertical jump	<	
				ball throwing	<	
	New Guinea	6-16	b-g	dash	=	size =
				vertical jump	=	
				ball throwing	>	
Malina et al. 1991	Mexico	9-14	b	grip strength	<	body weight =
						fat free mass <
Narvaez Perez et al. 1991	Argentina	9-13	b-g	40-s run	<	
				50-m dash	<	
				vertical jump	<	
Rocha-Ferreira cited in	Brazil	4-5	b-g	standing long jump	<	size <
				20-m dash	<	
Rocha-Ferreira et al. 1991	Brazil	8	b-g	long jump	<	
				50-m dash	<	
Sabogal et al. 1979	Guatemala	School children	b-g	grip strength	<	weight <
				grip strength	<	

Note. Undernourished girls (g) and boys (b). Comparisons of their performances with control groups of the same age indicate: < lower; = equal to; > higher than their well-nourished counterparts.

composition of fat-free mass, which is made up of viscera, bone tissue, and muscle, changes in malnourished subjects, who have a higher ratio of viscera and bone to muscle. Consequently, when Malina, Little, and Buschang (1991) corrected the strength developed during the handgrip test by using total fat-free mass, they misrepresented the comparison with normal children—all the more so since only a few muscles were involved in the arm exercise task. In fact, the methodological difficulty results from the lack of a valid method for easily measuring active muscle mass in multiarticular coordinated exercise; at present the best approximation, or at least the less inaccurate, would be muscle limb volumes when legs or arms are working. In contrast, the greater fatness observed in well-nourished children may exert a negative influence on events that require the displacement of body mass, for example dashes and jumps. However, all these comparisons tend to obscure the fact that in most cases the deficit is an absolute one, and the concept "small but healthy" claimed for chronically undernourished children must be rejected.

Evaluation of the physical fitness of undernourished children can also be distorted by the choice of the well-nourished "control" group. Thus racial, ethnic, geographical, and cultural differences should be taken into account for valid comparisons.

Laboratory Tests

To our knowledge, anaerobic performance on the cycle ergometer in malnourished children has been investigated only in our laboratory, in collaboration with the members of the Instituto Boliviano de Biologia de Altura in La Paz, Bolivia. Maximal anaerobic power (Pmax) evaluated by the force-velocity test and mean power (MP) developed during a 30 s Wingate test were compared between Bolivian boys (Obert et al. 1993) and girls (Blonc et al. 1996), 11 years of age, of high and low socioeconomic status and living at high and low altitudes. The low socioeconomic groups were considered marginally undernourished children on the basis of anthropometric measurements, nutritional intake, and biochemical and hematological analyses. Expressed in absolute values, Pmax and MP were lower in undernourished children (36% on average). Even when corrected by body mass, lean body mass, or muscle leg volume, anaerobic power remained lower for both undernourished boys and girls, whichever altitude they lived at (3600 m or 420 m). Therefore, next to quantitative changes (anthropometric characteristics and especially muscle mass) induced by malnutrition, qualitative muscle factors of either psychomotor, biochemical, or biomechanical origin can also play a role in the reduction in anaerobic power.

To clarify this issue, 11-year-old children from a poor socioeconomic background were compared to well-nourished children who were 2 years younger but exhibited the same anthropometric characteristics (i.e., same height, body mass, lean body mass, and muscle leg volume) (de Jonge et al. 1996). In spite of the strong relationship between body dimensions and short-term power output, Pmax and MP remained lower in the 11-year-old marginally malnourished boys and girls (see figure 15.1). Anthropometric characteristics explained only 67% of the variation of the Pmax values. The two different measurements for both boys and girls on the graph refer to two groupings of the children according to socioeconomic background. The white bar represents children from more affluent backgrounds and the cross-hatched bar, children from poorer backgrounds.

These results provide evidence that factors other than those related to body dimensions should account for the lower anaerobic performance in undernourished children. In line with some results obtained by field tests, these new data support the hypothesis of a deterioration of muscle function involved only in anaerobic processes (see figure 15.2).

In contrast, aerobic performance assessed by either field (9 min run, 12 min run) or laboratory tests ($\dot{V}O_2$max, physical work capacity [PWC 170], endurance test) is lower in children suffering from mild and moderate undernutrition, when expressed in absolute terms. However, in contrast to what is seen with anaerobic performance, this decrease is always found to be related to reduced body mass, and especially muscle mass (Parizkova 1987; Spurr 1983; Spurr and Reina 1995) (see figure 15.3).

At the present time there is no available information concerning oxygen debt or deficit and lactate or ventilatory anaerobic thresholds in undernourished children.

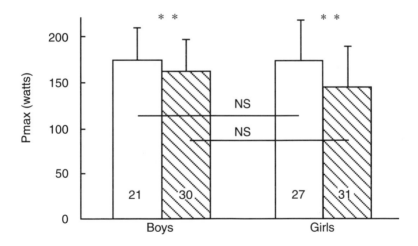

Figure 15.1 Maximal anaerobic power (Pmax) (means ± SD) developed during the force-velocity test by Bolivian children from high (□) and low socioeconomic (▧) backgrounds at low altitude (420 m). The boys and the girls of both groups demonstrated the same anthropometric characteristics, but because of their growth delay, the children living under deprived economic conditions were 2 years older than the control groups (9 vs. 11 years of age). NS: nonsignificant; ** p < 0.01,

Data from de Jonge et al. 1996.

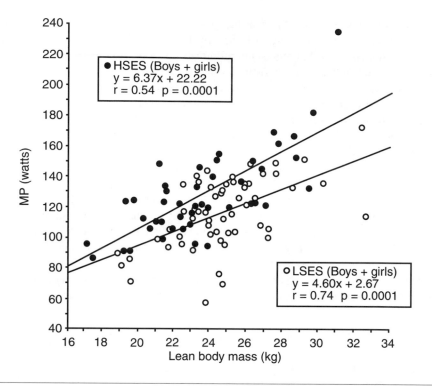

Figure 15.2 Relationship between mean anaerobic power (MP) developed during the Wingate test (30 s) and lean body mass (LBM) in boys and girls (9 to 11 years of age) of high (HSES) and low (LSES) socioeconomic status. Statistical analysis of the curves shows that MP was higher in HSES children but the slopes were the same

From unpublished data Coudert et al.

Underlying Mechanisms and Confounding Factors

As already emphasized, the decrease in anaerobic performance, even when adjusted for muscle mass, suggests that poor nutritional status can be responsible for muscle function deterioration.

Impaired Muscle Function

A direct consequence of malnutrition on muscle function in children appears to be supported by several studies that concentrated on the structural, metabolic, and functional changes occurring in human and animal skeletal muscle as a result of malnutrition or nutritional restriction (see references cited in Blonc et al. 1996; Obert et al. 1993).

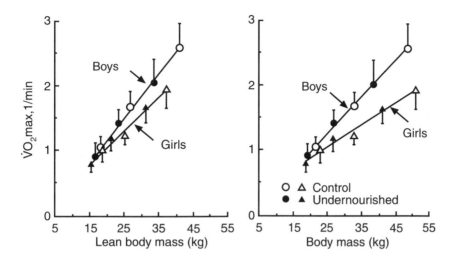

Figure 15.3 Maximal oxygen uptake ($\dot{V}O_2$max) of 6- to 16-year-old controls and marginally undernourished Colombian children as a function of lean body mass and body mass.

Adapted from Spurr and Reina 1995.

During severe nutritional deprivation in animals and humans (obese subjects during hypocaloric dieting and fasting, persons with anorexia nervosa, malnourished cancer and noncancer patients), the forces generated by the gastrocnemius, diaphragm, or adductor pollicis muscles in response to different electrical stimulations were modified. Nutritional deprivation resulted in lower maximal force at a high-frequency stimulation, increased muscle fatigability, and slower relaxation time. After refeeding, recovery of a normal pattern of muscle contraction and relaxation depended on the severity of the restriction and on age, and could have been significant before any changes in body composition could be detected.

In addition to muscle function, muscle biopsies in animals and adults showed that undernutrition led to muscular atrophy caused by a reduction in fiber diameter and in some cases a loss of fiber number. This effect was selective and concerned mainly the fast-twitch (FT) fibers, whereas the slow-twitch (ST) fibers were generally unaffected by undernutrition except in the case of very severe restriction. Since FT fibers have a higher glycolytic potential, a selective atrophy of FT fibers would be advantageous in terms of fuel economy because more costly anaerobic glycolysis and gluconeogenesis should be avoided when carbohydrate stores are depleted (Henriksson 1990). The mechanisms underlying the relative sparing of ST fibers as opposed to FT fibers are probably dependent on contractile activity (recruitment pattern). Since ST motor units are recruited earlier and more frequently than FT motor units, selective atrophy of FT fibers and muscle with nutritional deprivation can be caused by a lesser activity of the fast-twitch motor units. This hypothesis (Henriksson 1990) is in accordance with the lower spontaneous activity of a high intensity level reported by several authors (Kemper, n.d.; Spurr 1990). This "fiber adaptation" can be worsened by alterations in the responsiveness of inactive tissue to circulating hormones (Goldspink 1980). Inactive muscle becomes more responsive to catabolic hormones and less responsive to anabolic hormones. Unfortunately, undernutrition induces a decrease in insulin and insulin-like growth factor I and an increase in glucocorticoid concentrations (Henriksson 1990). Consequently, inhibition of protein synthesis and enhancement of protein breakdown induced by this hormonal environment are amplified by the relative inactivity of the FT fibers, in fact creating a vicious circle. However, it is questionable whether these results obtained in severely undernourished subjects and animals can be extrapolated to children suffering from marginal malnutrition.

Because of ethical limitations, no data on muscle biopsies from undernourished children are available, and extrapolation of mechanical power output measured during short-term maximal exercises to cellular metabolism or structural muscle is open to criticism. Nevertheless, the lack of difference between marginally malnourished and well-fed children at the optimal force for which Pmax was obtained could indicate a preferential alteration of FTa fibers (Blonc et al., 1996). However, the results on blood lactate concentration (L) measured after the Wingate test did not support the hypothesis of an altered glycolytic participation during the test (Fellmann, Beaune, and Coudert 1994). Values for L were lower in malnourished compared to normal children of the same chronological age, but when related to the power developed, L values were the same in both groups.

There is only one report of an indirect attempt to assess anaerobic capacity in chronically energy-deficient adults by measuring the postexercise recovery phase after VO$_2$max (Kulkarni, Kurpad, and Shetty 1993). The authors reported a rapid return of oxygen consumption to baseline values, in a single phase, in undernourished subjects. Consequently the total postexercise oxygen consumption was lower even when corrected for fat-free mass differences, while values for VO$_2$max expressed per kilogram fat-free mass were similar. These results could indicate a lower glycolytic participation in energy production. However, L was not measured in this study. Nevertheless, the malnourished subjects had lower resting plasma norepinephrine levels suggesting a reduced catecholamine response to heavy exercise. According to the authors this may be a contributing factor to the significantly reduced postexercise oxygen consumption in these subjects, and the small saving in energy during the postexercise recovery period may be an adaptive response.

Nevertheless, considering the difficulty associated with any prediction of anaerobic capacity from blood L and oxygen debt, this point needs to be pursued further. In addition, the delay in the growth spurt and in sexual maturation observed in malnourished children must be taken into account for the interpretation of L in circumpubertal boys, since testosterone level is positively correlated with L (Fellmann et al. 1988).

Factors Modulating the Effect of Malnutrition on Performance

To analyze the metabolic consequences of a shortage of food on performance, several factors must be taken into consideration.

Degree of Deficiency, Timing, and Duration of Malnutrition

The anaerobic metabolism seems to be more sensitive to the severity of malnutrition than the aerobic pathway. Anaerobic performances are altered by marginal or moderate malnutrition. In contrast, only severe or extreme malnutrition deteriorates aerobic capacity. Any correlation between $\dot{V}O_2max$ (relative to body mass) and hemoglobin concentration (range 94 to 157 g/L) was found in marginally malnourished children (Spurr et al. 1983). This suggests that the adaptation to chronic anemia (such as increase in arteriovenous oxygen extraction, modified blood flow distribution) is so complete that practically no impairment of exercise tolerance results from it (Spurr 1983). In more severe anemia (hemoglobin concentration equal to 80 g/L), the deficiency of the oxygen transport system induced lower aerobic work capacity, associated with a lower maximal heart rate (and consequently lower cardiac output), and a reduced plasma volume (Barac-Nieto et al. 1978).

The periods of gestation and lactation are particularly critical for the development of the fetus and the young child; there are very great weight and height gains during these periods of life. Unfortunately, maternal nutritional status is unknown in most studies. In the case of marginal undernutrition of the mother, it is likely that normal growth of the young child is preserved until weaning (which occurs more frequently in the second year of life for people from low socioeconomic and nutritional backgrounds). After this period, children are directly exposed to the effects of chronic malnutrition and the associated factors that worsen the nutritional deprivation.

Confounding Factors

Besides timing and duration as modulators of the severity of malnutrition, factors other than those associated with undernutrition can influence performance.

Parasitosis. Associated with low hygiene conditions, a high frequency of intestinal parasitosis *(Entamoeba, Giardia, Ascaridia, Anclyostoma, Strongyloides)* leads to a reduced absorption of nutriment that is already at an insufficient level. Few studies have focused on performance improvement after treatment of intestinal parasitosis. After a few weeks, treatment of African children induced an increase in appetite and weight gain. Spontaneous activity and aerobic performance, evaluated by indirect tests, were also improved (Kvalsvig 1986; Latham et al. 1990). As of now, no data are available for anaerobic performance.

Cultural and Psychological Factors. As suggested by Bénéfice (1992), who studied the negative effect of malnutrition on Senegalese children, the lack of a high degree of motivation and sense of competition was often encountered in children who came from low socioeconomic backgrounds. This effect is more marked in girls who are constrained to behave in a "lady-like fashion," a kind of "cultural squelch" of their natural exuberance (Spurr 1990). This cultural aspect has been discussed by Malina et al. (1987), who compared undernourished children from contrasting cultures: one sample from a rural area of Mexico and the other one from coastal Papua New Guinea. The running and jumping performances of children from the agricultural community were considerably below those of the children from the coastal fishing community, while the two groups had the same growth delay when compared to better-nourished American children. When corrected for body size, throwing and sprinting performances of the boys and, more surprisingly, of the girls from Papua New Guinea were better than those of the well-nourished group (table 15.1). According to the authors, the pattern of physical activity and the types of activities, which were different in the three groups, explained the results. Children of both sexes from the coastal community spent a considerable amount of time spearing fish, punting canoes around the lagoon, and swimming, at about 4-5 years of age. In the Mexican community, physical education was taught one day a week, and on school days and during school breaks, most of the children engaged in a variety of activities (e.g., soccer, basketball) that were very different from those of the other undernourished children. This study stresses, in fact, that cultural and physical activity aspects are closely linked and must be considered together when samples from different cultures are compared.

Spontaneous Physical Activity.   In addition to the direct effect of undernutrition on performance, reduced spontaneous physical activity as an adaptation to malnutrition, combined with some unfavorable environmental conditions (heat and humidity), can lower performance.

Marginally undernourished adults tend to become more sedentary than well-nourished persons and to limit their leisure-time activities at home and in social contexts, for example soccer playing (Shetty 1993). In malnourished children, restricting physical activity can also be an important strategy for saving energy. However, because reduced activity probably does not represent a large conservation of energy, it can be assumed that the first line of adaptation to moderate restricted energy intake is growth retardation, and the decrease in activity level may be seen only at a more serious degree of dietary deficit (Spurr 1990). These results agree with those from a more recent study in Bolivian children (Kemper et al. 1996). The physical growth of marginally malnourished boys and girls (10-12 years of age) was delayed by approximately 2 years. However, the children from low socioeconomic backgrounds spent more time at between 50% and 85% of heart rate reserve than their higher-socioeconomic-level counterparts; the boys were more physically active than the girls. The finding that children of low socioeconomic status were more active than their higher-socioeconomic-status peers might be explained by the fact that they had to participate more in household activities (e.g., carrying water in jerricans) and walk to and from school. Children from upper socioeconomic backgrounds were usually transported to and from their private school by car, and spent considerable amounts of time playing with their computers.

However, another observation made by Satyanarayana, Nadamuni, and Narasinga (1979) cannot rule out a salutary contribution of physical activity on aerobic performance. These authors assessed habitual physical activity status by questionnaire in 14- to 17-year-old Indian boys and demonstrated that malnourished children who were physically active had better physical performances than their less active malnourished peers. Habitual physical activity explained 10% of the variation in physical work capacity (PWC 170), while the difference in body mass explained about 64% of the variable.

Nevertheless, the apparent normal daily energy expenditure and physical activity of undernourished children in free-living conditions can mask their inability to keep up in situations of artificially increased activity levels above the usual. Indeed, Spurr and Reina (1995) showed that a group of undernourished Colombian boys were unable to keep up with their control counterparts in various athletic activities during a summer camp measurement of energy expenditure. Whether this apparent inability had an effect on their development was questioned by the authors.

Motor Learning. Next to lesser motivation and less desire to cooperate with others, children from low socioeconomic backgrounds experienced some problems when the tests for delivering external work required more technique and coordination. These children were not used to participating in physical education events and were less experienced cyclists. Bénéfice (1993) reported that Senegalese children did not have the technique to start a race efficiently when compared to African American children of the same age. And, when adjusted for body mass, there was no improvement in 33 m dash running results in contrast to long jump or throwing performance. Similarly, we observed in Bolivia that children of low socioeconomic status, especially girls, experienced some difficulties cycling in a coordinated manner. They produced great force on the pedals when these were not optimally positioned to accelerate the flywheel; therefore their feet were strapped firmly to the pedals to prevent them from slipping. These observations suggest that prior learning in advance of the actual tests would be useful in limiting the technical differences between high and low socioeconomic groups.

In conclusion, the effect of malnutrition on performances in children, as in adults, cannot be isolated from associated factors that worsen the nutrient deprivation. While the lower aerobic performance in children suffering from marginal malnutrition is mainly related to their lower muscle mass, factors other than body dimensions are probably responsible for their lower anaerobic aptitude. The qualitative muscle composition and motor learning involved in anaerobic power development would seem to be more sensitive indexes of low socioeconomic status and marginal undernutrition than the parameters implicated in aerobic capacity. Only serious or extreme malnutrition deteriorates maximal oxygen consumption and aerobic power. Attempts at dietary repletion of malnourished children indicate that the recovery process for aerobic capacity is long (Spurr 1983): After 3 years of an adequate diet without intestinal parasitosis treatment between 3 and 6 years of age, the supplemented groups had still lower maximal aerobic power than the control subjects. The timing of dietary intervention must also be taken into account: early nutritional improvement has been demonstrated to induce long-lasting effects on physical performance (Hass et al. 1995). Guatemalan subjects (14-19 years of age) exposed to high-energy, high-protein supplementation throughout gestation and the first 3 years of life improved $\dot{V}O_2$max, with a significant positive relationship between the amount of supplement administered and $\dot{V}O_2$max.

Directions for Future Research

From our perspective we look forward to further studies on the following topics:

- The effect of undernutrition on FT fiber muscle. Up to now this selective alteration has not been confirmed by direct observation in children because of ethical limitations. However, with the advent of nuclear magnetic resonance spectroscopy and imaging, it could become possible to investigate the contractile machinery in more detail.
- The mechanism underlying selective atrophy of FT fibers. We recently demonstrated in Bolivian girls of low socioeconomic status that serum insulin-like growth factor (Ig-FI) was an explanatory factor for their lower Pmax as compared to that of their counterparts of a high socioeconomic level (Beaune et al. 1997). Since Ig-FI is known to stimulate glycolysis, the lower serum Ig-FI levels found in these girls support the hypothesis of an action of this peptide on anaerobic power through the regulation of both muscle mass and muscle function (energy supply, contraction). Understanding of the mechanisms involved in such regulation is needed to clarify target sites of Ig-FI, but also of other metabolic hormones in this tissue.
- The effects of nutritional supplementation associated with antiparasitic treatment on the recovery process for anaerobic performance. Parasites are a common cause of chronic intestinal malabsorption of protein and other nutrients. Moreover, because of their bulk, some parasites require sizable quantities of nutrients that must be obtained from the same source available to host cells. Intestinal bleeding in hookworm infection also increases fecal protein loss. Consequently, protein intake evaluated by dietary inquiries underestimates the real quantity of nutrients absorbed and utilized. In these conditions, correction of dietary deficiencies by diet alone, while parasitic infections persist, is likely to be difficult. Therefore specific antiparasitic treatment in association with an appropriate nutritional regimen should be required. The length of recovery period necessary to improve the anaerobic performance needs to be investigated.

Summary

Reduced body size with a decrease in fat and muscle mass, and decreased spontaneous physical activity as an adaptation to marginal malnutrition, have a negative effect on the physical fitness and performance of undernourished children. Compared to adequately nourished peers of the same age, children suffering from marginal malnutrition have lower anaerobic performance, even when related to their lower muscle mass, whereas only serious or extreme malnutrition deteriorates maximal oxygen consumption and aerobic power. This indicates that factors other than body dimensions should be responsible for their lower anaerobic aptitude. The qualitative muscle composition (lower percentage and relative area of FT fibers, lower glycolytic potential) and motor learning involved in anaerobic power development would seem to be more sensitive indexes of low socioeconomic status and marginal undernutrition than the parameters implicated in aerobic performances.

In addition, the effect of malnutrition alone on performances in children, as in adults, cannot be isolated from the associated factors that worsen nutrient deprivation (low hygienic conditions associated with high incidence of infectious disease and intestinal parasitosis, which lead to malabsorption of food; social and cultural factors).

Attempts at dietary repletion of malnourished children indicate that the recovery process for aerobic capacity is long. At present, the effects of nutritional supplementation and/or treatment of intestinal parasitosis on anaerobic metabolism and performances remain unknown.

References

Acevedo, M. 1955. Contribucion al estudio de medidas antropometricas en al escola Chileno. *Revista Chilena de Education Fisica* 22: 1101-1104.

Barac-Nieto, M., Spurr, G., Maksud, G.M., and Lotero, H. 1978. Aerobic capacity in chronically undernourished adult males. *J. Appl. Physiol.* 44: 209-215.

Beaune, B., Blonc, S., Fellmann, N., Bedu, M., and Coudert, J. 1997. Serum insulin-like growth factor I and physical performance in prepubertal Bolivian girls of a high and low socio-economic status. *Eur. J. Appl. Physiol.* 76:98-102.

Bénéfice, E. 1992. Physical activity and anthropometric and functional characteristics of mildly malnourished Senegalese children. *Ann. Trop. Paediatr.* 12: 55-66.

Bénéfice, E. 1993. Physical activity, cardiorespiratory fitness, motor performance, and growth of Senegalese pre-adolescents. *Am. J. Hum. Biol.* 5: 653-667.

Blonc, S., Fellmann, N., Bedu, M., Falgairette, G., de Jonge, R., Obert, P., Beaune, B., Spielvogel, H., Tellez, W., Quintela, A., San Miguel, J.L., and Coudert, J. 1996. Effect of altitude and socio-economic status on $\dot{V}O_2$max and anaerobic power in prepubertal Bolivian girls. *J. Appl. Physiol.* 81: 2002-2008.

Dehkar, N. 1991. Growth, nutrition and physical performance in Algeria. In *Human growth, physical fitness and nutrition,* ed. R. Shephard and J. Parizkova. Basel: Karger.

FAO/WHO/UNU. 1985. *Energy and protein requirements.* Tech. report 724. Geneva: World Health Organization.

Fellmann, N., Beaune, B., and Coudert, J. 1994. Blood lactate after maximal and supramaximal exercise in 10- to 12 year-old Bolivian boys: effects of altitude and socio-economic status. *Int. J. Sports Med.* 15(suppl. 2): 90-95.

Fellmann, N., Bedu, M., Spielvogel, H., Falgairette, G., Van Praagh, E., Jarrige, J.F, and Coudert, J. 1988. Anaerobic metabolism during pubertal development at high altitude. *J. Appl. Physiol.* 64: 1382-1386.

Ghesquiere, J., and Eeckels, R. 1984. Health, physical development and fitness of primary school children in Kinshasa. In *Children and Sport,* ed. J. Ilmarinen & I. Valimäki. Berlin: Springer-Verlag.

Goldspink, D.F. 1980. The influence of contractile activity and the nerve supply on muscle size and protein turnover. In *Plasticity of muscle,* ed. D. Pette. Berlin: W. de Gruyter.

Haas, J., Martinez, E., Murdoch, S., Conlisk, E., Rivera, J., and Martoull, R. 1995. The effects of improved nutrition in early childhood: the Institute of Nutrition of Central America and Panama (INCAP) follow-up study. *J. Nutr.* 125(suppl.): 1078S-1089S.

Henriksson, J. 1990. The possible role of skeletal muscle in the adaptation to periods of energy deficiency. *Eur. J. Clin. Nutr.* 44(suppl. 1): 55-64.

de Jonge, R., Bedu, M., Fellmann, N., Blonc, S., Spielvogel, H., and Coudert, J. 1996. Effect of anthropometric characteristics and socio-economic status on physical performances of pre-pubertal children living in Bolivia at low altitude. *Eur. J. Appl. Physiol.* 74: 367-374.

Kemper, H.C.G., Spekreijse, M., Slooten, J., Post, B., and Coudert, Y. 1996. Physical activity in prepubescent children: relationship with residential altitude and socioeconomic status. Pediatric Exerc. Sci. 8: 57-68

Kulkarni, R., Kurpad, A., and Shetty, P. 1993. Reduced postexercise recovery oxygen consumptions: an adaptative response in chronic energy deficiency? *Metabolism* 42: 544-547.

Kvalsvig, J. 1986. The effects of schistosomiasis haematobium on the activity of school children. *J. Trop. Med. Hyg.* 89: 85-90.

Latham, M., Stephenson, L., Kurz, K., and Kinoti, S. 1990. Metrifonate or praziquantel treatment improves physical fitness and appetite of Kenyan schoolboys with schistosoma haematobium and hook worm infections. *Am. J. Trop. Med. Hyg.* 43: 170-179.

Malina, R. 1990. Growth of Latin-American children: socio-economic, urban-rural and secular comparisons. *Revista Brasileira de Ciencia e movimiento* 4: 46-75.

Malina, R., and Buschang, P. 1985. Growth, strength and motor performance of Zapotec children, Oaxaca, Mexico. *Hum. Biol.* 57: 163-181.

Malina, R., Little, B., Schoup, R., and Buschang, P. 1987. Adaptive significance of small body size: strength and motor performance of school children in Mexico and Papua, New Guinea. *Am. J. Phys. Anthropol.* 73: 489-499.

Malina, R.M., Little, B.B., and Buschang, P.H. 1991. Estimated body composition and strength of chronically mild-to-moderately undernourished rural boys in Southern Mexico. In *Human growth, physical fitness and nutrition,* ed. R. Shephard & J. Parizkova. Basel: Karger.

Narvaez Perez, G., D'Angelo, C., and Zabala, R. 1991. Physical fitness in children and adolescents from differing socio-economic strata. In *Human growth, physical fitness and nutrition,* ed. R. Shephard and J. Parizkova. Basel: Karger.

Obert, P., Bedu, M., Fellmann, N., Falgairette, G., Beaune, B., Quintela, A., Van Praagh, E., Spielvogel, H., Kemper, H., Post, B., Parent, F., and Coudert, J. 1993. Effect of chronic hypoxia and socio-economic status on $\dot{V}O_2$max and anaerobic power of Bolivian boys. *J. Appl. Physiol.* 74: 888-896.

de Onis, M., Montero, C., Akre, J., and Clugston, G. 1993. The worldwide magnitude of protein-energy malnutrition: an overview from the WHO Global Database on child growth. *Bull. World Health Org.* 71: 703-712.

Parizkova, J. 1987. Growth, functional capacity and physical fitness in normal and malnourished children. *World Rev. Nutr. Diet.* 51: 1-44.

Rocha Ferreira, M., Malina, R., and Rocha, L. 1991. Anthropometric, functional and psychological characteristics of eight year-old Brazilian children from low socio-economic status. In *Human growth, physical fitness and nutrition,* ed. R. Shephard and J. Parizkova. Basel: Karger.

Sabogal, F., Malina, B., and McVean, R. 1979. Desarollo fisico y cognotivo de ninos Guatemaltecos en function del nivel socio-economico y del sexo. *Revista Latino-Americana de psicologia* 11: 229-247.

Satyanarayana, K., Nadamuni, N., and Narasinga, R. 1979. Nutritional deprivation in childhood and the body size, activity, and physical work capacity of young boys. *Am. J. Clin. Nutr.* 32: 1769-1775.

Shetty, P.S. 1993. Chronic undernutrition and metabolic adaptation. *Proc. Nutr. Soc.* 52: 267-284.

Spurr, G. 1990. Physical activity and energy expenditure in undernutrition. *Prog. Food Nutr. Sci.* 14: 139-192.

Spurr, G.B. 1983. Nutritional status and physical work capacity. *Yearbook Phys. Anthrop.* 26: 1-35.

Spurr, G.B., and Reina, J. 1995. Undernutrition, physical activity, and performance of children. In *New horizons in pediatric exercise science,* ed. C. Blimkie and O. Bar-Or. Champaign, IL: Human Kinetics.

Spurr, G.B., Reina, J.C., Dahners, H.W., and Barac-Nieto, M. 1983. Marginal malnutrition in school-aged Columbian boys: functional consequences in maximum exercise. *Am. J. Clin. Nutr.* 37. 834-847.

Torun, B., Schutz, Y., Viteri, F., and Bradfield, R.B. 1979. Growth, body composition and heart rate/$\dot{V}O_2$ relationships changes during the nutritional recovery of children with two different physical activity levels. In *Nutritional aspects of physical performance,* ed. Somagyi and de Wijn. Basel: Karger.

16

CHAPTER

High Altitude and Anaerobic Performance During Growth

Mario Bedu
Jean Coudert

This chapter focuses on the following objectives:

- Discussing the connection between anaerobic performance and hypoxia
- Describing the methodological aspects of studying this connection
- Comparing the effects of high altitude on children and adults

It has been well known since the publication of *La Pression Barométrique* by Paul Bert (1878) that most of the deleterious effects of high altitude (HA) on humans are caused by hypoxia. This in turn is a direct result of the reduction in atmospheric pressure. Although most of the undesirable effects of HA are due to hypoxia, under some circumstances additional deterioration results from cold, dehydration, and solar and even ionizing radiations. Furthermore, most of the HA areas of the world are in the least economically developed regions, and for this reason, some effects attributed to HA could be the result of other factors such as nutritional deprivation (see Fellmann and Coudert in this book).

The effects of hypoxia and the responses of organisms to it depend on the severity and the rate at which hypoxia is imposed, among other parameters. Broadly speaking, the responses can be divided into two categories according to the duration of hypoxia: acute hypoxia, lasting from a few seconds to 1 or 2 hr, and chronic hypoxia, lasting from a few hours to many years. This includes lifelong hypoxia, that is, persons who were born in and have always lived at altitude. For HA residents, 5500-6000 m represents the highest acceptable level for permanent habitation. At greater altitudes, physical and mental deterioration occurs (Pugh 1967).

The changes induced by hypoxia of HA are numerous and take place over a period of hours to months. These changes, termed *acclimatization,* occur in different systems of the body (respiratory and cardiovascular systems, kidneys, blood). Changes that take place over decades, or are the result of having been born and bred in the mountain environment, are termed *adaptation*. Many of these changes can be considered an attempt to mitigate the effect of low inspired O_2 on the tissues by reducing the loss of O_2 partial pressure at each stage in the O_2 transport system from ambient air to tissue cells.

The decrease in maximal aerobic power ($\dot{V}O_2$max) during both acute and chronic HA exposure is well documented in adults (Cerretelli and di Prampero 1985). A similar decrease has been reported in children (Fellmann et al. 1986; Greksa et al. 1982). Conflicting studies of the effects of HA on anaerobic metabolism have been reported in adults (Coudert 1992). There is little information available concerning the influence of altitude on the anaerobic metabolism of children.

Anaerobic Performance and Hypoxia

For more than 10 years, in collaboration with the members of the Instituto Boliviano de Biologia de Altura in La Paz (3700 m, Pb = 495 mmHg, Bolivia), we have investigated the effect of acute hypoxia at low altitude (LA) or acute normoxia at HA and the effect of chronic hypoxia on O_2 debt, ventilatory threshold, performances on field tests, maximal anaerobic power (peak power, PP) during force-velocity tests or mean power (MP) during Wingate tests, and blood lactate concentration after different types of exercise.

Effects of Acute Hypoxia

The effect of acute hypoxia (FIO2 = 13.7%, simulated altitude of 3700 m) at LA and acute normoxia (FIO2 = 30.6%, simulated sea level) at HA (3700 m) on performance during a 30 s Wingate test has been investigated in prepubertal (Tanner stage 1) boys (Blonc et al. 1994). Compared to normoxia, acute hypoxia at LA did not alter PP (293 ± 40 vs. 302 ± 56 W, not significant [NS]) and MP (226 ± 30 vs. 227 ± 32 W, NS). Similarly, compared to chronic hypoxia, acute normoxia at HA did not modify these parameters (PP: 292 ± 69 vs. 289 ± 86 W, NS; MP: 213 ± 54 vs. 216 ± 49 W, NS). Moreover, change in blood lactate concentration after the Wingate test was neither significantly modified by acute hypoxia at LA (5.3 ± 1.7 vs. 4.8 ± 1.7 mmol · L^{-1}) nor by acute normoxia at HA (3.4 ± 1.3 vs. 3.3 ± 1.0 mmol · L^{-1}).

Effects of Chronic Hypoxia

The effect of chronic hypoxia was investigated on altitude-resident children who had lived at La Paz more than 3 years.

Field Tests

To appreciate the effect of chronic hypoxia on field performances in children, Falgairette et al. (1994) compared prepubescent (10-11 years old) and pubescent (13-15 years old) boys at HA and LA. At similar ages, there was no significant difference between HA and LA boys for the mean running velocity in a 30 m sprint (respectively, 5.26 ± 0.42 vs. 5.29 ± 0.39 m $\cdot$ s^{-1} at 10-11 years old and 5.85 ± 0.40 vs. 6.02 ± 0.48 m $\cdot$ s^{-1} at 13-15 years old). Moreover, the average speed calculated in a 30 s shuttle run (subjects ran forward and backward over a 30 m distance for 30 s) was slightly (3-4%) but significantly ($p < 0.05$) lower in HA than in LA boys (respectively, 4.20 ± 0.23 vs. 4.37 ± 0.30 m $\cdot$ s^{-1} for 10-11-year-olds and 4.68 ± 0.29 vs. 4.83 ± 0.33 m $\cdot$ s^{-1} for 13-15-year-olds).

Oxygen Debt

Oxygen debt after supramaximal (115% VO_2max) or inframaximal (50 W during 5 min) exercise was not significantly different between HA and LA children (Fellmann et al. 1986) (respectively, 1.64 ± 0.14 vs. 1.73 ± 0.16 L and 0.73 ± 0.19 vs. 0.71 ± 0.20 L). Oxygen debt increased with intensity of exercise in HA and LA. When intensity was expressed in absolute terms, HA children exhibited larger O_2 debt than LA children. But when related to percentage of VO_2max (taking into account the decrease in VO_2max at HA), all O_2 debt values from HA and LA subjects fell on the same line, and no difference was observed for supramaximal debt (Fellmann et al. 1986).

Ventilatory and Lactic Anaerobic Threshold

Ventilatory and lactic anaerobic thresholds were detected at approximately 70-75% $\dot{V}O_2$max at LA in 10- to 13-year-old boys and girls as well as in HA children (Fellmann et al. 1986).

Force-Velocity Test

The results obtained in children resident at high and low altitudes are summarized in figure 16.1. No significant difference was found in PP, expressed either in absolute terms or relative to body mass, between Bolivian boys at HA and European boys at LA (Bedu et al. 1991) or between Bolivian boys at HA and LA (Obert et al. 1993). This was true regardless of age or socioeconomic status (Obert et al. 1993). In girls, PP normalized for body mass was higher at HA (see figure 16.1) (Blonc et al. 1996).

Wingate Test

In a study of Bolivian boys from a high socioeconomic background at HA and European boys at LA (Bedu et al. 1991), MP was significantly reduced at HA for

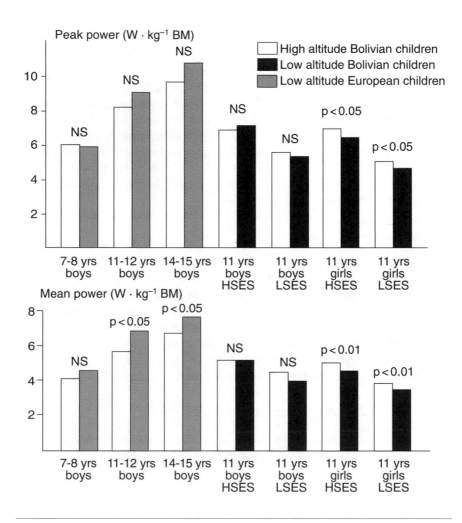

Figure 16.1 Peak power (force-velocity test) and mean power (Wingate test) at high and low altitudes. HSES, high socioeconomic status; LSES, low socioeconomic status.

11- to 15-year-olds (figure 16.1). In 11-year-old prepubertal boys from Bolivia, when comparisons between HA and LA were made, no significant difference was observed in MP, whatever the socioeconomic level (Obert et al. 1993). The difference in the results of the two studies may be explained by the fact that in the 11-12-year-old group in the first study, puberty had already started in some boys. In fact, the difference between HA and LA boys appeared with the onset of puberty and increased in puberty (Bedu et al. 1991). For 11-year-old European boys, MP was higher (248 ± 30 W and 6.9 ± 1.0 W $\cdot$ kg^{-1} BM (body mass) than in a high socioeconomic group at LA in Bolivia (183 ± 29 W and 5.2 ± 0.7 W $\cdot$ kg^{-1} BM). This difference probably can be explained by differences in the boys' level of physical activity as will be discussed further on. In girls, irrespective of socioeconomic status, MP was higher at HA (figure 16.1) (Blonc et al. 1996).

Furthermore, PP during force-velocity tests and MP during the Wingate tests increased, respectively, by 70-80% and 0.5 W · kg⁻¹ BM a year in boys between 7 and 15 years of age at both altitudes. These increases are close to those reported by other authors in boys at LA (Bar-Or 1983; Inbar and Bar-Or 1986; Mercier et al. 1992).

Blood Lactate Concentration

The results for blood lactate concentration (collected from the earlobe after 2 min of recovery) are summarized in table 16.1 for girls and table 16.2 for boys. Except in one study, in which other results can be explained by differences in sexual maturation, blood lactate concentration was lower at HA.

Methodological Aspects of Studying the Effects of Altitude

In order to study the effect of chronic hypoxia, especially in lifelong hypoxia, it is necessary to compare two different groups of subjects, one to be studied at HA and the other at LA. Thus it is difficult to isolate only the relevant factors pertaining to the effect of hypoxia.

Table 16.1 Postexercise (2 min) Blood Lactate at High and Low Altitudes in Girls

Altitude	Age	n	Lactate (mmol·l⁻¹)	%	P	Population	Type of exercise	Ref.
HA	11	27	5.7±1.7	-10%	NS	Bolivian		
LA	11	32	6.3±1.1		NS	HSES	VO₂max	Blonc 1996
HA	11	34	5.4±1.3	-5%	NS	Bolivian		
LA	11	31	5.7±1.4			LSES		
HA	11	27	5.2±1.5	0%	NS	Bolivian		
LA	11	32	5.2±1.5			HSES	Wingate	Blonc 1996
HA	11	34	3.6±1.3	-3%	NS	Bolivian		
LA	11	31	3.7±1.2			LSES		

Table 16.2 Postexercise (2 min) Blood Lactate at High and Low Altitudes in Boys

Altitude	Age	n	Lactate (mmol·l^{-1})	%	P	Population	Type of exercise	Ref.
HA	10-13	11	7.6±0.6	+17%	NS	Bolivian	115% $\dot{V}O_2$max	Fellmann et al. 1986
LA	10-13	13	6.5±0.6			European		
HA	10-13	11	6±0.3	-10%	NS	Bolivian	$\dot{V}O_2$max	Fellmann et al. 1986
LA	10-13	13	6.7±0.5			European		
HA	11-13	14	9.2±0.5	+35%	0.005	Bolivian	$\dot{V}O_2$max	Fellmann et al. 1988
LA	10-13	20	6.8±0.5			European		
HA	11-12	15	5.7±1.8	-19%	NS	Bolivian	$\dot{V}O_2$max	Bedu et al. 1991
LA	11-12	13	7±1.7			European		
HA	14-15	13	7±1.3	-11%	NS	Bolivian	$\dot{V}O_2$max	Bedu et al. 1991
BA	14-15	15	7.9±2			European		
HA	11	23	4.9±1.5	-34%	0.001	Bolivian HSES	VO_2max	Obert et al. 1993
BA	11	48	7.4±2.1					
HA	11	44	4.8±1.4	-24%	0.001	Bolivian LSES	VO_2max	Obert et al. 1993
BA	11	30	6.3±1.5					

Group	Age	N	Value ± SD	%	p	Population	Test	Reference
HA	7-8	12	3.4±1.5	-48%	0.001	Bolivian	Wingate	Bedu et al. 1991
LA	7-8	26	6.5±2.2			European		
HA	11-12	15	6.4±1.4	-17%	NS	Bolivian	Wingate	Bedu et al. 1991
LA	11-12	13	7.7±2.3			European		
HA	14-15	13	7.5±2	-9%	NS	Bolivian	Wingate	Bedu et al. 1991
LA	14-15	15	8.2±1.3			European		
HA	11	23	5.1±1	-18%	0.001	Bolivian	Wingate	Obert et al. 1993
LA	11	48	6.2±1.4			HSES		
HA	11	44	4.6±1	-13%	0.001	Bolivian	Wingate	Obert et al. 1993
LA	11	30	5.3±1.4			LSES		
HA	10-11	16	6.2±1.5	-10%	0.01	Bolivian	Field test 30 s dash	Falgairette et al. 1994
LA	10-11	28	6.9±16			European		
HA	13-14	12	6.8±1.3	-20%	0.01	Bolivian	Field test 30 s dash	Falgairette et al. 1994
LA	13-14	41	8.5±2.3			European		
HA	10-11	16	4.7±1.3	-27%	0.001	Bolivian	Shuttle run	Falgairette et al. 1994
LA	10-11	28	6.4±1.9			European		
HA	13-14	12	6.1±2.1	-9%	0.001	Bolivian	Shuttle run	Falgairette et al. 1994
LA	13-14	41	6.7±1.7			European		

Habitual Physical Activity

Differences between high- and low-altitude performances may be the result of the difference in the level of physical activity. Ambient conditions at HA in La Paz (cold and dry climate) may lead to an increase in daily physical activity. Conversely, Santa Cruz, at LA in Bolivia, is located in a tropical zone and has a very hot and humid climate for 9 months of the year. This could induce a reduction in physical activity. Moreover, at HA in La Paz, children have to climb up and down the slopes between home and school. Nevertheless, regular physical activity, obtained by 24 hr heart rate monitoring, was not significantly different in HA and LA boys (Slooten et al. 1994). Moreover, when 24 hr heart rate was expressed as the time subjects spent above the aerobic training threshold of 50% of heart rate reserve, LA boys (70-80 min) were physically more active than HA boys (15-60 min) (Slooten et al. 1994). As a result, the differences between HA and LA boys in the study of Obert et al. (1993) could perhaps have been minimized. In contrast, in girls, the habitual physical activity, measured with the same methodology, was significantly higher at HA (45 min) than at LA (30 min). This could explain why maximal anaerobic performances were higher at HA in girls (Blonc et al. 1996).

However, it seems unlikely that a 15 to 30 min difference in intense daily physical activity can induce a change in physical performance. In fact, in prepubertal European boys (11 years old), VO_2max, PP, and MP were not significantly different between active (7 hr of physical activity) and nonactive boys (3 hr/week) (Falgairette et al. 1993).

Growth and Development

Numerous studies have shown that maximal anaerobic power during the force-velocity test (Bedu et al. 1991; Crielaard and Pirnay 1985; Sargeant and Dolan 1986) or MP during the Wingate test (Bar-Or 1983; Inbar and Bar-Or 1986), expressed in absolute terms or relative to body mass, increases with age, especially during puberty (Mercier et al. 1992). Therefore, it is essential to compare subjects at HA and LA of the same chronological and biological age. Moreover, an age-related difference in anaerobic performance cannot be explained merely by differences in body size or in active muscle mass (Mercier et al. 1992). If this is the case, then age-related differences in anaerobic performance must be explained by qualitative characteristics of the muscle. One reason is the lower activity of the rate-limiting enzyme in glycolysis, phosphofructokinase. In fact, maximal muscle lactate or in vitro phosphofructokinase activity has been found to be related to the level of sexual maturation in boys (Eriksson 1980). Also, close correlations have been observed in children between blood lactate and serum (Mero 1988) or saliva testosterone (Fellmann et al. 1986) concentration. Furthermore, effects of testosterone on anaerobic muscle metabolism have been observed in animals (Beaune, Fellmann, and Coudert 1994; Krotkiewski, Kral, and Karlsson 1980). From these studies it seems that anaerobic lactacid metabolism was not completely functional in prepubertal children. Thus, it is possible that HA hypoxia has no effect in prepubertal children (when anaerobic lactacid metabolism is not totally functional) as observed by Obert et al. (1993).

Ergometry and Learning Effects

Most of the studies cited in the preceding section were carried out using a cycle ergometer, which is useful for bioenergetic measurement in children but is not commonly used in Bolivia at either HA and LA. Many children could not pedal properly, particularly at high velocity. Many of them had never cycled and had problems of coordination. This was, however, true for both altitudes and cannot be disputed when children originating from the same country were studied. However, this could explain why MP during the Wingate test was lower at HA when comparisons were made between Bolivian children at HA and European children at LA (Bedu et al. 1991) and not significantly different when comparisons between HA and LA were made in children from Bolivia (Obert et al. 1993). In fact, for 11-year-old boys, PP and MP in European boys (Bedu et al. 1991) were higher (respectively, 9.1 ± 1.3 and 6.9 ± 1 W $\cdot$ kg^{-1} BM) than in subjects from high socioeconomic groups, at approximately the same age, at LA (Obert et al. 1993) in Bolivia (7.1 ± 1 and 5.2 ± 0.7 W $\cdot$ kg^{-1}).

However, the ergometer used cannot explain all the difference observed between HA and LA, because differences persist in running field tests (Falgairette et al. 1994).

Comparing the Effects of Altitude on Children and Adults

It is difficult to extrapolate mechanical power output measured during short-term maximal exercises to cellular metabolism or structural muscle. The biochemical significance of the performance during force-velocity and 30 s Wingate tests remains unclear because all the energy sources (phosphagen depletion, anaerobic glycolysis, and aerobic metabolism) are involved.

Alactacid Metabolism at High Altitude

In spite of a glycolysis participation (Jacobs et al. 1983; Mercier, Mercier, and Préfaut 1991), it is generally acknowledged that short-term maximal exercise (force-velocity, 30 m field test) depends mainly on the available stores of adenosine triphosphate (ATP) and phosphocreatine sources. In boys, PP during the force-velocity test (Bedu et al. 1991; Obert et al. 1993) and performance in a very short dash exercise (30 m running) (Falgairette et al. 1994) were not affected by hypoxia. This is in agreement with data reported in adults. In fact, PP during the vertical jump was not impaired by acute or chronic hypoxia (di Prampero, Mognoni, and Veicsteinas 1982; Ferretti, Hauser, and di Prampero 1990; Narici et al. 1992). In acute hypoxia (Blonc et al. 1994; McLellan, Kavanagh, and Jacobs 1990) such as after acclimatization (di Prampero, Mognoni, and Veicsteinas 1982), PP during short, intensive cycle ergometer exercise was unchanged. Moreover, after 24 or 48 hr at simulated hypobaric altitude of 4570 m (Young et al. 1980) or after 4 weeks' acclimatization to 5050 (Narici et al. 1992), isometric contraction force was not affected by hypoxia.

Anaerobic Glycolysis at High Altitude

The main problem at altitude is associated with the glycolytic pathways. In adults, conflicting studies of the effect of HA on glycolysis have been reported (Coudert 1992). These discrepancies depend on the different experimental conditions and on the indirect parameters measured to assess this metabolism.

From records at the Mexican Olympic Games, altitude 2270 m, short-distance performances (< 400 m) were not altered when the reduction in air density is taken into account (Péronnet, Thibault, and Cousineau 1971).

In acute hypoxia in adults at a simulated altitude of 3400 m, O_2 debt after maximal exercise did not change (Linnarson 1974); at altitudes above 4000 m, O_2 debt increased (Asmussen, Döbeln, and Nielsen 1948; Knuttgen and Saltin 1973). In chronic hypoxia, O_2 debt was unchanged at LA (<3000 m) (Cunningham and Magel 1970; Pugh 1967) and decreased or was unchanged at 3700 m (Raynaud et al. 1974).

In adults, after 3 weeks at 6542 m, MP during the Wingate test decreased significantly from 453 ± 107 W to 406 ± 141 W, but remained unchanged according to body mass (loss of 6.3 kg) (Richalet et al. 1992). In six high-altitude-adapted Andean natives (Matheson et al. 1991) (lifetime residents at 3700-4500 m), MP (341 ± 18 W and 5.7 ± 0.3 W $\cdot$ kg^{-1}) was significantly lower compared to that of sedentary, power-trained, or endurance-trained subjects (6.5 ± 0.5, 8.8 ± 0.5, and 8.2 ± 0.6 W $\cdot$ kg^{-1}, respectively). In students (24 years old) lifetime resident in La Paz, we measured (unpublished observation), during the Wingate test, a MP of 7.1 ± 1.2 W $\cdot$ kg^{-1}, which was lower than the value observed in students of the same age at sea level: 8.3 ± 0.5 W $\cdot$ kg^{-1}. A possible explanation for a lower MP during the Wingate test under chronic hypoxia is a reduced aerobic participation. The relative energy contribution of aerobic metabolism during this test was high (25-30%), particularly in children (Van Praagh et al. 1991), and the difference in MP between HA and LA was associated with a decrease in O_2 consumption (Bedu et al. 1991). In acute hypoxia, MP during the Wingate test and also O_2 consumption remained unchanged (Blonc et al. 1994).

Another important observation at HA is a lower blood lactate concentration postexercise. This was not observed in acute hypoxia (Bender et al. 1989; Blonc et al. 1994), but occurred during acclimatization (Bender et al. 1989). This reduction in peak lactate accumulation in blood was observed in adults (Cerretelli, Veicsteinas, and Marconi 1982; Kayser et al. 1993) and also in children (tables 16.1 and 16.2) during recovery after different types of exercise (maximal or supramaximal exercises, Wingate test, field tests). Studies using measurements of net lactate flux (Bender et al. 1989) or isotopic tracers (Brooks et al. 1992) support lower muscle lactate production under chronic hypoxia. Several hypotheses have been put forward to explain this phenomenon. One of these is restriction of the maximal flux of substrates along the glycolytic pathway. However, in most studies, the maximal potential activity of key glycolytic enzymes was unchanged in chronic hypoxia compared with normoxia (Howald et al. 1990; Reynafarge 1962; Young et al. 1984). A second possibility is reduced blood buffering capacity. Cerretelli, Veicsteinas, and Marconi (1982) hypothesized that the reduced maximal glycolytic flux could be associated with a reduced buffer capacity consequential to renal compensation of the respiratory alkalosis secondary to hypoxic hyperventilation. The reduced blood buffering capacity was observed in altitudes above 5000 m, but for altitudes under 4000 m the decrease in bicarbonate buffering capacity was compensated by an increase in hemoglobin buffering capacity (Lefrançois et al. 1972). Moreover, lactate concentration did not change after the administration of $NaHCO3$ (Grassi et al. 1995; Kayser et al. 1993). Finally, in the presence of a presumably normal maximal potential activity of glycolytic enzymes, Grassi et al. (1995) hypothesized that the reduced lactate concentration is indicative of an upstream inhibition of glycolysis at altitude. This could be a decrease in β-adrenergic stimulation of glycolysis (Bender et al. 1989; Young et al. 1991) or a reduction in neuromuscular activation (Kayser et al. 1994).

Hochachka and coworkers (Hochachka et al. 1991) have postulated that high-altitude natives may have undergone a number of functional and structural adaptations, namely by maximizing (a) the amount of ATP obtained per mole of fuel substrate metabolized (decreased contribution of anaerobic pathways); (b) the amount of ATP obtained per mole of O_2 consumed (preferential use of carbohydrate); and (c) the work achieved per mole ATP used (increased work efficiency). But these assumptions are subject to controversy (Favier et al. 1995).

In conclusion, anaerobic metabolism during short, intense exercise is not affected at an altitude of 3700 m in prepubertal boys and girls when other factors such as nutritional deprivation or levels of physical activity are taken into account. The effect of HA hypoxia in postpubescent children requires further investigation. The lower postexercise blood lactate concentration observed in children and adults in chronic HA hypoxia has received no valid explanation.

Directions for Future Research

In prepubertal boys and girls, performance during short, intense exercise is not affected by lifelong hypoxia. However, anaerobic metabolism is not completely functional in prepubertal children. Thus it is possible that HA hypoxia could have an effect on postpubertal children and adolescents.

Some differences are observed with regard to the effect of chronic hypoxia between boys and girls. More studies on girls are needed.

Strength trainability during childhood has been studied at sea level, but no data exist on the effect of training at HA in pre- and postpubescent children.

The lower postexercise blood lactate concentration observed in children and in adults in chronic HA hypoxia has received no valid explanation. Now, it is possible with nuclear magnetic resonance spectroscopy to investigate the lactate metabolism in situ during exercise. Studies on children have been conducted in La Paz at 3700 m. More data are needed at greater altitude.

Summary

The decrease in maximal aerobic power, during both acute and chronic HA exposure, is well documented in adults, as in children. Conflicting studies of the effect of HA on anaerobic metabolism have been reported in adults. In collaboration with the members of the Instituto Boliviano de Biologia de Altura in La Paz (3700 m), we have investigated the effect of chronic hypoxia on parameters related to anaerobic metabolism.

At similar ages (10-15 years old), there was no significant difference between HA and LA boys in mean running velocity in a 30 m sprint. However, the average speed calculated in a 30 s shuttle run was significantly lower in HA than in LA boys.

When related to percentage VO_2max, the O_2 debt of 50 boys and girls aged 10 to 13 years who had been born at HA was similar to that of 25 French children at LA. Ventilatory and lactic anaerobic threshold were detected approximately at 70-75% VO_2max at both altitudes.

No significant difference was found in PP (force-velocity test) expressed either in absolute terms or relative to body mass between Bolivian boys at HA and European boys at LA, or between Bolivian boys at HA and LA. Moreover, MP (Wingate test) was significantly reduced at HA for 11- to 15-year-old boys. However, in 11-year-old prepubescent boys from Bolivia, no significant difference was observed in MP, whatever the socioeconomic level.

As in adults, we observed that postexercise (2 min) blood lactate concentration was lower at HA, in children, whatever the type of exercise (field test, VO_2max, Wingate test).

In conclusion, anaerobic metabolism during short, intense exercise is not affected at an altitude of 3700 m in prepubescent boys. The effect of HA in postpubescent children requires further investigation.

References

Asmussen, E., Döbeln, W.V., and Nielsen, M. 1948. Blood lactate and oxygen debt after exhaustive work at different oxygen tensions. *Acta Physiol. Scand.* 15: 57-62.

Bar-Or, O., ed. 1983. *Pediatric sports medicine for the practitioner. From physiologic principles to clinical application.* New York: Springer-Verlag.

Beaune, B., Fellmann, N., and Coudert, J. 1994. Effects of orchiectomy on EDL muscle ultrastructure and energy-supplying enzymes in the growing male guinea pig. *Am. J. Physiol.* 256, *Cell Physiol.* 35: C143-C148.

Bedu, M., Fellmann, N., Spielvogel, H., Falgairette, G., Van Praagh, E., and Coudert, J. 1991. Force-velocity and 30s Wingate tests in boys at high and low altitudes. *J. Appl. Physiol.* 70(3): 1031-1037.

Bender, P.R., Groves, B.M., McCullough, R.E., McCullough, R.G., Trad, L., Young, A.J., Cymerman, A., and Reeves, J.J. 1989. Decrease exercise muscle lactate release after high altitude acclimatization. *J. Appl. Physiol.* 67(4): 1456-1462.

Bert, P. 1878. *La pression barométrique.* Paris: Masson.

Blonc, S., Falgairette, G., Bedu, M., Fellmann, N., Spielvogel, H., and Coudert, J. 1994. The effect of acute hypoxia at low altitude and acute normoxia at high altitude on performance during a 30-s Wingate test in children, *Int. J. Sports Med.* 15(7): 403-407.

Blonc, S., Fellmann, N., Bedu, M., Falgairette, G., de Jonge, R., Obert, P., Beaune, B., Spielvogel, H., Tellez, W., Quintela, A., San miguel, J.L., and Coudert, J. 1996. Effect of altitude and marginal malnutrition on maximal oxygen uptake and anaerobic power in prepubertal Bolivians girls. *J. Appl. Physiol.* 80(6): 2002-2008.

Brooks, G., Wolfel, E., Groves, B., Bender, P., Butterfield, G., Cymerman, A., Mazzeo, R., Sutton, J., Wolfe, R., and Reeves, J. 1992. Muscle accounts for glucose disposal but not blood lactate appearance during exercise after acclimatization to 4,300m. *J. Appl. Physiol.* 72: 2435-2445.

Cerretelli, P., and di Prampero, P.E. 1985. Aerobic and anaerobic metabolism during exercise at altitude. In *High altitude deterioration,* ed. E. Jokl and M. Hebbelinck, 1-19. Basel: Karger, Medicine and Sport Science.

Cerretelli, P., Veicsteinas, A., and Marconi, C. 1982. Anaerobic metabolism at high altitude: the lactacid mechanism. In *High altitude physiology and medicine,* ed. W. Brendel and R.A. Zink, 94-102. New York: Springer-Verlag.

Coudert, J. 1992. Anaerobic performance at altitude. *Int. J. Sports Med.* 13(suppl.): S82-S85.

Crielaard, J.M., and Pirnay, F. 1985. Etude longitudinale des puissances aerobie et anaérobie alactique. *Med. du Sport* T591: 4-6.

Cunningham, D.A., and Magel, J.R. 1970. The effect of moderate altitude on post exercise blood lactate. *Internationale Zeitschrist Für Angeewandte Physiology* 29: 94-100.

di Prampero, P.E., Mognoni, P., and Veicsteinas, A. 1982. The effect of hypoxia on maximal anaerobic alactic power in man. In *High altitude physiology and medicine,* ed. W. Brendel and R.A. Zink, 88-93. New York: Springer-Verlag.

Eriksson, B.O. 1980. Muscle metabolism in children. A Review. *Acta Paediatr. Scand.* 283(suppl.): 20-27.

Falgairette, G., Bedu, M., Fellmann, N., Spielvogel, H., Van Praagh, E., Obert, P., and Coudert, J. 1994. Evaluation of physical fitness from field tests at high altitude in circumpubertal boys, comparison with laboratory data. *Eur. J. Appl. Physiol.* 69: 36-43.

Falgairette, G., Duche, P., Bedu, M., Fellmann, N., and Coudert, J. 1993. Bioenergetic characteristics in prepubertal swimmers: comparison with active and non active boys. *Int. J. Sports Med.* 14(7): 444-448.

Favier, R., Spielvogel, H., Desplanches, D., Ferretti, G., Kayser, B., and Hoppeler, H. 1995. Maximal exercise performance in chronic hypoxia and acute normoxia in high altitude natives. *J. Appl. Physiol.* 78(5): 1868-1874.

Fellmann, N., Bedu, M., Spielvogel, H., Falgairette, G., Van Praagh, E., and Coudert, J. 1986. Oxygen debt in submaximal and supramaximal exercise in children at high and low altitude. *J. Appl. Physiol.* 601: 209-215.

Fellmann, N., Bedu, M., Spielvogel, H., Falgairette, G., Van Praagh, E., Jarrige, J.F., and Coudert, J. 1988. Anaerobic metabolism during pubertal development at high altitude. *J. Appl. Physiol.* 64(4): 1382-1386.

Ferretti, G., Hauser, H., and di Prampero, P.E. 1990. Maximal muscular power before and after exposure to chronic hypoxia. *Int. J. Sports Med.* 11(1): 531-534.

Grassi, B., Ferretti, G., Kayser, B., Marzorati, M., Colombini, A., Marconi, C., and Cerretelli, P. 1995. Maximal rate of blood lactate accumulation during exercise at altitude in human. *J. Appl. Physiol.* 79(1): 331-339.

Greksa, L.P., Haas, J.D., Leatherman, T.L., Spielvogel, H., Paz zamora, M., Paredes fernandez, L., and Moreno-black, G. 1982. Maximal aerobic power in trained youths at high altitude. *Ann. Hum. Biol.* 9: 201-209.

Hochachka, P.W.C., Stanley, C., Matheson, G.O., McKenzie, D.C., Allen, P.S., and Parkhouse, W.S. 1991. Metabolic and work efficiencies during exercise in Andean natives. *J. Appl. Physiol.* 70: 1720-1730.

Howald, H., Pette, D., Simoneau, J.A., Uber, A., Hoppeler, H., and Cerretelli, P. 1990. Effects of chronic hypoxia on muscle enzymes activities. *Int. J. Sports Med.* 11: 510-514.

Inbar, O., and Bar-Or, O. 1986. Anaerobic characteristics in male children and adolescents. *Med. Sci. Sports Exerc.* 18(3): 264-269.

Jacobs, I., Tesch, P.A., Bar-Or, O., Karlsson, J., and Dotan, R. 1983. Lactate in human skeletal muscle after 10 and 30s of supramaximal exercise. *J. Appl. Physiol.* 55(2): 365-367.

Kayser, B., Ferretti, G., Grassi, B., Binzoni, T., and Cerretelli, P. 1993. Maximal lactic capacity at altitude: effect of bicarbonate loading. *J. Appl. Physiol.* 75: 1070-1074.

Kayser, B., Narici, M., Binzoni, T., Grassi, B., and Cerretelli, P. 1994. Fatigue and exhaustion in chronic hypobaric hypoxia: influence of exercising muscle mass. *J. Appl. Physiol.* 76: 634-640.

Knuttgen, H.G., and Saltin, B. 1973. Oxygen uptake, muscle high energy phosphates and lactate in exercise under acute hypoxia condition in man. *Acta Physiol. Scand.* 87: 368-376.

Krotkiewski, M., Kral, J.G., and Karlsson, J. 1980. Effects of castration and testosterone substitution on body composition and muscle metabolism in rats. *Acta Physiol. Scand.* 109: 233-237.

Lefrançois, R., Gauthier, H., Pasquis, P., Cevaer, A.H., Hellot, M.F., and Leroy, J. 1972. Chemoreflex ventilatory response to CO_2 in man at low and high altitudes. *Resp. Physiol.* 14: 296-306.

Linnarson, D. 1974. Muscle metabolites and oxygen deficit with exercise in hypoxia and hyperoxia. *J. Appl. Physiol.* 36(4): 399-402.

Matheson, G.O., Allen, P.S., Ellinger, D.C., Hanstock, C.C., Gheorghin, D., McKenzie, D.C., Stanley, C., Parkhouse, W.S., and Hochachka, P.W. 1991. Skeletal muscle metabolism and work capacity: a 31P-NMR study of Andean natives and lowlanders. *J. Appl. Physiol.* 70: 1963-1976.

McLellan, T.M., Kavanagh, M.F, and Jacobs, I. 1990. The effect of hypoxia on performance during 30s or 45s of supramaximal exercise. *Eur. J. Appl. Physiol.* 60: 155-161.

Mercier, B., Mercier, J., Granier, P., Le Gallais, D., and Préfaut, C. 1992. Maximal anaerobic power: relationship to anthropometric characteristics during growth. *Int. J. Sports Med.* 13: 21-26.

Mercier, J., Mercier, B., and Préfaut, C. 1991. Blood lactate increase during the force velocity exercise test. *Int. J. Sports Med.* 12: 17-20.

Mero, A. 1988. Blood lactate production and recovery from anaerobic exercise in trained and untrained boys. *Eur. J. Appl. Physiol.* 57: 660-666.

Narici, M., Kayser, B., Cibella, F., Grassi, B., and Cerretelli, P. 1992. No changes in body composition and maximum alactic anaerobic performance during a 4 week sojourn at altitude. *Int. J. Sports Med.* 13: 87.

Obert, P., Bedu, M., Fellmann, N., Falgairette, G., Beaune, B., Quintela, A., Van Praagh, E., Spielvogel, H., Kemper, H., Post, B., Parent, G., and Coudert, J. 1993. Effect of chronic hypoxia and socioeconomic status on $\dot{V}O_2$max and anaerobic power of Bolivian boys. *J. Appl. Physiol.* 74(2): 888-896.

Péronnet, F., Thibault, G., and Cousineau, D.D.L. 1971. A theoretical analysis of the effect of altitude on running performance. *J. Appl. Physiol.* 70: 399-404.

Pugh, L.G.C.E. 1967. Athletes at altitude. *J. Physiol.* (London) 192: 619-646.

Raynaud, J., Martineaud, J.P., Bordachar, J., Tillous, M.C., and Durand, J. 1974. Oxygen deficit and debt in submaximal exercise at sea level and high altitude. *J. Appl. Physiol.* 37: 43-48.

Reynafarge, B. 1962. Myoglobine content and enzymatic activity of muscle and altitude adaptation. *J. Appl. Physiol.* 17: 301-305.

Richalet, J.P., Marchal, M., Lamberto, C., Letronc, J.L., Anthezana, A.M., and Cauchy, E. 1992. Alteration of aerobic and anaerobic performance after 3 weeks at 6542m (Mt Sajama). *Int. J. Sports Med.* 13: 86.

Sargeant, A.J., and Dolan, P. 1986. Optimal velocity of muscle contraction for short term (anaerobic) power output in children and adults. In *Children and exercise XII*, ed. J. Rutenfranz, R. Mocellin, and F. Klimt, 39-42. Champaign, IL: Human Kinetics.

Slooten, J., Kemper, H.C.G., Post, G.B., Lujan, C., and Coudert, J. 1994. Habitual physical activity in 10 to 12-year-old Bolivian boys: the relation between altitude and socioeconomic status. *Int. J. Sports Med.* 15(suppl. 2): S106-S111.

Van Praagh, E., Bedu, M., Falgairette, G., Fellmann, N., and Coudert, J. 1991. Oxygen uptake during a 30s supramaximal exercise in 7 to 15 year old boys. In *Children and exercise XV,* ed. R. Frenkl and I. Szmodis, 281-87. Budapest: Nevi.

Young, A.J., Evans, W.J., Fisher, E.C., Sharp, P.L., Costill, D.L., and Maher, J.T. 1984. Skeletal muscle metabolism of sea level natives following short term altitude residence. *Eur. J. Appl. Physiol.* 52: 463-466.

Young, A.J., Wright, J., Knapik, J., and Cymerman, A. 1980. Skeletal muscle strength during exposure to hypobaric hypoxia. *Med. Sci. Sports Exerc.* 12(5): 330-335.

Young, A.J., Young, P.M., McCullough, R.E., Moore, L.G., Cymerman, A., and Reeves, J.T. 1991. Effect of ß-adrenergic blockade on plasma lactate concentration during exercise at high altitude. *Eur. J. Appl. Physiol.* 63: 315-322.

17

CHAPTER

Trends and Future Research Directions in Pediatric Anaerobic Performance

Emmanuel Van Praagh

This volume constitutes a concerted effort by leading pediatric research scientists to summarize the available literature and introduce new concepts, methodologies, and results with respect to developmental anaerobic performance. In anaerobic tasks or sports events such as sprint running, swimming, cycling, jumping, or throwing, the child's performance is distinctly lower than that of the adult. This partly reflects the child's lesser ability to generate mechanical energy from chemical energy sources during short-term intensive work or exercise. Anaerobic fitness and performance are quantitative traits influenced by several factors such as age, sex, motivation, training, and physical environment. However, anaerobic performance is also determined by innate biological and mechanical variables.

General Trends in Research: What Is Known

As has been shown throughout this text, much progress has been made in understanding and assessing the research that has been done in the area of pediatric anaerobic performance. Significant findings have contributed to greater knowledge of this often overlooked but important area of study.

Developmental Issues

Recent research on developmental issues has shown that the wide variation in anaerobic fitness among children and adolescents can be attributed largely to inheritance. Genetic factors account for approximately 50% of the total variance in anaerobic performance phenotype. It has been well documented that the child's growth is not only determined by genetic factors but is also reliant on mechanical ones. The interaction of biological and mechanical constraints is of considerable importance in shaping the infant's motor performance. Physical growth signifies changes in mass, mass distribution, and the forces associated with moving masses. It can be shown that relief from biomechanical demands leads to precocious movement behavior. Thus, the latter enlarges the infant's motor repertoire and must be viewed as an important step in a young person's increasing ability to functionally employ and master muscular and nonmuscular forces (e.g., motion-dependent forces and gravitational forces).

As muscle fibers increase in length, growth occurs due to an increase in the number of sarcomeres, which appear to be added to the ends of the myofibrils. Animal studies have shown that muscle immobilization in a lengthened position produces 20% to 30% more sarcomeres in series and thus more power, whereas immobilization in a shortened position results in a loss of 40% of the muscle's sarcomeres in series, accompanied by a substantial power loss. It is therefore important to increase flexibility during the growing years. In a population of over 1500 children, it was observed that those exhibiting continual low back pain were also those associated with a decrease in lumbar extension and straight leg raising. In the increasing number of youth competitions, such as those in gymnastics, dance, ice skating, and diving, a full range of movement is necessary not only for peak athletic performance, but also for prevention of joint and muscle injuries. Anaerobic performance increases continuously with age, reaching peak levels in the second or third decade of life. Sex differences are evident in late childhood and early adolescence.

Physiological Assessment

The increase of anaerobic capabilities during development and maturation is a fundamental aspect of the child's physical capacity. In the past, however, its measurement and interpretation were relatively neglected in comparison with aerobic power. In adults, impressive progress has been made in understanding muscle mechanics and energetics. It has now become possible to show that a complex set of genes control the expression of contractile properties. For example, it is the (iso-)form of the myosin heavy chain that is expressed that seems to be the primary determinant of muscle fiber's maximum shortening and hence defining power. Undoubtedly, the development of more sophisticated equipment (e.g., magnetic resonance imaging [MRI] and spectroscopy [MRS]) will allow pediatric exercise scientists to approach the relationship between anaerobic function and growth at a molecular level.

Over the years, various attempts have been made to quantify the anaerobic energy yield in short-term exercise, but many assumptions have had to be made with respect to mechanical efficiency, lactate turnover, dilution space for lactate, and so on. Measurement of the accumulated oxygen deficit at the onset of exercise has been used as an alternative method to estimate the anaerobic capacity of the individual. Despite some methodological difficulties, this method seems promising and appropriate, especially for untrained and pediatric populations. The assumed lower glycolytic response to maximal and supramaximal exercise during growth is manifested by a lower postexercise lactate concentration in muscle or blood. Blood lactate illustrates all those processes by which lactate is produced and eliminated. Therefore, postexercise blood lactate provides only a qualitative indication of the degree of stress placed on anaerobic metabolism by a particular exercise bout, not a quantitative measure of glycolysis. In the intact human, making direct measurements on the rate or capacity of anaerobic pathways for energy turnover presents several ethical and methodological difficulties. Thus, rather than measure energy supply, investigators have concentrated on measuring force or short-term power by means of standardized tests.

Isokinetic strength-testing equipment is often employed to obtain quantitative information with respect to the muscle contraction capabilities of the child and adolescent. The isokinetic parameters most frequently assessed are maximum joint moment, reciprocal muscle group ratio, bilateral muscle group ratio, and muscle endurance. Isokinetic dynamometry allows accurate objective quantification of muscle strength. Anaerobic tests, which use mechanical power as their criterion, can be divided in two categories: (1) maximal short-term power (MSTP) tests, those that measure mechanical energy yield during overall exercises (jumping, cycling, running, etc.) of very short duration (ranging from a few milliseconds to 40 s) and (2) maximal short-term athletic power (MSTAP) tests, those that measure mechanical energy yield during specific sport patterns (ball throwing, ball kicking, sprint starts, "dunks," high jump, etc.).

Anaerobic Trainability

In recent years, chronic physiological responses of children engaged in anaerobic training programs have received increasing interest from both practitioners and scientists. As children are more and more involved in training and competitions, it is important to screen not only the child's training potential but also the long-term effects of excessive training procedures, for example. Overuse injuries due to repetitive microtrauma represent a new spectrum in this area. Recognition of the risk factors of injury, combined with appropriate modification, diversification of training programs, and adequate conditioning, allows adolescents to compete effectively and safely in anaerobic events. Carefully supervised strength training has the potential of improving sports performances, enhancing body composition, and reducing sports injury rates and rehabilitation time following injury.

With appropriate technical instruction, proper exercise prescription, and supervision, strength training does not appear to be a particularly dangerous activity for most children in terms of health or injury risk. However, caution is warranted for disabled children. This group should be closely supervised and monitored by a physician trained in pediatric sports medicine. Moreover, strength training should be recommended as only one of a variety of physical activity and sport pursuits for the child. Direct observations on prepubertal children during leisure-time activities or games have shown that the average duration of these short-burst spontaneous activities is only of about 6 s. The average recovery interval between these short-term activities is only three times longer. Coordination, motor skills, speed, and power improve significantly during childhood, together with the rapid development of the nervous system. In spite of limited research, it is apparent that training accelerates speed and power improvement during puberty. Increasing training and competitions in organized sports puts enormous physical and psychological pressure on youngsters. The adolescent athlete can achieve levels of performance equal to or better than those of many adult counterparts.

Clinical and Environmental Limitations

Exertion can be deleterious to a child's health under certain circumstances. In some types of disease, parents or patients assume that exercise entails a risk that in fact is minimal or nonexistent. Even when some risk is involved, the detrimental psychological and physical effects of inactivity probably outweigh those of activity. This is particularly important for the sick or disabled child, where physical hypoactivity may render the child irreversibly immobile. It is well known that children with a neuromuscular disease have significantly lower endurance capacities compared with the general child population. In contrast, there are very little data regarding their lower anaerobic fitness. The latter probably sets greater limitations on their daily activities and physical abilities. Participation in physical education classes or athletic training of the asthmatic child is among the everyday concerns of educational and health care professionals. Even if recent reports have shown that the percentage of asthmatic athletes participating in elite sport events is continually increasing, parents and most physicians are still reluctant to allow the asthmatic child to try to enhance his or her anaerobic fitness.

Current investigations into the effects of anaerobic training during growth have shown an increase in muscle power, greater postexercise bronchospasm control, and an improved self-image. Chronic undernutrition of a moderate nature is a widespread problem in many parts of the world. In these undernourished children, reduced size, linked with decreased fat and muscle mass, has a negative effect on physical anaerobic fitness. However, factors other than body size alone should be taken into account in relation to this lower anaerobic ability during growth and development. Lower qualitative muscle composition, poor hygienic conditions associated with high incidence of infectious disease and intestinal parasitosis, and social and cultural factors may all partially explain the significant diminution of anaerobic fitness. In children as in adults, it is well known that maximal aerobic power is decreased during both acute and chronic high-altitude exposure. In adult studies, conflicting results have been reported concerning the effect of high-altitude stress on anaerobic metabolism. However, very little research has been undertaken into children who are physiologically adapted to living at altitudes of more than 3500 m. It is suggested in this volume that high-altitude stress does not affect the anaerobic fitness of the young child.

Directions for Future Research: What We Would Like to Know

There are many determinants of anaerobic performance, and pediatric exercise scientists have devoted considerable efforts toward understanding phenotypic variation in size and body composition, strength, velocity, power, and capacity. These efforts include not only the effects of training and practice, but also age- and sex-associated variations. Of course, training and practice are important environmental components of the genotype-environment interaction. However, little research has been done on the contribution of genes to anaerobic performance phenotypic characteristics.

To encompass the accumulated knowledge on anaerobic function during growth is no small task when one considers the scope of the few published research documents in this area. Investigations range from systematic observations of functional adaptations in response to the stress of anaerobic exercise, to assessment of morphological changes following physical training. Recent investigations in genetics, structural adaptations at the cellular level, motor development, and the like have added new dimensions to our understanding of the physiological adjustments in pediatric populations.

The pediatric exercise scientist must work within two major constraints, one ethical and the other methodological. Not all techniques justifiable for use with adults can be applied to children. Therefore, in the healthy child, noninvasive techniques and procedures that will not induce any pain or damage must be developed. Whereas muscle biopsy is often used in adult athletic populations, very few investigators would dare to use it with healthy children. Fortunately, amazing progress is being made at the moment in the development of molecular biology tools that can be used in, for example, the genetic dissection of human performance phenotypes. Noninvasive power tools like MRI and MRS are presently used by research scientists to assess fiber type in skeletal muscles, for example, or to determine possible differences in phosphorus compounds between fast-glycolytic and slow-oxidative fiber types. Undoubtedly these tools will give us more information in the near future regarding the anaerobic capabilities of the growing child.

To conclude, I hope that the publication of this book will fill an apparent need for current information and give the reader more insight into this particularly exciting education and research domain.

Index

A

acceleration, in sprint running, 164-165
acclimatization, 337-338
accumulated oxygen deficit (AOD)
  advantages of testing with children, 131-133
  aerobic and anaerobic contributions to, 124-126
  measurement issues, 121-124, 126-127, 129-131, 131 table 6.3
  as measure of capacity, 120, 126
  results with pediatric subjects, 127, 128 table 6.2
  sample calculation of, 122 fig. 6.2
  and supramaximal work, 123 fig. 6.3, 130-131
accumulated oxygen demand, 125 fig. 6.4
active tension, 103
acute hypoxia, 338
acute plasticity, 111
acute traumatic dislocations, 278-281
acute traumatic injuries, 271, 276-281
adaptation, 338
adenosine diphosphate (ADP), 98
adenosine triphosphate (ATP), 98-99, 106, 119-120, 156, 251
aerobic contribution
  to accumulated oxygen deficit (AOD), 124-126
  to energy supply, 99-100, 100 fig. 5.1
aerobic fitness, in asthmatic children, 315
age
  AOD results profile by, 127-129
  and flexibility, 87
  isokinetic dynamometry and, 236
  peak anaerobic power differences with, 54
  peak power increases with, 47-49
  and postexercise lactates, 146-147
  strength development differences, 194-195
alactacid metabolism, 345-346

alternate stepping, in infants, 36-38
altitude. *See also* high altitude
  child-adult effects comparisons, 345-347
  studying effects of, 341-345
American Academy of Orthopaedic Surgeons, 70-71, 73-74, 82
American Alliance for Health, Physical Education, Recreation and Dance (AAHPERD)
  Fitness Test Manual (1984), 76-77
  Health Related Fitness Test, 66, 80
amperometric assays, 140
anaerobic alactic energy, 99
anaerobic capacity
  definition of, 45-46, 119-120
  direct measurements of, 157
  measurement methods, 46
  physiological assessment, 354-355
  profiles in pediatric populations, 127-129
  testing children and youth, 46-47
anaerobic contribution
  to accumulated oxygen deficit (AOD), 124-126
  to energy supply, 99-102, 100 fig. 5.1
anaerobic glycolysis
  as anaerobic lactic energy, 99
  in asthmatic children, 312
  at high altitude, 346-347
  and phosphofructokinase (PFK), 55
anaerobic lactic energy, 99
anaerobic performance
  child-adult comparisons, 54-55
  determinants of, 55-60
  heritability of, 6-8, 8-15, 16-18
  and hypoxia, 338-341
  and malnutrition, 321-326
  and neuromuscular diseases, 291-293, 293-297, 299-300
  training effects on, 15-16
  variance components of phenotypes, 18 fig. 1.7

About the Editor

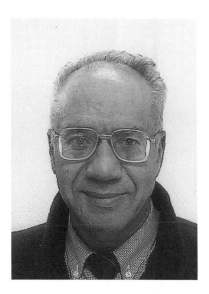

Emmanuel Van Praagh, PhD, is a professor of exercise physiology at the Université Blaise Pascal in Clermont-Ferrand, France. His major research interest lies in the field of children's cardiorespiratory and anaerobic fitness, and he has published more than 100 research and scholarly articles on these subjects.

Dr. Van Praagh served as chair of the anaerobic metabolic sessions during several Pediatric Work Physiology Congresses. He is a journals referee for the *International Journal of Sports Medicine, Pediatric Exercise Science,* and *Science & Sport.* He is also a Fellow of the American College of Sports Medicine and the European College of Sport Science as well as a member of the French Société de Physiologie, the European Group of Pediatric Work Physiology, and the North American Society of Pediatric Exercise Medicine.

A former French champion and record holder in the 400-meter hurdles, Dr. Van Praagh was selected for Olympic and European track and field events. In 1988 he received his PhD in physiology from the Université de Poitiers. He lives near Clermont-Ferrand in the heart of France, where he enjoys running, cross-country skiing, golfing, and playing jazz guitar.

About the Contributors

Neil Armstrong is Professor of Health and Exercise Sciences and Director of the Children's Health and Exercise Research Centre at the University of Exeter. Professor Armstrong is a Fellow of the British Association of Sport and Exercise Sciences (BASES), the European College of Sports Science, and the American College of Sports Medicine. A former Chair of BASES, he has edited five books on physical education and pediatric exercise science and co-authored *Young People and Physical Activity* with Dr. Joanne Welsman. On the topics of physical education and pediatric exercise science, Professor Armstrong has published almost 300 papers and made over 300 presentations at national and international conferences.

Vasilios Baltzopoulos completed his PhD in Biomechanics on Dynamic Knee Joint Function Modeling in Isokinetics in the Department of Movement Science in the Faculaty of Medicine at the University of Liverpool. His is currently a Reader in Biomechanics in the Department of Exercise and Sport Science at the Manchester Metropolitan University and is leader of the biomechanics group. His main research interests include biomechanical data processing and musculoskeletal modeling, most specifically in modeling of dynamic joint and muscle function using different imaging techniques, such as video x-ray, magnetic resonance imaging, and ultrasonography. He has written review papers and book chapters on isokinetic dynomometry and various research papers on muscle and joint function as well as in biomechanical data processing.

Oded Bar-Or is a Professor of Pediatrics and Director of the Children's Exercise and Nutrition Centre at McMaster University in Hamilton, Ontario. He was the founder and director of the Department of Research and Sports Medicine at the Wingate Institute in Israel, where he led the team that developed the Wingate Anaerobic Test. He has published extensively on responses of children to exercise in health and disease and has written and edited several books.

Mario Bedu is a specialist in respiratory physiology and sports medicine. He is an associate professor in the Department of Physiology and Sports Biology at the Faculty of Medicine at the University of Clermont-Ferrand, France. Professor Bedu is a member of the French Société de Physiologie and also of the European Group of Pediatric Work Physiology. His pastimes include hiking, collecting fungus, canoeing, and woodworking.

Sig Berven is a senior resident in the Harvard Combined Orthopaedic Program. His research interests have included the genetic basis of adolescent idiopathic scoliosis and the molecular basis of osteanagenesis in limb lengthening. He recently completed a Moseley Fellowship for research in orthopaedics conducted at the Nuffield Orthopaedic Center in Oxford, England. In the future, he will be training as a fellow in spine surgery at the University of California at San Francisco.

Cameron J. R. Blimkie has just recently been appointed Professor and Foundation Chair of Pediatric Sport and Exercise Science at the Children's Hospital Institute of Sports Medicine, the New Children's Hospital, and the Australian Catholic University, all in Sydney, Australia. His research interest has, and continues to center on, the effects of physical activity, exercise, and sport on growth and development of the neuromuscular, skeletal, and cardiovascular systems both in healthy children and in children with various pediatric diseases and disabilities. He hopes to apply recent advances in magnetic resonance imaging and spectroscopy to investigate ultrastructural and biomechanical adaptations of bone and muscle, respectively, in exercising children.

Krisanne Bothner received her PhD in motor control from the University of Oregon where her research focused on the kinetics of postural recovery following disturbances of balance. Currently, Dr. Bothner is a clinical biomechanist at the Center for Human Kinetic Study, a gait laboratory affiliated with Mary Free Bed Hospital and Rehabilitation Center and Grand Valley State University in Grand Rapids, Michigan.

Claude Bouchard is a professor in the Division of Kinesiology and Department of Social and Preventive Medicine at Laval University in Quebec City, Canada. He is a fellow of the American College of Sports Medicine and of several professional societies in the fields of obesity, genetics, and health. He is an author and co-author of more than 500 publications, including several books. His research focuses on the genetic and molecular basis of physical performance, obesity, and cardiac disease and diabetes risk factors.

David A. Brodie, educated at the University of Nottingham and Loughborough University, is currently Professor and Head of the Department of Movement Science and Physical Education at the University of Liverpool. He has published nine books, 94 peer-reviewed papers, 14 chapters in books, 23 peer-reviewed abstracts, 34 published proceedings, 11 articles, and 21 poster publications. Professor Brodie's research interests are in body composition, pediatric work physiology, and cardiac rehabilitation. He is involved in research training for BSc Movement Science students and MSc Health Science students.

John S. Carlson is the inaugural holder of the Jack Refshauge Chair in Movement Sciences at Victoria University in Melbourne, Australia. Professor Carlson is also the Director of the Research Centre for Rehabilitation, Exercise, and Sport Science.

He has published and presented his work in pediatric exercise science in many international forums. His research has focused on the growing child and the many facets of growth that are influenced by physical activity and sport.

Jean Coudert is a specialist in high altitude physiology and sports medicine and is the former Director of the High Altitude Laboratory in La Paz, Bolivia. He is head of the Department of Physiology at the University of Clermont-Ferrand, France. He is also doing work with the Human Nutrition Research Institute. Professor Coudert is a member of the French Société de Physiologie, the European Group of Pediatric Work Physiology, and is a fellow of the European College of Sport Science. In his leisure time he enjoys jogging, mountain climbing, and cross-country skiing.

François-Pierre J. Counil is a specialist in the field of Pediatric Pulmonology and Cardiology. He is an assistant professor at the Faculty of Medicine of Montpellier, France. Dr. Counil is a member of the French Pediatric Society and the French-speaking Pediatric Pulmonary Society. In his leisure time he enjoys jogging, tennis, and playing music.

Nicole Fellman has specialized in energy expenditure during ultra-endurance events, particularly in hormonal and hydromineral regulations, and in nutrition. She is an associate professor in the Department of Physiology and Sports Biology at the University of Clermont-Ferrand, France. She is a member of the French Société de Physiologie and also of the European Group of Pediatric Work Physiology. In her free time, she enjoys jogging, tennis, cross-country skiing, and mountain climbing.

Nanci M. França is a doctoral student in the Department of Exercise Physiology at the Université Blaise Pascal in Clermont-Ferrand, France. She is involved in the study of pediatric exercise physiology. Her main research involves the study of growth and development of children in developing countries. She is editor-in-chief of the Brazilian Journal of Science and Movement. In her leisure time she enjoys jogging and bicycling.

Jody L. Jensen is an associate professor in the Department of Kinesiology and Health Education at the University of Texas at Austin where she directs changes in motor control across the life span with specific emphasis on the contribution of muscular and nonmuscular forces to the development of movement control and coordination. Dr. Jensen was the 1995 recipient of the Early Career Distinguished Scholar Award from the North American Society for Psychology of Sport and Physical Activity.

Eleftherios Kellis received his PhD in movement sciences from the University of Liverpool and is a Lecturer in Sport Biomechanics in the Division of Sport and Recreation at the University of Northumbria in Newcastle. Professor Kellis has authored and co-authored books and articles on isokinetic dynamometry. He enjoys playing basketball, listening to music, and playing with his one-year-old daughter.

Robert M. Malina is Professor of Physical Education and Exercise Science and Director of the Institute for the Study of Youth Sports at Michigan State University. He holds PhD degrees in both physical education and anthropology and was awarded an honorary doctorate by the Katholieke Universiteit Leuven in Belgium. He has done extensive research on the growth, maturation, and performance of children and adolescents in the United States and several countries in Europe and Latin America. Dr. Malina is the co-author of *Growth, Maturation, and Physical Activity,* and *Genetics of Fitness and Physical Performance.*

James C. Martin is a professional engineer and has also earned a master's degree in exercise science. He is presently completing his PhD in exercise science at the University of Texas at Austin. The primary focus of his research is changes in maximal neuromuscular power across the life span.

Antti Mero is an associate professor in the Department of Biology of Physical Activity at the University of Jyväskaylä, Finland. He earned his PhD in Exercise Physiology in 1987. Since then, he has done considerable research in both biomechanics and exercise physiology. He has written 90 international scientific publications and three training books. He is a member of the International Society of Biomechanics and the American College of Sports Medicine.

Lyle J. Micheli is director of the Division of Sports Medicine at Children's Hospital and Associate Clinical Professor of Orthopaedic Surgery at Harvard Medical School in Boston. He is a past president of the American College of Sports Medicine (1989-1990). He is the author of over 100 scientific articles and reviews related to sports injuries (particularly for children), scoliosis and other disorders of the spine, and medical problems of dancers. Dr. Micheli's present research activities are focused on the prevention of sports injuries in children, as well as assessment of dysfunctions of the shoulder in children and young adults.

Geraldine Naughton is the Director of the Pediatric Exercise Research Unit at Victoria University and the consulting Exercise Physiologist to the Obesity Clinic at the Royal Children's Hospital in Melbourne. Her research in the area of anaerobic performance and development in children is internationally recognized as some of the most unique work conducted on children. Dr. Naughton, through her research, is dedicated to providing the scientific foundations underlying the roles that participation in sport and physical activity play in the lives of children.

Christian G. Préfaut is a specialist of physiology and pathophysiology of exercise, including training programs in cardiorespiratory patients. He is head of the Department of Physiology at the Faculty of Medicine of Montpellier, France. Dr. Préfaut is a member of numerous scientific societies including the American Physiological Society and the American Thoracic Society. He is the author of more than 150 published research articles. In his free time he enjoys bicycling, walking outdoors, and playing table tennis.

Jon Royce undertook his MSc by research at the University of Liverpool. His research mainly focused on measurement of and changes in flexibility in schoolchildren. He now lives in the South of England where he combines teaching physical education with coaching youth hockey at the international level.

Digby G. Sale is a professor in the Department of Kinesiology at McMaster University in Hamilton, Ontario. He has researched neuromuscular adaptation to resistance exercise since the mid-1970s. His recent work focuses on adaptations to "ballistic" training and the influence of training on posttetanic potentiation.

Anthony Sargeant is a fellow of the American College of Sports Medicine, a founding member of the European College of Sports Science, and a member of the Physiological Society. Over a 30-year career of research, Dr. Sargeant has published papers on many aspects of fundamental and applied physiology, including pediatric exercise physiology. In recent years, his work has focused on muscle function and, in particular, on acute and chronic plasticity of the neuromuscular system. Current funded projects include studies of muscle plasticity, spinal cord injuries, post-polio syndrome, and the effects of fatigue and temperature on muscle properties and mechanical performance.

Jean-Aimé Simoneau is an exercise physiologist and is specialized in skeletal muscle histochemistry and biochemistry. He is an associate professor in the Division of Kinesiology and Department of Social and Preventive Medicine at Laval University in Quebec City, Canada. Professor Simoneau is an associate editor of the Canadian Journal of Applied Physiology and an author or co-author of approximately 85 publications and 150 communications on the skeletal muscle metabolic capacity and its potential role in health-related risk factors, such as obesity, as well as in exercise performance. In his free time he enjoys fly-fishing and golf.

Joanne Welsman joined the Children's Health and Exercise Research Centre at the University of Exeter in England at its inception in 1987. Since completion of her PhD in 1990, Dr. Welsman has held the position of Research Fellow at the Centre. She has published widely in pediatric exercise science, contributing nearly 80 papers, book chapters, and scientific reports and has made almost 100 presentations at national and international conferences. Dr. Welsman recently co-authored *Young People and Physical Activity* with Professor Neil Armstrong.

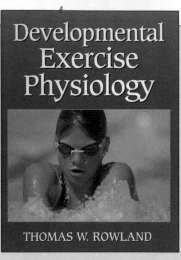
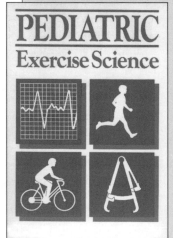